# Hospitals in Iran and India, 1500–1950s

# Iran Studies



VOLUME 7

*The titles published in this series are listed at brill.nl/is*

# Hospitals in Iran and India, 1500–1950s

*Edited by*

Fabrizio Speziale

BRILL

LEIDEN · BOSTON
2012

*Cover illustration*: The main building of the Niẓāmiyya ṣadr šifā-ḫāna (1926–1939) in Hyderabad seen from the Čār Mīnār (picture by F. Speziale).

Library of Congress Cataloging-in-Publication Data

Hospitals in Iran and India, 1500–1950s / [edited] by Fabrizio Speziale.
p. cm. — (Iran studies ; v. 7)
In English and French.
Includes bibliographical references and index.
ISBN 978-90-04-22829-0 (hbk. : alk. paper) 1. Hospitals—Iran—History. 2. Hospitals—India—History. 3. Medicine—Iran—History. 4. Medicine—India—History. 5. Iran—Social conditions. 6. India—Social conditions. I. Speziale, Fabrizio, 1968–

RA990.I6H66 2012
362.110954—dc23

2012004418

This book is copublished with the Institut Français de Recherche en Iran (IFRI) as no. 74 in the *Bibliothéque Iranienne* series.

ISSN 1569-7401
ISBN 978 90 04 22829 0 (hardback)
ISBN 978 90 04 22919 8 (e-book)
ISBN 978 2 909961 50 7 (IFRI)

CONTENTS

CONTENTS

# LIST OF ILLUSTRATIONS

*Willem Floor*

*Figures*



*Maps*



*Omid Rezai*

*Cristiana Bastos*



*Fabrizio Speziale*

*Figures*



*Plan*

## ACKNOWLEDGMENTS

Some of the articles gathered in this volume were presented at the conference on *Hôpitaux en Iran et en Inde des Safavides aux Pahlavi*, which was held at the National Museum of Medical Sciences History of Tehran on 25 January 2007. This conference was organized by the Institut Français de Recherche en Iran (IFRI), the National Museum of Medical Sciences History, and the Research Institute for Islamic and Complementary Medicine (RICM) of the Iran University of Medical Sciences. This conference was part of the activities organized within the IFRI research program on The History of Medicine in Iran and India in the Modern Period. These proceedings also include articles from scholars who were unable to participate in the Tehran conference, and whose writings enrich the topics examined in this work with important contributions. For other reasons, it was unfortunately not possible to include some contributions presented at the Tehran conference.

I would like to thank the directors of the institutions that supported the realization of this congress in particular: Christian Bromberger (IFRI), Shams Shariat Torbaghan (National Museum of Medical Sciences History), and Ashrafodin Gooshegir (RICM). I likewise thank Philippe Rochard, who has taken over direction of the IFRI. I am grateful to Amir Mehdi Taleb and Alireza Parsapoor for their help in organizing the conference. I would especially like to thank Farid Ghassemlou for his contribution to the activities of the IFRI program on the History of Medicine.

I would like to thank Yann Richard for supporting the publication of this work in the *Iran Studies* collection, and for his reading of the chapters in French. I further thank Brill editors, Nicolette van der Hoek and Ingrid Heijckers-Velt, and the IFRI publishing team, especially Catherine Azarnouche and Annette Caracache. I likewise thank Yolande Momtaz for her cooperation in the translation of the articles of Hasan Tadjbakhsh and Omid Rezai from Persian; and Vincent Bensaali, Denis Hermann, Delfina Giovannozzi, and Alessandra Marchi for their reading of some texts. I likewise thank Dominik Wujastyk for his observations on Ayurvedic institutions, and for having allowed me to consult his copy of the volumes edited by N. S. Mooss.

Fabrizio Speziale
Paris, October 2011

# INTRODUCTION

Fabrizio Speziale

The history of medicine and science in the post-medieval Muslim world remains a lightly explored subject in comparison to studies of the preceding period, which is considered the golden age of Avicennian medicine. The same is true for the historiography of scientific institutions. This work presents a significant panorama of studies on the history and role of hospitals in the Indo-Iranian world during the early modern and the modern periods, that is, beginning in the 16th century. The contributions gathered into this volume study the hospital from various perspectives, both as a scientific institution and in function of its social utility. The portrait that emerges from these studies is not homogeneous, but is instead an ambivalent and contrasting image of these establishments. Hospitals can be seen as powerful symbols of the piety of Muslim rulers or of the Muslim scientific civilization, and then of the triumph of modern western medicine. Nevertheless, the hospital remained an institution relegated to the fringes of society for quite a long period—it was regarded with suspicion and was usually reserved for the poor.

The period this work explores is notably characterized by a substantial transformation in the scientific identity of this institution, which occurred along parallel paths in Iranian and Indian cities. In Iran during the Safavid period (1501–1722) and in India during the Mughal period (1526–1857), the hospital remained an institution that was still tied to the Avicennian tradition of medicine. In Iran during the Qajar period (1794–1925) and in British India (1858–1947), the hospital instead became one of the important instruments for the spread of modern western medicine in these regions. The history of hospitals thus reflects the state of, and the fundamental changes to, medical knowledge during this period, which is divided between the continuation of tradition, and a break with it that is determined by the eruption of modernity. At the same time, the history of these institutions constitutes a fundamental lens through which one may look at these questions.

One should note that the most common term employed to designate hospitals in post-medieval Iran and India is not the Persian word *bīmāristān* (from *bīmār*, "sick", and the locative suffix *stān*), which had been the most used term in the medieval Muslim world. In fact, a number of equivalent terms were used in the Indo-Iranian world, especially *dār al-šifā, marīż-ḫāna* and *šifā-ḫāna*. The frequency of these terms changes with time. The Arabic expression *dār al-šifā* (house of healing) was most often used in the Safavid and Mughal period; while *marīż-ḫāna* (house of the sick) became more common in the Qajar period in Iran, and *šifā-ḫāna* (house of healing) was used in colonial India. It however appears that these terms were not exclusively used to designate hospitals, but that they were also used at certain dispensaries—although there were other terms to designate dispensaries, such as *šarbat-ḫāna* and *dawā-ḫāna*.

## The Hospital and Other Muslim Institutions

The hospital, like the madrasa, the hammam, or the caravansary, is one of the typical establishments of Muslim cities. The development of hospitals is among the contributions that Muslim culture brought to Indian society, where hospitals were apparently not extremely common institutions at the time that Muslims arrived.[1] Nevertheless, as various facts analyzed in this work show, one should not exaggerate the importance of this institution. One must first of all consider the place of hospitals in comparison to other Muslim institutions, as well as the relations that they entail. The number of hospitals founded during the Safavid-Mughal period is incomparably lower than that of other establishments, such as the madrasa or the hammam. In comparison to other Muslim scientific establishments, the number of hospitals surpasses only that of astronomical observatories. During the Safavid-Mughal period, hospitals were often attached to other establishments, such as a mosque, a mausoleum, a madrasa, a hammam, or a caravansary. Examples of this for Iran can be found in the hospital of the shrine of Imam ʿAlī al-Rižā (d. 203/818) and the one built at Isfahan by Šāh ʿAbbās I (r. 1588–1629); and for India, in the hospital built at Hyderabad by the Shiite sultan Muḥammad Qulī Quṭb Šāh (r. 1580–1612) and that built at Delhi by the Mughal Šāh Jahān (r. 1628–1658). This is a model that dates from the medieval period, as the hospitals founded during the Seljuk period in Turkey, at Kayseri (beginning of the 13th century) and Divriği (1228–1229) show, as does the celebrated al-Manṣūrī hospital

1 See Basham 1998, pp. 34–36.

complex of Cairo, established in 1284, as well as the hospital established at Bursa during the Ottoman period, in 1399.

Several hospitals were thus established adjoined to religious institutions. The most important case in Iran is certainly that of the shrine of Imam al-Rižā at Mashhad, which became one of the most important Shiite pilgrimage sites from the Safavid period on. Religious establishments usually had much more property and revenue than hospitals, and it was sometimes possible for these to be used to maintain hospitals and dispensaries. Thus, in 19th century India, part of the revenues from certain Sufi shrines (*dargāh*) in Awrangabad were assigned to hospitals and other charitable works.[2] In Iran during the Qajar period, a few clinics were established within *takya*, places where Shiite mourning rituals take place.[3]

One should not think, however, that the hospital in the Muslim world was itself a religious institution. Hospitals in Muslim cities were not founded or directed by religious in particular, unlike numerous hospitals in the Christian world. Further, hospitals of traditional medicine were not the only ones associated with religious institutions. There were a few hospitals of allopathic medicine in Tehran until the end of the Qajar period that were attached to a mosque, a madrasa, or a tomb. Likewise, in 19th century British India, the civil hospital in Ahmadnagar was located in the eastern part of the Kamānī mosque (16th century), and, in 1876–77 during a famine and a smallpox epidemic, a hospital for men and children was opened within the Farhādḫān mosque (16th century). The two mosques were still used for prayer when these colonial hospitals were established.[4]

References to the teaching of medicine in the hospitals of Safavid and Mughal cities are quite rare. In his article, Willem Floor mentions the case of the hospital of Astarabad, where during the 16th century a part of the endowment was dedicated to a medical professor and his students. There were madrasas next to some hospitals, as in the cases of Tabriz, Isfahan, Hyderabad and Delhi. In the district of Birbhum, in the Bengal Presidency, there were two cases of madrasas whose endowments were used to maintain hospitals until 1830.[5] Nevertheless, it does not appear

[2] *Gazetteer of Aurangabad*, 1884, p. 323.

[3] Ebrahimnejad 2004, p. 74.

[4] *Gazetteer of the Bombay Presidency, vol. XVII, Ahmadnagar*, 1884, pp. 680, 682, 700. In modern Pakistan, the government directly supported the opening of allopathic hospitals in Sufi shrine complexes, Buehler 1998, p. 230.

[5] Adam 1838, p. 68.

that there were madrasas attached to a hospital and exclusively dedicated to teaching medicine (*ṭibb*) during the Safavid-Mughal period in Iran or India, although the madrasa of the Hyderabad hospital has often been presented as a medical school. During that period, medical formation was based on private teaching and the transmission of the profession within families. It is nevertheless probable that certain medical texts, such as Avicenna's (d. 1037) *Qānūn* and its commentaries, were taught along with other subjects in some madrasas next to hospitals. It is known that the curriculum of madrasas in India included the rational sciences and medicine from the Akbar (r. 1556–1605) period on.[6] These subjects were later included in the *dars-i niẓāmī*, which became the dominant program for Indian madrasas from the 18th century on. It seems that certain medical texts, such as the *Qānūn* and Nafīs ibn 'Iważ al-Kirmānī's commentary of the *Kitāb al-asbāb wa al-'alāmāt* by Najīb al-Dīn al-Samarqandī (d. 1222), were also read in Iranian Shiite madrasas.[7]

## *Waqf*s for Hospitals

Various hospitals in the Muslim world were founded through the establishment of a *waqf* (or *vaqf*), that is, a "pious endowment".[8] Assets and their revenues were endowed as *waqf* to found and maintain religious and charitable institutions such as mosques, madrasas, shrines, and hospitals. Omid Rezai's article studies this type of endowment in particular, as well as its legal acts (*waqf-nāma*). The sources that Omid Rezai presents show that the *waqf*s established to build and maintain hospitals in Qajar Iran integrated numerous kinds of properties and buildings, such as a caravansary, a garden, or a water reservoir, as well as revenues from villages, lands, *qanāt* (underground irrigation canal), and mills. Local nobility and prominent citizens were the sponsors of these charitable works, while hospitals were notably designed to offer medical assistance to the poor. One should however note that *waqf*s were not founded for pious motives alone, but were also a means to protect the properties that were part of

[6] See Abū al-Fażl, 2001, vol. 1, p. 289.

[7] Tunakābunī 1353/1974, pp. 54–56.

[8] For a description of *waqf*s established for Cairo hospitals in the medieval period, see Bey 1928, pp. 55–57, 61–72, 78.

the *waqf*.[9] The *waqf* was in fact managed by an administrator (*mutawallī*) who was appointed by the donor (*wāqif*).

*Waqfs* for hospitals were certainly fewer and less enduring than those for other Muslim establishments, such as mosques and shrines. The *waqfs* established for hospitals generally did not survive political turmoil, even though *waqfs* should be permanent (*mu'abbad*) endowments. *Waqfs* for medical establishments were founded until the 20th century. The Hamdard, which became a *waqf* in 1953, is an important and fairly recent case. It should be underscored that during the Modern period, *waqfs* were no longer only consecrated to establishments of traditional medicine, like the Hamdard, an institution that aimed to reform Avicennian medical tradition, and whose history is described in the article by Anna Vanzan. In Qajar Iran, numerous *waqfs* began to be established for the foundation of hospitals of allopathic medicine, as Omid Renzai's article shows. One can also mention a recent case of a medical center with twenty beds, which was established by the Karnataka Board of Waqfs and adjoined to the *dargāh* of Ḥamīd Šāh in Bangalore.[10]

One should however specify that the sources only rarely mention whether or not a hospital was founded through a *waqf*. On the other hand, it is certain that there were hospitals that were not maintained through a *waqf*. The case of the Mughal empire from the 17th century on is quite important for this subject. Emperor Jahāngīr (r. 1605–1627) decreed that all the expenses of the hospitals in Mughal cities were to be funded from the *ḫāliṣa*, that is, lands directly managed by the imperial government.[11] The new institutions of *yūnānī* medicine[12] created during the colonial period in India were generally not founded through *waqfs*, as in the case of the Niẓāmiya Ṣadr Šifā-Ḫāna hospital which was established in Hyderabad under the last Niẓām, Mīr 'Uṯmān 'Alī Ḫān (r. 1911–1948), whose administration and funds depended on the new department of *yūnānī* medicine created by the State.

---

9 Cf. Werner 2000, pp. 103–122.

10 See Ahmed – Khan 1418/1997, p. 122.

11 Jahāngīr, 1978, p. 9.

12 *Yūnānī* (Greek)—or *unani* according to English pronunciation—is the term used in India to designate the Avicennian medical tradition practiced by Muslim physicians, see Speziale 2005.

## Hospitals in Society

The foundation of hospitals in the Muslim world was primarily linked to individual efforts and donations—those of sovereigns and nobles in particular. Many hospitals thus received their name from their founder. Hospitals were part of the public institutions founded by sultans, particularly in the capitals and urban areas of their kingdoms. Numerous wealthy individuals established hospitals in Iran and India into the Qajar-colonial period. Omid Rezai's article analyzes this phenomenon toward the end of the Qajar period. The Parsees of Bombay provide us with another example with their establishment of hospitals there during the colonial period—the first of which was established in the mid-19th century, and is named after its founder, Sir Jamshedji Jijibhai (d. 1859), a wealthy merchant.[13] Towards the end of the century, another Zoroastrian merchant, referred to by Willem Floor in his article, provided buildings in the city of Yazd for the foundation of a hospital, which was to be managed by the British Church Missionary Society. In colonial India, private physicians, such as Ḥakīm ʿAbd al-Majīd, the founder of the Hamdard, and Ajmal Ḫān (d. 1927), provided a fundamental contribution to the creation of new *yūnānī* institutions.

The fact that hospitals were established by nobles did not mean that these institutions were then used by their founders or by others of their social status. Hospitals were in fact mainly used by the poor until the Qajar-colonial period.[14] When members of other classes were ill, they were treated at home by private doctors. Only those who could not be treated at home, such as the poor, vagabonds, pilgrims, and soldiers, went to hospitals. The situation was not that different in Europe where, until the beginning of the 19th century, the hospital, with a few exceptions, was an inn for the poor and destitute.[15] The plaque at the entry of San Gallicano hospital in Rome, established in 1725 by Pope Benedict XIII, indicates this: *Neglectis rejectisque ab omibus*, "For those neglected and rejected by all". The hospitals of Tabriz in the Safavid period, such as the one in Ardabil near the shrine of Šayḫ Safī al-Dīn (d. 735/1334), were primarily known as places where free meals were distributed to the poor and to pilgrims.[16]

---

[13] See Arnold 1993, pp. 271–272; Burdett 1893, pp. 227–228.

[14] See Dols 1987, pp. 370–371; Arnold 1993, pp. 249–250; Ebrahimnejad 2004 pp. 82–83; Harrison 2009, p. 14.

[15] Catananti 2002, pp. 137, 140–141.

[16] Chardin 1811, vol. 2, p. 324; Elgood 1970, p. 29.

According to a mid-18th century source that describes the administration of Gujarat, hospitals were established for the treatment of the sick and those who were not even able to buy their own food.[17] This state of affairs only gradually changed during the Qajar-colonial period. When a hospital was opened by missionaries at Miraj (Maharashtra) en 1894,[18] for example, only lower caste men were willing to go there at first, while certain establishments in British India are described as places that were mainly frequented by beggars and prostitutes.[19]

A strategy in India to overcome the upper classes' mistrust for these institutions introduced separated services, based on one's social class and religion. As Cristiana Bartos shows in her article, in the mid-19th century, segregation measures of this sort were used in the Portuguese hospital of Goa to garner the trust of Hindu patients. Around the same time, separate services for upper caste Hindus were created in certain hospitals of British India.[20] In the Jamshedji Jijibhai hospital of Bombay, there was a section for Parsees as well, beyond the services for Hindus and Muslims.[21] Likewise, separate hospitals for local troops were established in the British army.[22] Paying rooms for wealthy Muslim patients were even planned in the new *yūnānī* hospital of Hyderabad, the Niẓāmiya Ṣadr Šifā-Ḫāna.[23]

The Portuguese and British hospitals were not however the first to introduce separate services for Hindus. In certain hospitals founded by Muslims in India, Ayurvedic (*vaidya*) physicians were employed. This was not the first known case of this kind: During the Abbassid period, the Indian physician Ibn Dahn is mentioned by the Barmakid Vizier Yaḥyā ibn Ḫālid as the director of the hospital, which was founded before 187/803 in Baghdad.[24] As has been observed by Basham, it is quite plausible that

---

17 Ḫān 1930, p. 186.

18 The Woman's Foreign Missionary Society of the Presbyterian Church, 1908, p. 10.

19 Arnold 1993, p. 250.

20 Arnold 1993, pp. 250–251; Harrison 2009, p. 30. For separation measures based on religion and social class in insane asylums of British India, see Ernst 2006, pp. 142–143, 150–151, 163.

21 Burdett 1893, p. 227; Arnold 1993, p. 271.

22 The quality of these establishments was obviously lower than that in hospitals for British troops : "They are generally nothing but a shed perhaps a "gun-shed", or a "cattle shed" as at Kolapore, converted into a hospital, where the sick receive nothing but medicine. The patients cook their own diets [...] There are no conveniences; sometimes the sick go home to wash", Nightingale 1863a, pp. 145 f.

23 See Fārūqī 1356/1937, p. 200.

24 According to the *Fihrist* of Ibn al-Nadīm (d. around 995), Manka, another Indian physician, translated a medical text from Sanskrit in the same hospital. The text was probably that of Suśruta. See Ibn al-Nadīm, 1970, vol. 2, pp. 589–590, 710; Dols 1987, pp. 382–384.

the *vaidyas* in the hospitals established by the Muslims in India were at the service of Hindus who would have otherwise been polluted by contact with the impure.[25] The first reference to this subject regards the hospital established in the mid-15th century at Bidar (Deccan), the capital of the Bahmanid sultanate.[26] Under Šīr Šāh Sūrī (r. 1540–1545), separate services for Hindus were introduced in caravansaries established along Indian roads and financed by the State.[27] During the Awrangzīb (r. 1658–1707) period, the physicians Kanwal Nain, Sukhānand, and Nainsukh were employed at the hospital founded in Etawah (in present day Uttar Pradesh) by a Muslim nobleman.[28] Another case of this type can be found a little later at Gujarat, where two Ayurvedic physicians, whose stipends were paid by the government, worked at the *dār al-šifā* of the Šāh Wajīh al-Dīn (d. 1589) shrine in Ahmadabad. ʿAlī Muḥammad Ḫān, a historian of Gujarat and a Mughal dignitary, communicates this to us in the mid-18th century, and specifies that the Ayurvedic doctors were at the service of Hindus, whose treatments they knew well.[29] It is also very plausible that the provision of medicines in these hospitals was essentially based on the medicines available on the local market.

## The Safavid-Mughal Period

During the Safavid-Mughal period, there were hospitals in numerous Iranian and Indian cities. The sources regarding these hospitals are however fairly limited and contain few details. Many are not contemporary to the foundation of these establishments, but written in later periods. Hospital buildings dating from this period that survive today are also very rare. In Deccan, one can still see the hospital building founded at the end of the 16th century in Hyderabad and described in my article. Hospital buildings from the Safavid-Mughal period in Iran and India have not been preserved as well as those of the same period in the Ottoman world, such as that established in Edirne by Bāyazīd II (r. 1481–1512), and *dār al-šifā*, founded in 1555, which was part of sultan Sūleymān's *külliye* in Istanbul.

[25] Basham 1998, p. 40.
[26] Firišta 1290/1874, vol. 1, p. 333.
[27] Sarwānī 1865, pp. 147–148.
[28] Fārūqī 1356/1937, pp. 114–115.
[29] Ḫān 1930, p. 187.

Most hospitals from the Safavid-Mughal period were located in the principal cities, although some establishments were also located in smaller urban centers. According to the Capuchin Raphaël du Mans (d. 1696), who lived in Iran for a long time, there were one or two hospitals in each large city of the country.[30] Nevertheless, there is not more specific information other than for a limited number of these establishments: at Tabriz, Qazvin, Mashhad, Isfahan, Shiraz, Ardabil, Yazd, Astarabad, Damghan, in the village of Ben Isfahan, and perhaps in Ashraf. In his memoirs, the Mughal Bābur (d. 1530) speaks of the existence of a hospital in Herat which he had visited in 1506, four years before the city was conquered by the Safavids.[31] The sources that describe the hospitals in Safavid cities are presented in the articles of Hassan Tadjbakhsh and Willem Floor. Tadjbakhsh underscores that prominent physicians of the period were employed in these institutions, notably during the periods of Šāh Ṭahmāsp (r. 1524–1576) and Šāh ʿAbbās I (r. 1588–1629). ʿImād al-Dīn Maḥmūd Šīrāzī was certainly the most important of these doctors. He was the author of several medical works in Persian, and was employed at the hospital of Mashhad during the period of Šāh Ṭahmāsp. According to Willem Floor, the study of sources demystifies the usual conception of the Safavid period as characterized by a considerable decline in the establishment of hospitals in comparison to earlier centuries. Nevertheless, according to Floor, these institutions probably had a rather limited effect on the general situation of public health in Safavid Iran. The condition of these establishments were described by some European travelers who visited Iran after the period of Šāh ʿAbbās I, and their descriptions of the hospitals they visited are rather dark. Some of these establishments undoubtedly had a bad reputation among the Iranians, especially the hospital of Isfahan, which, instead of being called *dār al-šifā*, "house of healing", was ironically called *dār al-marg*, "house of death" by the locals.

Some hospitals had already been established in Indian sultanates before the Mughal period: in Delhi during the 14th century, and during the following century in Bidar and Mandu. The *dār al-šifā*s founded in Srinagar by sultan Sikandar (r. 1389–1413) were probably still open at the beginning of the 17th century.[32] For the Mughal period, we have references to

30 Richard 1995, vol. 2, p. 171.

31 This hospital was part of a complex that included the tomb of Mīr ʿAlīšīr Beg (d. 906/1500), a madrasa, a mosque and a hammam, Bābur 1998, p. 306.

32 See the anonymous *Bahāristān-i šāhī*, a history of Kashmir until 1023/1614, *Bahāristān-i šāhī* 1991, p. 45.

hospitals having been established in Agra, Fatehpur Sikri, Ahmadabad,[33] Surat,[34] Delhi, Awrangabad, and in smaller centers such as Etawah and Chiniot; the *dār al-šifā* of Hyderabad date from this period as well. In some Mughal cities, such as Agra, Ahmadabad, and Delhi, there were probably more than one of these establishments—either hospitals or dispensaries.[35] The precise date of the establishment of the first hospitals of the Mughal period is not clear.[36] A hospital established in Fatehpur Sikri dates from the Akbar (r. 1556–1605) period, as does perhaps another, founded in Agra.[37] After his enthronement, Jahāngīr (r. 1605–1627) promulgated an edict ordering the construction of hospitals in all the cities of the empire, the assignment of physicians to them, and that their expenses be taken from the *ḫāliṣa*.[38] It is unknown how successful this project was after this. Around 1060/1650, Šāh Jahān (1628–1658) built a *dār al-šifā* against the northwest corner of the Jāmi' Masjid in Delhi, where there was also a madrasa.[39]

Numerous Iranian physicians migrated to India during this period, where they were often employed in local Muslim courts.[40] Some Iranian physicians and scholars are associated with hospital establishment and activity in India. According to the version described by the historian Abū al-Fażl (d. 1011/1602), Ḥakīm Abū al-Fatḥ Gīlānī (d. 997/1589), an Iranian Shiite physician in service to Akbar who had occupied important positions in the Mughal administration, urged Akbar to establish hospitals.[41] The Hyderabad hospital project is associated with the activity of another Shiite scholar, Mīr Mu'min Astarābādī (d. around 1034/1625), who became a highly influential figure in the court of sultan Muḥammad Qulī Quṭb Šāh

33 See Ḫān 1930, pp. 186–187; Ḥasanī 1977, p. 191; Fārūqī 1356/1937, p. 109.

34 See Awrangzīb 1908, p. 124; Ḥasanī 1977, p. 191.

35 On Agra, Fatehpur Sikri, and Ahmadabad see Ḥasanī 1977, pp. 190–191; on Delhi during the period of Muḥammad Šāh (r. 1719–1748) see Fārūqī 1356/1937, p. 119, who speaks of small hospitals (*šifā-ḫāna*) beyond the Jāmi' Masjid.

36 'Abd al-Razzāq praises the Mughal Humāyūn (r. 1531–1540 and 1555–1556) in a verse of the introduction to his treatise on anatomy, and mentions having worked in the *dār al-šifā sulṭānī*, without specifying where it was; this establishment does not appear to be mentioned by other sources, see 'Abd al-Razzāq, *Ḫulāṣat al-tašrīḥ*, MS. Hyderabad, Salar Jung Oriental Library, *ṭibb* 72, ff. 2r, 3r.

37 Ḥasanī 1977, pp. 190–191; Khan 1983, p. 206; Fārūqī 1356/1937, p. 106.

38 Jahāngīr, 1978, p. 9.

39 Sayyid Aḥmad Ḫān (d. 1898) reports that this hospital building still existed when he published his history of Delhi monuments, in 1846, although it was no longer used as a hospital, see Ḫān 1979, p. 59.

40 See Speziale 2009.

41 Abū al-Fażl 2000, vol. 3, p. 560.

(r. 1580–1612). Until 1702, Muḥammad Taqī Šīrāzī was the head physician of the hospital of Ahmadabad, which had been established in 1622.[42]

The annual budget of the hospital of the Jāmiʿ Masjid in Delhi during the period of Muḥammad Šāh (r. 1719–1748) was 300,000 rupees.[43] In regard to the salary of physicians (*ḥakīm*) employed in these establishments, during the period of Awrangzīb, that of superintendent (*dāroġa*) of the hospital of Awrangabad, Muḥammad Zamān, was 136 rupees net (180 gross) monthly, and was paid by the treasurer (*ḫazānčī-i ḫizāna-yi ḫarč-i kull*).[44] The sum was calculated on a daily basis, and for this reason the physicians who worked in hospitals were required to procure an attestation of presence (*taṣdīq-i ḥāżirī*), as a document of this type delivered in 1068/1657 to Muḥibb ʿAlī, *dāroġa* of the hospital of Awrangabad witnesses to.[45] Nadeem Rezavi has shown in his study that the salary of the *dāroġa* of a hospital was higher than that of other local officials in the Mughal administration,[46] although it was much lower than the salary of physicians employed in Mughal courts.[47] Nevertheless, a hospital position must have been considered sufficiently sought after, since it led an important religious of Surat to write letters to emperor Awrangzīb in order to recommend that a certain physician be hired in the hospital of that city.[48] A head physician of one of these establishments could also hope for the rank of imperial officer (*manṣabdār*) in the Mughal administration: in 1692, a superintendent of a dispensary had the eighteenth rank (*manṣab*)—out of thirty three—a rank whose maximum annual salary was 27,500 rupees.[49]

Some hospitals were founded by the nobles of the Mughal period. ʿAlīm al-Dīn Wazīr Ḫān (d. 1050/1640–41)—who was learned in medicine and had also been the governor of Panjab under Šāh Jahān—built a hospital, a madrasa, and other establishments in his home town of Chiniot (Panjab).[50] The hospital of Etawah was founded during the Awrangzīb

---

42 Ḥasanī 1977, p. 191.

43 Fārūqī 1356/1937, p. 119.

44 Khan 1958, pp. 122–123.

45 See Yahya 1950, pp. 211–212; Khan 1958, p. 122, and the study of Rezavi 2001, p. 48.

46 Rezavi 2001, p. 62, note 67.

47 For example, the Iranian physician Ruknā Kāšī (d. 1656), who was in India during the Jahāngīr and Šāh Jahān periods, received a salary of 24,000 rupees a year, see Fārūqī 1356/1937, p. 107. Manucci reports that the annual salary of the head physician of the court of the Mughal prince Šhāh ʿĀlam (d. 1712) was 100,000 rupees, while that of a newly recruited physician was only 300 rupees a month, Manucci, vol. 4, pp. 205, 210.

48 Awrangzīb 1908, p. 124.

49 Sharma 1937, p. 23.

50 Nawāz Ḫān, 1999, vol. 2, pp. 982–983.

period by the *nawāb* Ḫayr Andīš Ḫān, for the care of the poor. Eight doctors were employed there—five who were Muslim, and three who were Ayurvedic.[51]

There are no references to insane asylums established under the Savafids and the Mughals. In 849/1445, eighty years before the beginning of the Mughal period, a hospital that included service for lunatics had been established in Mandu by the sultan Maḥmūd Ḫalǧī,[52] but it is unknown whether this remained active during the Mughal period. European travelers did not make the same remarks about the hospitals in Mughal cities as those about the hospitals of Savafid Iran. Gemelli Careri (d. 1725) recounts that European soldiers hesitated to enroll in the Mughal army because it did not have hospitals for the wounded.[53] Beginning in the 17th century, European travelers such as Jean-Baptiste Tavernier (d. 1689) and John Fryer (d. 1733) described the animal hospitals (*pinjrāpol*)—which were notably managed by the Jains—of the urban centers of western India, such as in Ahmadabad, Bombay, and Kerala. Tavernier writes that there were two or three houses in Ahmadabad that served as hospitals, for cows, bulls, and swans in particular, as well as for other sick animals.[54]

## Hospitals in the Modern Period

Europeans had already established hospitals and dispensaries in Iran and India during the Safavid-Mughal period. In the beginning, these hospitals were primarily planned for European and military needs, since many of them became sick in the colonies.[55] The first hospitals founded by the Europeans were in centers under Portuguese control. During the first decades of the 16th century, the Portuguese established hospitals on the island of Hormuz and in Goa. Cristiana Bastos' article focuses on the hospital of Goa, and notably manifests the evolutions of this institution, which in the beginning was reserved to Christian military elite, and then,

[51] Fārūqī 1356/1937, pp. 114–115.

[52] Firišta 1290/1874, vol. 2, p. 249.

[53] Gemelli Careri 1949, p. 247.

[54] Tavernier, Jean-Baptiste, 1676, p. 48; Fryer 1698, p. 53; Rousselet 1875, pp. 17–18.

[55] The military death rate was high: in 1863, Florence Nightingale observed that there were still "very much doubts that an army of seventy thousand men can be kept up in India, with the present death-rate", Nightingale 1863b, p. 3. At the end of the 19th century, venereal disease was the first cause (31%) of the admission of European soldiers to hospitals, *The Imperial Gazetteer of India*, 1909, vol. I, p. 532.

during the 19th century, attempted to Indianize itself and thus adopted reserved spaces for Hindu patients.

The first military and civil hospitals of British India were established during the 17th and 18th centuries: at Madras in 1679, in Calcutta, and in Bombay.[56] The Dutch established hospitals during the Mughal period as well, in Colombo and Jaffna;[57] the French established a hospital in Pondicherry;[58] and the Danes in Tranquebar. Some of these establishments were of fairly modest dimensions. In the 18th century, the hospital of Tranquebar had two Danish doctors in all—a chief surgeon and an assistant surgeon—and some local auxiliaries.[59] In 1934, the colonial hospital of Pondicherry had only two military doctors, who were also the teachers of the medical school, and a pharmacist, who was also responsible for three other government pharmacies of the colony.[60]

The number and impact of modern western hospitals was fairly limited before the 19th century in both Iran and India. This situation changed slowly throughout the 19th century, and it was only in the second half of this century that more significant changes occurred. The limits of government activity played a critical role in both India and Iran. There was no modern hospital in Tehran, the new Qajar capital, until 1852. Government hospitals were established in Tehran at this point, but no plan was developed under the Qajars to establish a system of public hospitals in the rest of the country. Outside the capital, the hospitals founded during the Qajar period were generally established by westerners and some Iranian individuals, and not by the Qajar government. In India, the British colonial authorities hesitated to establish hospitals, above all in adequate proportion to the population.[61] In British India of 1902 there were more than 2,400 hospitals and dispensaries under government control (there were 1,211 in 1880), 480 private establishments, and 506 managed by the police, the railroads, and other institutions. This is certainly a large number, but is only one dispensary for every 330 square miles.[62] The British

---

56 *The Imperial Gazetteer of India*, 1909, vol. IV, p. 461.

57 Reddy 1975, pp. 87–89.

58 Ramanathan, 1962; for the hospital's location, see the map of Croisey 1764.

59 Jensen 2005, pp. 492, 495, 496.

60 *Etablissements français dans l'Inde, exposé des motifs du projet de budget de l'exercice 1935*, p. 51.

61 Arnold 1993, pp. 247, 249.

62 Further, more than one sixth of the budget of hospitals and clinics under government control was derived from "subscriptions, endowments, fees and other sources", *The Imperial Gazetteer of India*, 1909, vol. IV, pp. 462, 480.

administration reports note that the progress in this regard were slow for quite some time, and that major developments only occurred during the last decades of the 19th century. The principal causes cited are the lack of funds and doctors, as well as local populations' mistrust of these institutions, who preferred to seek care with traditional physicians.[63] The reports on Indian colonial hospitals often deplore the bad conditions of many of these establishments.[64]

Despite this, hospitals and dispensaries progressively made an important contribution, both for the spread of western medicine in the country and for improving access to medical services, especially for urban populations. Hospitals also played an important role in the modernization of medical teaching during this period. This is true for traditional medicine as well, as the case of the college of the Niẓāmiya Ṣadr Šifā-Ḫāna at Hyderabad shows. Colonial hospitals became the place where information was recorded and investigations took place, including on Indian *materia medica*. Before the establishment of a meteorology department in 1874–75, meteorological information was recorded in numerous hospitals of British India, even if the information was often of low quality.[65] Sir Ronald Ross (d. 1932) discovered the malaria parasite in 1897 while conducting research at the hospital of Secunderabad, for which he won the Nobel prize for medicine in 1902.[66]

In Tehran during the Qajar period and in the Indian Princely States, as in Ottoman Turkey, medical modernization was not the result of colonial constraint, but of a process that was supported by local powers and the local elite. Emblematic examples are offered to us by the Niẓāms of Hyderabad and the Begums of Bhopal, the two principal Muslim Princely States of the colonial period. Claudia Preckel's article explores the development of hospitals and medical institutions in Bhopal, as well as the active role of the Begums within this process. The Begums and Niẓāms provided ample support for *yūnānī* medicine and for efforts to renew the tradition

---

63 *The Imperial Gazetteer of India*, 1909, vol. IV, pp. 461–462.

64 See Nightingale 1863a, pp. 133–155. In 1904, the surgical equipment of numerous Bengali hospitals was considered "... defective: instruments being of antiquated patterns: means of sterilisation imperfect or non-existent; and operating rooms very unsatisfactory", "Hospitals Reports", 1094, p. 474. Twenty years later, the primary hospital of Multan was described as: "... neither spacious enough nor adequately equipped for the needs of a large town. The site is cramped and shut in by surroundings dwellings of insanitary type; the buildings are old and in a bad repair, while the operation room is badly constructed and lighted.", *Punjab District Gazetteers, Multan District, 1923–24*, p. 263.

65 *The Imperial Gazetteer of India*, 1909, vol. I, pp. 105–106.

66 Aladin 1998, pp. 31–35.

through the creation of new institutions. At the same time however, they favored medical modernization, carried out vaccination campaigns and, created modern hospitals that were larger and more expensive than the *yūnānī* ones.

In India, especially in the beginning, local populations were suspicious of western hospitals and medicine, and of surgery in particular.[67] Members of high social classes and women were among the most hesitant to go to hospitals in British India. Cristiana Bastos indicates that a similar situation existed in Portuguese Goa in the 19th century, where most of the local population preferred to go to local healers. Hostile reactions to European hospitals were also observed in Iran, above all by the ulama. As Willem Floor reports, in Isfahan, toward the end of the 19th century, the ulama managed to temporarily shut the clinic established by British missionaries in the Armenian quarter of Jolfa. Omid Rezai highlights that some Iranian nobles who established hospitals during this period were motivated by ulama's exhortations, in order to oppose the Christian missionary hegemony in this domain. This attitude changed during the course of the 19th century. The Iranian ulama's preoccupations obviously witness to the fact that western hospitals and dispensaries were gaining the trust of local populations. British reports state that, thanks to its results, surgery had become a highly important part of hospital activities in India at the beginning of the next century, and that popular prejudices against it had been largely overcome.[68]

Qajar Iran is analyzed from different perspectives by Willem Floor and Omid Rezai. Willem Floor's contribution offers a broad overview of the development of modern hospitals during this period. There were hospitals and dispensaries in numerous Iranian cities, although Floor's analysis indicates that these institutions still had a fairly limited impact on Iranian society during the Qajar period, since there were too few of them in comparison to the population's size and health requirements. Omid Rezai's article studies the hospitals founded by prominent Iranians during the first decades of the 20th century. Many of these institutions were established in the country's provincial cities, where there was the greatest lack of medical services. The author shows the role that the establishment of *waqfs* still played at this time, as well as the relationships between these benefactors and the ulama, as in the case of the *waqf* for the hospital of

[67] Cf. especially Arnold 1993, pp. 182, 220–221, 223, 252.
[68] *The Imperial Gazetteer of India*, 1909, vol. IV, p. 465.

Isfahan, whose legal act (*waqf-nāma*) was redacted by an influential religious of the city.

Western missionaries, above all the Protestant ones, provided an important contribution to the development of medical services. Until the middle of the 19th century however, Protestant missionaries did not particularly insist on medical practice. Before that, the Jesuits had managed hospitals in India, such as the *Hospital dos pobres* in Goa during the 16th century, and the Chandannagar (Bengal) hospital during the 18th century;[69] while the Augustinian fathers had managed the hospital of Hormuz until the beginning of the 17th century.[70] It was not until the second half of the 19th century that medical missions gradually became an important instrument of Protestant missionary proselytism.[71] The participants in medical missions made an effort to show that their activities were conformed to the teaching in Sacred Scripture, and to Jesus, "the Great Physician", in particular.[72] Numerous Zanana missions,[73] which were administered by women, were established—primarily in India—to overcome indigenous women's resistance to going to western hospitals.[74] Women's conditions in Indian society and customs such as *satī* were presented as an incontestable reason for the importance of the Zanana missions.[75] Irene Barnes, a member of the Church of England Zanana Missionary Society, provided an example of the evangelization strategies used by these missions when she explained that Gospel tracts that had been translated into Bengali were printed on the back of prescriptions.[76] Despite the multiplication of medical missions and their efforts, it appears that they were not able to significantly increase conversions in either Iran or India.

During the second half of the 19th century, these services were often provided by missionaries who did not have formal medical degrees. This became necessary for work in medical missions in 1892–93, following accusations of charlatanism in regard to unqualified missionaries.[77] There were medical missions in both India and Iran, but there were far more of

---

[69] See Županov 2008; Launay 1898, p. xliv.

[70] Elgood 1951, p. 512.

[71] Fitzgerald 2006. On medical missions, see especially the work of John Lowe, whose first edition appeared in 1886, Lowe 1903.

[72] See Barnes 1901, p. 134; Wilson 1849; Gauld 1886; Lowe 1903, pp. 11–23.

[73] From the Persian *zanāna*, the adjectival form of *zan*, "woman".

[74] On the activity of these missions, see Armstrong-Hopkins 1898; Barnes 1901; Lowe 1903, pp. 175–198; Pitman n. d.

[75] Pitman n. d., pp. 5–19.

[76] Barnes 1901, p. 147.

[77] Fitzgerald 2006, pp. 102–111, 126; Hardiman 2009, pp. 201–202.

them in India than in Iran. According to 1916 statistics, Protestant medical missions in Iran included 10 hospitals and 17 dispensaries with 500 beds total; 19 foreign doctors, including 6 women; 7 foreign nurses; and 1 local doctor and 49 auxiliaries, half of whom were women. In India, on the other hand, they managed 183 hospitals with 3,348 beds and 376 dispensaries, which employed 281 foreign doctors, 159 of whom were women; 108 foreign nurses; 51 local doctors; and 289 male and 461 female auxiliaries.[78]

The efforts to improve female health conditions and medical education were not only by westerners. Claudia Preckel examines an important case for this subject, that of the Bhopal Princely State. Beginning in the 19th century, Bhopal was governed by women, the Begums, two of whom in particular, Šāh Jahān Begum (r. 1868–1901) and Sulṭān Jahān Begum (r. 1901–1926), were quite active in the education of Muslim women and its reform. They wrote texts on this subject that were influenced by the Indo-Muslim educational reformism of the colonial period. The education of traditional midwives (*dā'ī*) and of nurses was institutionalized under Sulṭān Jahān, with courses for the women of the city offered at the hospital. As Preckel shows, the development of medical services for women had to adapt to the local traditions of *zanāna* and *parda*. This was clearly a compromise that medical services provided by westerners also had to conform to, despite their criticisms of women's conditions in India.

Medical institutions established by westerners employed and formed local personnel. As Willem Floor notes, medical missions in Iran mainly employed Iranian Christians, while Indian assistants also worked for British consulate medical services. In British India, most of the local personnel employed by the Indian Medical Service were Hindu, but there were also some Muslims, Christians, and Parsees.[79] In the region of Ahmadnagar, numerous members of the Barber caste (*nhavi*) were employed in hospitals as "wound dresser[s], surgery with some being an hereditary calling".[80]

In some regards, the boundary between modern and traditional medical knowledge was not absolute during this period. Local physicians who were also experts in traditional medicine worked in modern hospitals in Iran. There were several attempts in hospitals of British India to use

[78] These numbers from the 1916 *World Statistics of Christian Mission* are provided by Lambuth 1920, pp. 226–227. These statistics are perhaps incomplete, see Fitzgerald 2006, p. 127, who cites numbers for India from *Medical Missions in India*, 1912, 68, p. 145.

[79] *The Imperial Gazetteer of India*, 1909, vol. IV, p. 460.

[80] *Gazetteer of the Bombay Presidency, vol. XVII, Ahmadnagar*, 1884, p. 146.

drugs from the local *materia medica*, while modern subjects were taught in the new colleges of *yūnānī* medicine. Local drugs were also used in other establishments founded by westerners in India. The high costs of importing drugs from Europe pushed the British in particular to seek out local substitutes.[81] This situation was clearly analogous to the one Muslims experienced when they arrived in India. Muslim physicians in India had particular difficulties in finding the substances mentioned in their books, which pushed them to seek out local substitutes and to compose numerous works in Persian on Indian medicine and its pharmacopoeia.[82] Around the end of the 18th century, Francis Gladwin (d. 1812) redacted an English adaptation of the *Alfāẓ al-adwiya*, a Persian dictionary of drugs that had been written in 1628–29 by Nūr al-Dīn Šīrazī, a physician of the Mughal court. Gladwin, who was not a physician, specified that the English version was executed on the request of the hospital board of Fort William in Calcutta, "... for the use of the Honourable Company".[83] The official *Pharmacopoeia of India* was published in 1868, whose introduction explained that one of the "primary objects" of the work was the insertion of indigenous products into the European medicine of the country's hospitals and clinics.[84] The *Pharmacopoeia of India* gave several results from local drug tests carried out in Indian hospitals.[85] At the beginning of the 20th century, the British still encouraged the use of drugs that could be purchased in the Indian market.[86]

## Traditional Medicine

The supremacy of modern western medicine did not therefore lead to the loss of traditional medical knowledge and practice, although it did relegate it to a subordinate role in comparison to colonial science. In 19th century Iran, Avicennian traditional medicine was still fairly popular, especially if one takes into account the access limits to modern medicine. Along with traditional physicians, there was a growing number of

[81] See Arnold 2000, pp. 68–70; Harrison 2006, pp. 67–68.
[82] See Speziale 2010.
[83] Šīrāzī 1793.
[84] Waring 1868, p. ix.
[85] Waring 1868, pp. 10, 53, 60, 118, 142, 151, 228; cf. also Alavi 2007, pp. 171–174.
[86] During this period, hospitals "... make their own arrangements for the supply of indigenous drugs purchasable locally. The use of such drugs is encouraged, and there is a permanent committee for investigating [...] their properties.", *The Imperial Gazetteer of India*, 1909, vol. IV, p. 463.

Iranian physicians formed both in western and traditional medicine.[87] Beginning in 1860, Avicennian medicine was taught at Dār al-funūn college of Tehran, which was founded in 1268/1851 and marked the official beginning of modern scientific education in Iran. Mirzā ʿAlī Akbar Nafīsī (d. 1924) and Muḥammad Kirmānšāhī (d. 1908), the directors of the state hospital of Tehran between 1873 and 1886, had also studied traditional medicine. The first was a member of a prominent family of traditional physicians from Kerman, the Nafīsī, who descended from Nafīs ibn ʿIważ al-Kirmānī (15th century), the court physician of Uluġ Beg (d. 1449) and author of an important commentary on al-Samarqandī's *Kitāb al-asbāb wa al-ʿalāmāt*, which was also widely read in India.[88] There were also a few Iranian physicians who contested the influence of European knowledge, such as Muḥammad Taqī Šīrāzī Malik al-Aṭibbā (d. after 1866), the author of *Risāla-yi jawhariya*—a work that refuted western drugs.[89] Nevertheless, these tendencies did not lead to a movement in Qajar Iran that would have aimed at the creation of new institutions exclusively consecrated to traditional medicine, as did occur in India beginning in the end of the 19th century.

Traditional medicines went through a phase of reforms in India during this period, which led to the creation of a considerable number of new colleges, pharmacies, associations, journals, and a few hospitals as well.[90] The reform of the *yūnānī* tradition—as in the case of Ayurvedic medicine—occurred through the incorporation of elements of western medicine and colonial medical institutions. This is most pronounced in the disciplines of *yūnānī* medicine that were most contested by modern scientific thought such as surgery, anatomy, or pathology. At the same time, these reforms determined a gradual exclusion of those aspects of the tradition that did not agree with the new scientific criteria of the colonial period. New influential institutions were founded and run by private physicians, who were often members of families of medical scholars—such as the Šarīfī of Delhi, the ʿAzīzī of Lucknow, and the Hamdard. The contribution of these private initiatives was obviously more important in cities such as Delhi and Lucknow, which were under British control. Significant reforms of *yūnānī* institutions occurred in some Muslim Princely

87 See Tadjbakhsh 2003, pp. 275–280; Ebrahimnejad 2004, pp. 88–111.

88 Storey 1971, pp. 307–308; Tadjbakhsh 2003, pp. 279–280; Ebrahimnejad 2009, p. 264.

89 Elgood 1951, p. 511; Floor 2004, pp. 182–184.

90 On hospitals of Ayurvedic medicine established during this period cf. Mooss 1937, pp. 18a, 53–54, 67–72, 83 f.; Mooss 1949, pp. 47–48, 57–58, 77, 82–83, 85, 130–132.

States, which were heirs to the Mughal tradition of patronage of Muslim and Indian arts and learning. Two contributions to this work treat Hyderabad, under the Niẓāms, and Bhopal, under the Begums, where the birth of new institutions of *yūnānī* medicine was supported and promoted by the State.

A few *yūnānī* hospitals were founded during this period. The creation of hospitals was part of the efforts to provide *yūnānī* medicine with new and more modern establishments that would be capable of adapting the tradition to the changing conditions of colonial India's scientific environment. Further, there were many initiatives to open new dispensaries of *yūnānī* medicine. In 1911, one of the points in the program of the Association (*anjuman*) of *yūnānī* physicians of Lucknow was the creation of charitable hospitals and dispensaries of *yūnānī* medicine.[91] Nevertheless, hospitals—no doubt due to their costs—played a decisively smaller role in this context than establishments such as dispensaries or colleges. The *dār al-šifā* that had been established during the Mughal period no longer played any role. All efforts were dedicated to the creation of new establishments whose model was no longer that of the Muslim *dār al-šifā*. One of the last establishments based on the *dār al-šifā* model was the hospital established in Lucknow next to the Imāmbāṛa,[92] and built in 1791 by the *nawāb* Āṣaf al-Dawla (r. 1775–1797).[93] The change is clear with the Šāhī šifā-ḫāna, the hospital founded in the same city in 1834 by Ḥakīm Mahdī ʿAlī Ḫān, a minister of Nāṣir al-Dīn Ḥaydar (r. 1827–1837). The Šāhī šifā-ḫāna was divided into two sections, one for *yūnānī* medicine and the other for western medicine, in which one of the first Muslim doctors to receive a degree at Calcutta Medical College worked.[94]

A section for hospitalized patients was established at the Ayurvedic and Yūnānī Ṭibbiya College (AYTC), which was opened in Delhi in 1921 by Ajmal Ḫān (d. 1927). Ajmal Ḫān, a member of the Šarīfī, was also active in politics, and was one of the most influential *yūnānī* physicians of the colonial period, as well as one of the great proponents of the efforts to modernize the *yūnānī* tradition. The AYTC included a surgery room, a service for patients who desired separate lodgings, and a service for the contagiously sick. In his inaugural discourse, Ajmal Ḫān especially

[91] Alavi 2007, p. 326.

[92] A Shiite place of worship where *Muḥarram* ceremonies took place.

[93] The complex, described by Abū Ṭālib Iṣfahānī (d. 1805), a historian from the period, included a mosque and a caravansary, Iṣfahānī 1885, pp. 91 ff.

[94] Alavi 2007, pp. 186–188, cf. also Ḥasanī 1977, p. 192.

highlighted the importance of the service for hospitalized patients for the practical instruction of the students of the college.[95] Modern anatomy and surgery were also taught at the college, as in that of Niẓāmiya Ṣadr Šifā-Ḫāna in Hyderabad. The AYTC was founded through contributions of numerous donors, among which were the Shiite *nawāb* of Rampur (who gave 50,000 rupees), who had used Ajmal Ḫān as his personal physicians; Sulṭān Jahān Begum of Bhopal (25,000 rupees), as well as the Maharajas of Patiala (25,000 rupees) and of Indore (5,000 rupees). Ayurvedic medicine was taught at the AYTC as well. Moreover, there was a *zanāna* college of obstetrics and female medicine. Hindus went there for Ayurvedic medical treatment. According to the numbers published by *al-Ḥakīm*—a journal of *yūnānī* medicine—the AYTC hospital treated 922 patients during the month of *Muḥarram* 1346/July 1927, 670 of whom received Ayurvedic treatment.[96] Another service for hospitalized patients was established in another important college of *yūnānī* medicine in northern India, the Ṭibbiya College of Aligarh, which opened in 1927. This college was founded within the Aligarh Muslim University—the institution that symbolized the modernization of Muslim education in South Asia—and included ʿAbd al-Laṭīf Falsafī (d. 1970) among its teachers, who was one of the most influential physicians from the ʿAzīzī family of Lucknow.

The contribution of Anna Vanzan and my own examine two other institutions which, like the Ṭibbiya Colleges of Delhi and Aligarh, are still active today. Anna Vanzan studies the history of the Hamdard, which was founded in Old Delhi by Ḥakīm ʿAbd al-Majīd (d. 1922) in 1906. During the 20th century, the Hamdard established itself as one of the leading institutions and enterprises of *yūnānī* medicine in South Asia. The Hamdard manages dispensaries and hospitals, and is especially known among the public for its traditional remedies. These are mass produced, includes a few Ayurvedic products, and are extensively advertised in Indian cities. One of the principal aims of these new establishments is to overcome the limits of the traditional pedagogy of *yūnānī* medicine, which was based on private teaching and transmission of the profession within families of physicians. Nevertheless, the Hamdard, like other *yūnānī* establishments of this period, remains an institution that was solidly based on the family, and which on the death of its founder was directed by his wife, and then by their sons. My contribution analyzes the development of *yūnānī*

95 Abdur Razzack 1987, pp. 27, 30, 36–37.
96 "Ṭibbiya Kālij Dihlī" 1927, p. 36.

institutions under state control in Hyderabad under the last two Niẓāms, which began at the end of the 19th century and culminated with the project of the Niẓāmiya Ṣadr Šifā-Ḫāna hospital. This hospital, with its large and elegant building built in the center of the old city, is one of the great symbols of the *yūnānī* revival of this period. Nevertheless, the completion of such an expensive project became a fairly involved affair. The hospital became the seat of the new *yūnānī* college, where several physicians formed in the *yūnānī* schools of northern India were called to teach. One such doctor was Ḥakīm Kabīr al-Dīn (d. 1976), who was favorable to the incorporation of elements taken from colonial science. Like other Indo-Muslim rulers before him,[97] the last Niẓām also supported Indian medicine, and between 1936–38 an Ayurvedic section was attached to the *yūnānī* department of Hyderabad. Claudia Preckel's article examines the role of *yūnānī* medicine in the Princely State of Bhopal. Under the Begums, new *yūnānī* dispensaries were created in Bhopal, as well as a college to regulate the education of *ḥakīms*, and a dispensary for women. These efforts especially show the priority given to the creation of these types of establishments in comparison to hospitals during this period.

Although this type of question goes beyond the topics treated in this volume, it is fitting to briefly reflect on the future of these institutions of traditional medicine. In India, the establishment and reform of *yūnānī* hospitals continued and accelerated during the post-colonial period, within the framework of state institutions dedicated to traditional medicines that were created after India's independence. There were seventy-four *yūnānī* hospitals in fourteen States at the beginning of the 21st century, with the greatest concentration in Uttar Pradesh, which had nineteen hospitals. India, where Muslims are a minority, today has the most advanced hospital system of traditional Avicennian medicine. It is important to note that the number of *yūnānī* hospitals today is twice that of recognized colleges, although it is far less than the number of *yūnānī* dispensary under State control, as there are more than one thousand of them in twenty Indian States.[98] In regard to Iran, a few new institutions dedicated to traditional medicine have been created in the last years, while courses in traditional medicine are offered in a few universities. These first efforts have not led to the creation of new hospitals of Avicennian medicine, but it is possible that services of traditional medicine could open in allopathic hospitals in the years to come.

---

97 See Speziale 2010.
98 *Unani Medicine in India*, 1997, pp. 32–35.

## Bibliography

'Abd al-Razzāq, *Ḫulāṣat al-tašrīḥ*, MS Hyderabad, Salar Jung Oriental Library, *ṭibb* 72.
Abdur Razzack, H. M., 1987, *Hakim Ajmal Khan. The Versatile Genius*. New Delhi, Central Council for Research in Unani Medicine.
Abū al-Fażl, 'Allāmī, 2000, *Akbar-nāma*, English translation: *The Akbarnama of Abu'l Fazl*, 3 vols., H. Beveridge, ed., Calcutta, The Asiatic Society, (1st ed. 1897–1921).
——, 2001, *Ā'īn-i Akbarī*, English translation: *The Ā-īn-i Akbarī*, 3 vols., H. Blochmann—H. S. Jarrett, eds., New Delhi, Low Price Publications, (1st ed. Calcutta, 1868–1894).
Adam, William, 1838, *Third Report on the State of Education in Bengal; including some account of the State of Education in Behar*. Calcutta.
Ahmed, Hasanuddin – Khan, Ahmedullah, 1418/1997, *Strategies to Develop Waqf Administration in India*. Jeddah, Islamic Research and Training Institute—Islamic Development Bank.
Aladin, Bilkiz, 1998, *Sir Ronald Ross: his life and work*. Hyderabad, Zen Publications.
Alavi, Seema, 2007, *Islam and Healing. Loss and Recovery of an Indo-Muslim Medical Tradition 1600–1900*. New Delhi, Permanent Black.
Armstrong-Hopkins, S., 1898, *Within the Purdah, also, in the Zenana homes of Indian princes... Being the personal observations of a medical missionary in India*. New York, Eaton & Mains.
Arnold, David, 1993, *Colonizing the Body. State Medicine and Epidemic Disease in Nineteenth-Century India*. Berkeley – Los Angeles, University of California Press.
——, 2000, *Science, Technology and Medicine in Colonial India*. Cambridge, Cambridge University Press (*The New Cambridge History of India*, III, 5).
Askari, S. H., 1957, "Medicines and Hospitals in Muslim India". *Journal of Bihar Research Society*, 43, pp. 7–21.
Awrangzīb, 1908, *Ruqā'āt-i 'Ālamgīrī*, English translation: *Ruka'at-i-Alamgiri or Letters of Aurungzebe*, J. H. Bilimoria, ed., London – Bombay.
Bābur, 1998, *Bābur-nāma*, English translation: *Bābur-nāma (Memoirs of Bābur)*, A. S. Beveridge, ed., Delhi, Munshiram Manoharlal (1st ed. London, 1921).
*Bahāristān-i šāhī*, 1991, English translation: *Bahāristān-i-Shāhī. A Chronicle of Medieval Kashmir*, K. N. Pandit, ed., Calcutta, KLM.
Barnes, Irene H., 1901, *Between Life and Death: The Story of the C. E. Z. M. S. Medical Missions in India, China and Ceylon*. London, Marshall Brothers—Church of England Zenana Missionary Society.
Basham, A. L., 1998, "The Practice of Medicine in Ancient and Medieval India", in: C. Leslie, ed., *Asian Medical Systems*. New Delhi, Motilal Banarsidass, pp. 18–43 (1st ed. Berkeley, 1977).
Bey, Issa, 1928, *Histoire des bimaristans (hôpitaux) à l'époque islamique*. Cairo.
Buehler, Arthur F., 1998, *Sufi Heirs of the Prophet. The Indian Naqshbandiyya and the Rise of the Mediating Sufi Shaykh*. Columbia, University of South Carolina Press.
Catananti, Cesare, 2002, "La nascita dell'ospedale moderno tra i '*lumi della ragione*' ed i '*fuochi della rivoluzione*' ". *Medicina nei secoli*, 14, 1, pp. 135–153.
Chardin, Jean, 1811, *Voyages du chevalier Chardin en Perse, et autres lieux de l'Orient*, L. Langles, ed., 10 vols. Paris, Le Normant, nouvelle édition.
Cloarec, Françoise, 1998, *Bîmâristâns, lieux de folie et de sagesse*. Paris, Harmattan.
Croisey, 1764. *Plan de la ville de Pondicheri*. Bibliothèque national de France. (see: http://gallica.bnf.fr/ark:/12148/btv1b59628855.r=pondichery.langEN, last access 5 March 2010)
Dols, Michael W., 1987, "The Origins of the Islamic Hospital: Myth and Reality". *Bulletin of the History of Medicine*, 61, 3, pp. 367–390.
Düzbakar Ömer, 2006, "Charitable Women and their Pious Foundation in the Ottoman Empire: the Hospital of the Senior Mother, Nurbanu Valide Sultan". *Journal of the International Society for the History of Islamic Medicine*, 5, 10, pp. 11–20.
Ebrahimnejad, Hormoz, 2004, *Medicine, Public Health and the Qājār State: Patterns of Medical Modernization in Nineteenth-Century Iran*. Leiden, E. J. Brill.

——, 2009, "Hospitals and Development of Medicine in Nineteenth-Century Iran", in: M. Harrison – M. Jonnes – H. Sweet, *From Western Medicine to Global Medicine. The Hospital Beyond the West*. New Delhi, Orient Blackswan, pp. 249–273.

Elgood, Cyril, 1951, *A Medical History of Persia and the Eastern Caliphate*. Cambridge, Cambridge University Press.

——, 1970, *Safavid Medical Practice*. London, Luzac & Co.

Ernst, Waltraud, 2006, "Colonial Lunacy Policies and the Madras Asylum in the Early Nineteenth Century ", in: B. Pati – M. Harrison, eds., *Health, Medicine and Empire. Perspectives in Colonial India*. New Delhi, Orient Longman, pp. 137–164 (1st ed. 2001).

*Etablissements français dans l'Inde, exposé des motifs du projet de budget de l'exercice 1935*, 1934. Pondichery, Government Press.

Fārūqī, Qāẓī Muʿīn al-Dīn Rahbar, 1356/1937, *Islāmī ṭibb šāhānah sarparastiyūn men*. Hyderabad (reprint: Hyderabad, Maktaba-yi ʿAīn al-ʿUlūm, 1420/1999).

Firišta, Muḥammad Qāsim, 1290/1874, *Tārīḫ-i Firišta*, 2 vols., Kanpur.

Fitzgerald, Rosemary, 2006, " 'Clinical Christianity': The Emergence of Medical Works as a Missionary Strategy in Colonial India, 1800–1914", in: B. Pati – M. Harrison, eds., *Health, Medicine and Empire. Perspectives in Colonial India*. Delhi, Orient Longman, pp. 88–136 (1st ed. 2001).

Floor, Willem, 2004, *Public Health in Qajar Iran*. Washington DC, MAGE.

Fryer, John, 1698, *A New Account of East-India and Persia, in Eight Letters. Being Nine Years Travels, Begun 1672. And Finished 1681*. London, Ri. Chiswell.

Gauld, William, 1886, "*Scriptural Warrant for Medical Missions*", in: *Proceedings of The Conference on Foreign Missions*. London, John F. Shaw, pp. 108–112.

*Gazetteer of Aurangabad*, 1884. Published under the orders of His Highness the Nizam's Government. Bombay, Times of India Press.

*Gazetteer of the Bombay Presidency, vol. XVII, Ahmadnagar*, 1884. Bombay, Government Central Press.

Gemelli Careri, Francesco, 1949, *Giro del mondo del dott. d. Gio. Francesco Gemelli Careri. Parte terza contenente le cose piu ragguardevoli vedute nell'Indostan*, English translation: *Indian Travels of Thevenot and Careri*, S. Sen, ed., New Delhi.

Hamarneh, Sami, "Development of Hospitals in Islam". *Journal of the History of Medicine and Allied Sciences*, 17, 3, pp. 366–384.

Ḫān, ʿAlī Muḥammad, 1930, *Ḫātima-yi Mir'āt-i Aḥmadi*, S. Nawāb ʿAlī, ed., Calcutta.

Ḫān, Sayyid Aḥmad, 1979, *Āṯār al-ṣanādīd*, English translation: *Monuments of Delhi: Historical Study*, R. Nath, ed., Delhi, Indian Institute of Islamic Studies.

Hardiman, 2009, "The Mission Hospital, 1880–1960", in: M. Harrison – M. Jonnes – H. Sweet, *From Western Medicine to Global Medicine. The Hospital Beyond the West*. New Delhi, Orient Blackswan, pp. 198–220.

Harrison, Mark, 2006, "Medicine and Orientalism: Perspectives on Europe's Encounter with Indian Medical Systems", in: B. Pati – M. Harrison, eds., *Health, Medicine and Empire. Perspectives in Colonial India*. Delhi, Orient Longman, pp. 37–87 (1st ed. 2001).

——, 2009, "Introduction" in: M. Harrison – M. Jonnes – H. Sweet, *From Western Medicine to Global Medicine. The Hospital Beyond the West*. New Delhi, Orient Blackswan, pp. 1–32.

Ḥasanī, ʿAbd al-Ḥayy, 1977, *Hindustān islāmī ʿahd men*, English translation: *India during Muslim rule*, Mohiuddin Ahmad, ed., Lucknow, Academy of Islamic Research and Publications.

"Hospitals Reports", 1904, *The Indian Medical Gazette*, 39, pp. 473–474.

Ibn al-Nadīm, 1970, *al-Fihrist*, English translation: *The Fihrist of al-Nadīm*, 2 vols., B. Dodge, ed., New York, Columbia University Press.

*The Imperial Gazetteer of India*, 1909, vol. I, The Indian Empire, Descriptive; vol. IV, The Indian Empire, Administrative. Oxford, Clarendon Press.

Iṣfahānī, Abū Ṭālib, 1885, *Tafẓīḥ al-ġāfilīn*, English translation: *History of the Ásafu'd Daulah Nawáb Wazír of Oudh*, W. Hoey, ed., Allahabad.

Jahāngīr, 1978, *Tūzuk-i Jahāngīrī*, English translation: The *Tūzuk-i-Jahāngīrī or Memoirs of Jahāngīr*, 2 vols., A. Rogers – H. Beveridge, eds., New Delhi, Munshiram, (1st ed. London, 1909–14).
Jensen, Niklas Thode, 2005, "The Medical Skills of the Malabar Doctors in Tranquebar, India, as Recorded by Surgeon T L F Folly, 1798". *Medical History*, 49, 4, pp. 489–515.
Jones, Margaret, 2009, "The Indian Immigrant Worker and the Development of Hospital Provision in Nineteenth-Century Ceylon" in: M. Harrison – M. Jonnes – H. Sweet, *From Western Medicine to Global Medicine. The Hospital Beyond the West*. New Delhi, Orient Blackswan, pp. 33–66.
Khan, Habib, 1983, "Early Hospitals in Muslim World". *Studies in History of Medicine*, VII, 3–4, pp. 196–208.
Khan, Yusuf Husain, ed., 1958, *Selected Documents of Aurangzeb's Reign*. Hyderabad, Central Records Office.
Lambuth, Walter R., 1920, *Medical Missions: the Twofold Task*. New York.
Launay, Adrien, 1898, *Histoire des missions de l'Inde*. Paris, Charles Douniol, vol. 1.
Lowe, John, 1903, *Medical Missions: Their place and Power*. New York, F. H. Revel (5th ed.).
Manucci, Nicolò, 1989, *Storia do Mogor*, English translation: *Moghul India 1653–1708 or Storia do Mogor*, 4 vols., W. Irvine, ed., New Delhi, Atlantic Publishers.
Mooss, N. S. [Vayaskara], 1937, *The All India Ayurvedic Directory*, vol. 1, Kottayam, The Vaidya Sarathy.
——, 1949, *The All India Ayurvedic Directory*, vol. 5, Kottayam, The Vaidya Sarathy.
Nawāz Ḫān, 1999, *Ma'āṯir al-umarā*, English translation: *The Maāthir-ul-umarā*, 2 vols., H. Beveridge – B. Prashad, eds., Delhi, Low Price Publications (1st ed. Calcutta, 1941–1952).
Nightingale, Florence, 1863a, *Notes on Hospitals*. London, Longman and Green.
——, 1863b, *How people may live and not die in India*. London, Emily Faithfull.
Pitman, Emma Raymond, n. d., *Indian Zenana Missions. Their Need, Origin, Objects, Agents, Modes Working and Results*. London, John Snow.
*Punjab District Gazetteers, Multan District, 1923–24*, 1926. Lahore.
Ramanathan, M. K., 1962, "French Hospital of Pondicherry during first half of Eighteenth Century". *Indian Journal of the History of Medicine*, 7, pp. 22–25.
Reddy 1975, "Health Hazards, Diseases, Hospitals & Physicians in East Indies and Ceylon in XVII century, based on Travels of Christopher Schweitzer". *Bulletin of the Indian Institute of History of Medicine*, 5, 2, pp. 80–91.
Rezavi, S. Ali Nadeem, 2001, "Physicians as Professionals in Medieval India" in: D. Kumar, ed., *Disease and Medicine in India: A Historical Overview*. New Delhi, Tulika – Indian History Congress, pp. 40–65.
Richard, Francis, ed., 1995, *Raphaël du Mans: missionnaire en Perse au XVII*[e] *s.*, 2 vols., Paris, Société d'Histoire de l'Orient—L'Harmattan.
Romani, Francesca Romana, 2002, "Sull'origine del modello islamico di ospedale". *Medicina nei secoli*, 14, 1, pp. 69–99.
Rousselet, Luis, 1875, *L'Inde des rajahs: voyage dans l'Inde centrale et dans les présidences de Bombay et de Bengale*. Paris, Hachette.
Sarwānī, 'Abbās Ḫān, 1865, *Tuḥfa-yi Akbar-šāhī*, French translation: *Un chapitre de l'histoire de l'Inde musulmane ou Chronique de Scher Schah, Sultan de Delhi*, G. de Tassy, ed., Paris.
Sharma, Sri Ram, 1937, "Organization of Public Services in Mughal India (1526–1707)". *Journal of the Bihar and Orissa Research Society*, 23, 2, pp. 1–57.
Šīrāzī, Nūr al-Dīn Muḥammad, 1793, *Alfāẓ al-adwiya*, English translation: *Ulfáz Udwiyeh, or the Materia Medica, in the Arabic, Persian, and Hindevy Languages*, F. Gladwin, ed., Calcutta.
Speziale, Fabrizio, 2005, "Linguistic strategies of de-Islamisation and Colonial science: Indo-Muslim physicians and the yūnānī denomination". *International Institute for Asian Studies Newsletter*, 37, p. 18. (online version: http://www.iias.nl/nl/37/IIAS_NL37_18.pdf).

——, 2009, "India xxxiii. Indo-Muslim Physicians". *Encyclopaedia Iranica*, (online version: www.iranica.com).

——, 2010, "Les traités persans sur les sciences indiennes: médecine, zoologie, alchimie" in: D. Hermann – F. Speziale, eds., *Muslim Cultures in the Indo-Iranian World during the Early-Modern and Modern Periods*. Berlin, Institut Français de Recherche en Iran – Klaus Schwarz Verlag, pp. 403–447.

Storey, C.A., 1971, *Persian Literature. A Bio-bibliographical Survey*, vol. II, pt. 2 E, London.

Tadjbakhsh, Hasan, 1379 h. š./2000, *Tārīḫ-i bīmāristānhā-yi Īrān*. Tehran, Pažūhišgāh-i ʿulūm-i insānī wa muṭālaʿāt-i farhangī.

——, 2003, *History of Medicine and Veterinary Medicine in Iran*. Lyon, Fondation Mérieux.

Tā'ib, Ḥasan, 1384 h. š./2005, *Bīmāristānhā-yi Rašt*. Rasht, Farhang-i Īliyā.

Tavernier, Jean-Baptiste, 1676, *Les six voyages de Jean-Baptiste Tavernier, … qu'il a fait en Turquie, en Perse, et aux Indes, … Seconde partie, Où il est parlé des Indes, et des Iles voisines*. Paris, G. Clouzier et C. Barbin.

"Ṭibbiya Kālij Dihlī", 1927. *Al-Ḥakīm*, September 1927, p. 36.

Tunakābunī 1353 h. š./1974, "Kutub-i darsī-i qadīm". *Farhang-i Īrān-zamīn*, 20, pp. 39–82.

*Unani Medicine in India*, 1997. New Delhi, Central Council for Research in Unani Medicine.

Waring, Edward John, 1868, *Pharmacopoeia of India. Prepared Under the Authority of Her Majesty's Secretary of State for India in Council*. London, W. H. Allen.

Werner, Christoph, 2000, *An Iranian Town in Transition. A Social and Economic History of the Elites of Tabriz, 1747–1848*. Wiesbaden, Harrassowitz.

Wilson, George, 1849, "On the Sacredness of Medicine as Profession", in: *Lectures on Medical Missions. Delivered at the Instance of the Edinburgh Medical Missionary Society*. Edinburgh, Sutherland and Knox, pp. 219–266.

The Woman's Foreign Missionary Society of the Presbyterian Church, 1908, *Hospitals in India*. Philadelphia.

Yahya, Y. H., ed., 1950, *Muntaḥab-i kāġazāt-i ʿahd-i Šāh Jahān—Selected Documents of Shāh Jahān's Reign*. Hyderabad, Daftar-i Dīwānī.

Županov, Ines G., 2008, "Conversion, Illness and Possession: Catholic Missionary Healing in Early Modern South Asia", in: I. Zupanov – C. Guenzi, eds., *Divins remèdes. Médecine et religion en Inde, Purusartha* collection, 27. Paris, Editions de l'École des Hautes Études en Sciences Sociales, pp. 263–300.

# HÔPITAUX ET MÉDECINS AVICENNIENS EN IRAN À L'ÉPOQUE SAFAVIDE[1]

Hasan Tadjbakhsh

Le propos de cet article est de donner une description des établissements hospitaliers en activité dans les villes d'Iran à l'époque safavide (1501–1722). Les sources disponibles sur le sujet sont en réalité assez limitées : en plus de quelques mentions dans les textes des auteurs musulmans on trouve des descriptions dans les récits des voyageurs européens qui visitèrent la Perse à cette époque. Ces sources attestent de l'existence de plusieurs hôpitaux (*dār al-šifā, šifā-ḫāna*), dans les villes les plus importantes sous le règne des Safavides, mais n'offrent que très peu de détails sur l'intérêt qui à cette époque était accordé par les souverains et les notables iraniens à la construction, à la restauration ou à l'entretien des établissements hospitaliers. Cependant, nous savons qu'à l'époque safavide des hôpitaux et des dispensaires existaient à Tabriz, Qazvin, Mashhad, Ispahan, Ardabil, Yazd et Téhéran. Certaines villes telles Tabriz et Ispahan avaient plus d'un hôpital en fonction à la même période.

Il faut remarquer que certains de ces hôpitaux employèrent des médecins éminents de l'époque. Parmi ceux-ci on trouve notamment des auteurs de textes médicaux, tels 'Imād al-Dīn Maḥmūd Šīrāzī, qui travailla au *dār al-šifā* de Mashhad et compte parmi les médecins plus illustres de la période safavide, et 'Alī Afżal Qāṭi' qui fut en service à l'hôpital de Qazvin. En outre, certains médecins en service dans ces hôpitaux et dispensaires œuvrèrent également comme médecins dans les cours et les camps royaux safavides de Šāh Ṭahmāsp et de Šāh 'Abbās, comme ce fut le cas pour Mīrzā Muḥammad Šīrāzī, 'Imād al-Dīn Maḥmūd, Ḥakīm Sayf al-Dīn Muẓaffar Kāšānī, Ḥakīm Šamsā Muḥammadā et Ḥakīm Nūr al-Dīn 'Alī[2]. A partir des sources disponibles, nous pouvons observer que la fondation et le patronage d'hôpitaux connaissaient une expansion durant la période allant du règne de Šāh Ṭahmāsp (r. 1524–1576) à celui de Šāh 'Abbās Ier (r. 1588–1629), or ensuite, comme en témoignent les voyageurs

---

[1] Traduction du persan de Yolande Momtaz et Fabrizio Speziale.

[2] Cf. Munšī 1350, vol. 1, p. 168, vol. 2, p. 1070; Qummī 1359, vol. 1, pp. 340–341.

européens, la situation de ces institutions sera fortement affectée par la décadence de la dynastie, après Šāh ʿAbbās.

Quelques hôpitaux de l'époque safavide se trouvaient à proximité d'institutions religieuses, tels les mosquées et les mausolées. Selon Elgood, un hôpital était en fonction à Ardabil, près de la mosquée et du mausolée de Šayḫ Ṣafī al-Dīn (m. 735/1334), maître d'un ordre soufi portant son nom et ancêtre d'Ismāʿīl Ier (r. 1501–1524), fondateur de la dynastie safavide. Elgood écrit qu'il était donné quotidiennement un repas gratuit à qui se présentait[3]. On peut en sus noter que vers l'époque de Šāh ʿAbbās Ier, le médecin et poète Ḥakīm Šaraf al-Dīn Šifāʾī avait son dispensaire dans la cour de la Mosquée du Vendredi d'Ispahan[4].

Le cas le plus important d'hôpital jouxtant une institution religieuse est celui de Mashhad. Le tombeau de l'Imam ʿAlī ibn Mūsā al-Riżā (m. 203/818) à Mashhad devint à l'époque safavide un lieu de pèlerinage chiite très important et nombre de notables s'honoraient de servir dans l'enceinte du sanctuaire, y compris dans son hôpital. Déjà auparavant, des sultans sunnites également, tels Maḥmūd de Ghazni (m. 421/1030) et le seldjoukide Sanjar (m. 552/1157) avaient favorisé l'expansion de ce lieu. Un hôpital fut fondé au sein du sanctuaire avant même l'époque safavide. On sait que l'ancien hôpital était situé à proximité de la mosquée principale, à savoir la mosquée Gawhar Šād, et que le lieu trop étroit était inadapté. Il fut abandonné par la suite[5]. L'institution d'hôpitaux dans ces lieux était très vraisemblablement aussi commandée par la nécessité de soigner les maux des nombreux pèlerins qui y affluaient. Quelques médecins éminents furent en service à l'hôpital du sanctuaire sous les Safavides. Sayyid Muʿizz al-Dīn Iṣfahānī (m. 950/1543), qui avait été un notable de la cour, s'y retira sous Šāh Ṭahmāsp. Le médecin Mīrzā Abū Ṭālib Iṣfahānī y exerça vers la fin de l'époque safavide[6]. Mais le plus célèbre médecin à s'être trouvé attaché au sanctuaire fut certainement Ḥakīm ʿImād al-Dīn Maḥmūd Šīrāzī, qui servit également à la cour de Šāh Ṭahmāsp et composa des monographies notoires en persan sur la syphilis (*Risāla-yi ātišak*), sur l'opium (*Risāla-yi afyūn*) et sur la squine (*Risāla-yi čûb-i čīnī*). ʿImād al-Dīn fut directement chargé de ce service par Šāh Ṭahmāsp, qui était particulièrement attaché au patronage du sanctuaire de l'Imam al-Riżā.

3 Elgood 1970, p. 29.
4 Tadjbakhsh 2003, p. 236.
5 Cf. Ḥasan Ḫān 1363, vol. 2, p. 525.
6 Cf. Qummī 1359, vol. 1, p. 313 ; Elgood 1970, pp. 28–29.

Iskandar Beg Munšī, l'historien de l'époque de Šāh ʿAbbās, nous a laissé la description suivante :

> *Puisque le roi bienheureux* [Šāh Ṭahmāsp] *accordait la plus grande attention à la splendeur et à la prospérité du sanctuaire sacré du saint Imam des esprits et des humains, il désignait à ses services les meilleurs de chaque corporation. Lui aussi* [Ḥakīm ʿImād al-Dīn] *à son tour, reçut la mission de se consacrer au service médical de ces lieux. Longtemps, il est resté dans la sainte ville de Mashhad afin d'y traiter les malades. En vérité, il était doté de toutes les qualités, étant le plus doué et le premier des érudits*[7].

Un hôpital, ou peut-être un dispensaire (*ṣiḥḥat-ḫāna*), était en fonction dans la ville de Yazd. Ici exerçait Ḥakīm Mīrzā Muḥammad Šīrāzī, un médecin renommé de l'époque de Šāh Ṭahmāsp. Muḥammad Šīrāzī était parent d'un autre médecin illustre, Ḥakīm Kamāl al-Dīn Ḥusayn Šīrāzī, qui avait été le médecin particulier de Šāh Niʿmatullāh Yazdī, un descendant du maître soufi Šāh Niʿmatullāh Valī (m. 1431). Muḥammad Šīrāzī était en service à l'établissement de Yazd une partie de l'année seulement, le reste du temps il exerçait comme médecin au camp royal de Šāh Ṭahmāsp[8].

ʿAlī Afżal Qāṭiʿ Qazvīnī, un médecin célèbre de l'époque, mentionne dans ses livres son activité hospitalière au sein du *dār al-šifā* (lit. maison de la guérison) de Qazvin, ville qui fut la capitale des Safavides dès 955/1548, sous le règne de Šāh Ṭahmāsp, et ce jusqu'au début de celui de Šāh ʿAbbās Ier[9]. Il existait à Qazvin un établissement hospitalier permanent, très probablement fondé par Šāh Ṭahmāsp. Il n'y a pas si longtemps, un quartier de cette ville, où se trouvait vraisemblablement autrefois l'hôpital en question, était encore appelé *dār al-šifā*. ʿAlī Afżal Qāṭiʿ travailla à l'hôpital de Qazvin vers la moitié du XVIIe siècle, lorsque la ville avait cessé d'être la capitale. Il était issu d'une famille de médecins et son arrière grand-père, Mawlānā Fażl Allāh Ṭabīb Tabrīzī, avait été au service de Tamerlan (m. 807/1405)[10]. Au terme de ses études de médecine à Qazvin, ʿAlī Afżal se rendit quelque temps à Herat. Il mentionne son activité à l'hôpital de Qazvin dans le *Manāfiʿ-i Afżaliya*, composé en 1501/1641–42, et le *Favāʾid-i*

---

7 Munšī 1350, vol. 1, p. 168.

8 Munšī 1350, vol. 1, p. 168 ; Elgood 1970, p. 29 ; Tadjbakhsh 2003, p. 239.

9 Dans le dispensaire du camp royal de Šāh Ṭahmāsp à Qazvin, travaillèrent également Ḥakīm Abū Naṣr Gīlānī et Mīrzā Muḥammad Šīrāzī, Munšī 1350, vol. 1, p. 168.

10 Sur Mawlānā Fażl Allāh Ṭabīb cf. Ḫvāndamīr 1353, vol. 3, p. 534. Il semblerait bien que des membres de la famille de ʿAlī Afżal se soient installés à Qazvin, d'où leur patronyme de Qazvīnī, à l'époque safavide, très probablement sous le règne de Šāh Ṭahmāsp, et que Muḥammad Amīn Qazvīnī, père de ʿAlī Afżal, fût lui aussi médecin, également versé dans la science vétérinaire.

*Afžaliya*, deux traités sur la médecine et la pharmacopée. Il s'agit en réalité de deux ouvrages très similaires, et souvent presque identiques[11].

Dans le quinzième paragraphe de la préface du *Manāfiʿ-i Afžaliya*, ainsi que dans le *Favāʾid-i Afžaliya*, ʿAlī Afžal décrit six cas relatifs à la différenciation à établir entre des maladies similaires, le sixième concernant la distinction entre l'apoplexie (*sakta*) et le décès. À ce propos, il affirme qu'il est fort possible qu'une personne victime d'une crise d'apoplexie, qui n'était pas décédée mais néanmoins considérée comme telle, fût inhumée vivante. Il relate qu'à Herat, en 1032/1622–23, il sauva ainsi un homme victime d'apoplexie et sur le point d'être inhumé. Puis, il raconte comment à l'hôpital de Qazvin, en 1051/1641–42 (année où il écrivait *Manāfiʿ-i Afžaliya*), il sauva la vie d'un serviteur géorgien :

> *Le sixième cas est le suivant : la plupart du temps, avant que ne survienne une crise d'apoplexie, apparaissent certaines affections d'origine cérébrale, comme des vertiges, étourdissements et maux ou lourdeurs de tête. Mais pouvoir distinguer une victime d'apoplexie d'un mort est indispensable car il arrive souvent que la première soit présumée décédée et inhumée. Ainsi, à Herat en 1032, informé de l'état d'un homme victime d'apoplexie* [...] *je suis parvenu à le rétablir en lui administrant des sternutatoires et des lavements. Puis, en 1051, lorsque j'étais en service à l'hôpital de Qazvin, j'ai traité* [...] *un serviteur géorgien en pratiquant sur lui une saignée et un lavement. Il incombe donc à tout médecin, à chaque fois qu'il constate qu'une personne non atteinte de maladie mortelle perd toute sensibilité et motricité, de faire tout son possible pour rechercher d'éventuels signes de vie. C'est pourquoi Galien a dit qu'il fallait attendre au moins 72 heures avant d'inhumer une victime d'apoplexie*[12].

À la fin du XVI^e^ siècle, Šāh ʿAbbās Ier transféra la capitale de Qazvin à Ispahan, où il fit édifier un hôpital (*dār al-šifā*), à proximité de l'actuelle place Naqš-i jahān. L'hôpital d'Ispahan était disposé autour d'un jardin. Comme l'explique Munšī, cet établissement fut édifié avec plusieurs autres bâtiments et ouvrages de bienfaisance :

> *Sur la mention des œuvres de bienfaisance et la construction de bâtiments* [...] *et tout ce qu'il a fait édifier de merveilleux à Ispahan :* [...] *une autre mosquée*

---

[11] *Favāʾid-i Afžaliya* fut réalisé à l'époque de Šāh ʿAbbās II (r. 1642–1666) et peut être considéré comme une version plus complète de *Manāfiʿ-i Afžaliya*. Ce qui diffère entre les deux ouvrages est l'ajout à *Favāʾid-i Afžaliya* de trois chapitres ainsi que de nombreuses pages préliminaires à la préface. La section finale de chacun des deux ouvrages comprend une partie donnant une description de la médecine du Prophète et des Imams, cf. Tadjbakhsh 2003, pp. 236–238.

[12] Qazvīnī, *Manāfiʿ-i Afžaliya*, ms. Téhéran, Bibliothèque Centrale de l'Université de Téhéran, pers. 13/d, p. 11 ; *Favāʾid-i Afžaliya*, ms. Téhéran, Bibliothèque Centrale de l'Université de Téhéran, pers. 3288, p. 253.

> *face à la cour du palais* [...], *une école théologique, un hôpital, des hammams, le bazar Qayṣariya, un bazar tout autour de la place* [...] *et des caravansérails* [...][13]

Parmi les médecins qui travaillaient à l'hôpital d'Ispahan à cette époque, on connaît Ḥakīm Sayf al-Dīn Muẓaffar Kāšānī, qui mourut en 1037/1627–28 à Sultaniya. Vers la fin de sa vie, Sayf al-Dīn, affaibli par la vieillesse, pratiquait beaucoup moins et délégua ses fonctions de médecin de l'hôpital et du camp royal de Šāh ʿAbbās à son fils Šamsā Muḥammadā[14]. Engelbert Kaempfer (1651–1716), médecin, naturaliste et voyageur allemand, visita Ispahan en 1684, avec la mission diplomatique suédoise, avant d'être employé pour quelques années dans le Golfe persique comme chirurgien de la Compagnie hollandaise des Indes orientales. Kaempfer écrit qu'à Ispahan il avait un hôpital (*nosocomium*), une centaine de mosquées et écoles, ainsi que d'innombrables hammams et hôtelleries pour voyageurs. Il observe que ces édifices publics manifestaient plus d'élégance que de technicité et de grandeur[15]. Il mentionne également les boutiques d'apothicaires de la ville : l'*ʿaṭṭār-ḫāna*, où les médicaments étaient préparés pour le souverain et pour les nobles par le pharmacien du roi, sous la direction d'un archiatre. Le *parhīzāna*, où pour les malades étaient préparés juleps et décoctions à base d'orge, de riz et de plantes médicinales, comme prescrit par le médecin[16].

On peut avancer l'hypothèse que ces hôpitaux étaient financés par des *vaqf* (fondation de mainmorte) similaires à ceux que les souverains et les notables iraniens fondaient habituellement pour l'institution et le fonctionnement de mosquées, mausolées, madrasas, hammams et autres établissements. Cependant, nous ne connaissons jusqu'à aujourd'hui que peu de documents (*asnād, vaqf-nāma*) à cet égard, pour ce qui concerne notamment l'époque safavide. Autre cas remarquable, celui du dispensaire de bienfaisance établi à Téhéran par un particulier, sous Šāh Ṭahmāsp : à cette époque Téhéran n'était qu'un centre de moyenne importance qui s'était développé à côté de l'ancienne ville de Rey et Ḥakīm Yār ʿAlī Tihrānī y avait fondé un dispensaire du nom de *šarbat-ḫāna-yi ḫayrī* dans lequel les médicaments étaient offerts aux pauvres. Ses œuvres pieuses lui valurent le surnom de Ḥakīm Ḫayrī (le médecin charitable). Voici le portrait qu'en donne Munšī :

---

13 Munšī 1350, vol. 2, p. 1110.

14 Munšī 1350, vol. 2, p. 1110.

15 « ... *plus referunt nitoris, quàm artis & magnificentiæ*. », Kaempfer 1712, p. 169.

16 Kaempfer 1712, p. 124.

> *Ḥakīm Yār ʿAlī Tihrānī, connu sous le nom de Ḥakīm Ḫayrī, était un homme de savoir, bien disposé,* […] *à qui le bienheureux roi portait le plus grand intérêt. Au service des sans-abri et des indigents qu'il soignait, il administrait lui-même le* šarbat-ḫāna […] *Ses fils* […], *tous deux compétents* […] *l'assistaient* […] *dans sa tâche*[17].

Yār ʿAlī Tihrānī avait probablement étudié la médecine à Chiraz et rédigea un texte sur la pharmacopée[18]. Lorsqu'il devint vieux, ses deux fils, Ḥakīm Nūr al-Dīn ʿAlī (m. 1032/1622–23, Karbala) et Ḥakīm Šaraf, également médecins, administrèrent le dispensaire de bienfaisance, dont les dépenses étaient approvisionnées par les revenus des propriétés immobilières et des exploitations agricoles de la famille. Nūr al-Dīn ʿAlī devint également l'un des médecins particuliers de Šāh ʿAbbās Ier [19].

Des voyageurs européens ayant visité la Perse à cette époque apportent quelques mentions et de brèves descriptions des hôpitaux situés dans diverses villes. Il faut en outre rappeler que dès l'époque safavide, les Européens fondèrent des établissements hospitaliers en Perse, précisément aux abords du Golfe persique. Les Européens donnent des descriptions qui sont souvent très négatives regardant l'état des hôpitaux dans les villes safavides. Tous ces voyageurs visitèrent la Perse après la période de Šāh ʿAbbās Ier (m. 1629), à une époque où le règne des Safavides entrait dans son déclin, ce qui affecta évidemment le patronage d'institutions comme les hôpitaux, qui tombèrent alors dans un état de négligence.

Le voyageur français Jean-Baptiste Tavernier (1605–1689) se rendit plusieurs fois en Perse entre 1632 et 1668, soit à une époque qui vit le règne de trois Safavides, Ṣafī I (r. 1629–1642), ʿAbbās II (r. 1642–1666) et Sulaymān (r. 1666–1694). Tavernier relate comme suit la piètre situation des hôpitaux iraniens :

> *Il n'y a point en Perse de magnifiques hôpitaux pour les malades comme en notre Europe. Ainsi, quand un malade n'a pas le moyen de faire venir le médecin chez lui, il monte sur un âne accompagné de deux ou trois hommes qui le soutiennent, ayant une serviette ou une écharpe au col, pour marque qu'il est malade*[20].

Jean Chardin (1643–1713), qui faisait commerce de diamants, se rendit en Perse à diverses reprises durant la deuxième moitié du XVIIe siècle, et

---

[17] Munšī 1350, vol. 1, p. 169.

[18] Cf. Tadjbakhsh 2003, p. 239.

[19] Nūr al-Dīn était lui aussi connu sous le nom de Ḥakīm Ḫayrī, cf. Munšī 1350, vol. 1, p. 169, vol. 2, p. 1010 ; Ṣafavī 1314, p. 137.

[20] Tavernier 1976, p. 639.

écrit qu'à l'hôpital d'Ispahan personne ne s'occupait des malades et des aliénés, si bien que les gens redoutaient ce lieu, dit *šifā-ḫāna* (maison de la guérison), et l'appelaient par dérision « établissement de mort » :

> *Les fous et les malades y sont extrêmement mal entretenus, et périssent de misère : ce qui fait dire aux Persans, par ironie, en parlant des hôpitaux, qu'on appelle habitation de santé : l'habitation de la santé est l'habitation de la mort*[21].

Chardin donne une description moins péjorative des établissements de Tabriz, où existaient divers hôpitaux. La ville avait été la capitale des Safavides de 1502 à 1548, sous Šāh Ismāʿīl Ier et pour la première partie du règne de Šāh Ṭahmāsp. L'un des hôpitaux dont Chardin fait mention, avait été édifié par Uzūn Ḥasan (m. 882/1478, aïeul du côté maternel de Šāh Ismāʿīl Ier), et fonctionnait dès l'époque de ce monarque. Chardin écrit :

> *Il y a trois hôpitaux dans la ville : ils sont assez propres, et bien entretenus. On n'y loge guère ; mais on y donne à manger deux fois le jour, à tous ceux qui y viennent. Les hôpitaux s'appellent à Tauris* [Tabriz] Ach-tacon, *c'est-à-dire lieux où l'on fait profusion de vivres*[22].

La description la plus détaillée que donne Chardin est celle de l'hôpital d'Ispahan. Il rapporte que Šāh ʿAbbās Ier l'avait fait édifier avec le caravansérail des chaudronniers, dont les revenus devaient approvisionner le budget de cet établissement de 80 lits. Le témoignage de Chardin est celui d'un lieu en état de négligence considérable, qui n'avait alors pour patients que huit aliénés enchaînés. Il fait mention du personnel qu'on y employait, médecin, apothicaire et autres, signalant l'absence de chirurgien. L'explication concernant l'absence de chirurgiens en Perse, remplacés par des barbiers, ne semble pas tout à fait exacte. Il est toutefois intéressant de remarquer la théorie de Chardin, selon laquelle la chirurgie ne s'est pas développée du fait de la clémence du climat se chargeant de guérir les plaies.

> Darelchafa, *l'habitation de la santé, qui ne ressemble en rien à nos hôpitaux ; car c'est un cloître autour d'un jardin, composé de petites chambres basses, à deux étages, assez jolies, au nombre d'environ quatre-vingt en tout. Je n'y ai jamais vu de malades, mais seulement sept ou huit fous enragés, qu'on enchaîne par les bras, par le corps et par le cou, entre quatre murailles sans le moindre meuble. L'hôpital est fort pauvrement fondé, n'ayant pas deux mille*

---

21 Chardin 1811, vol. 7, p. 391.
22 Chardin 1811, vol. 2, p. 324.

> *écus de rente pour la nourriture des malades, et même mal assignés ; outre dix-huit cents écus pour les gages des officiers, dont le fonds est plus solide ; car c'est le revenu d'un fort grand caravansérail, qui est tout joignant, qu'on appelle le caravansérail des potiers de cuivre, parce qu'il s'y vend toute sorte de chaudronnerie. Abas-le-Grand fit bâtir l'hôpital et le caravansérail tout à la fois, afin que le revenu du caravansérail entretînt les officiers de l'hôpital. Ils consistent en un médecin, un droguiste, un prêtre ou molla, un cuisinier, un portier, un balayeur. On trouvera étrange qu'il n'y ait point de chirurgien parmi ces officiers ; mais la chirurgie n'est pas une profession particulière en Orient, et même elle y est peu connue. Les barbiers sont ceux qui saignent ; et quant aux autres opérations de chirurgie, on s'en passe en Orient. La bonne constitution du climat guérit les plaies, qui n'étant d'ordinaire que des coups de sabre et de lance, il suffit de les tenir nettes, et d'y mettre un emplâtre sans autre façon. On ne sait point dans ces pays-là ce que c'est que trépaner, couper des bras et des jambes, scier des membres, tailler de la pierre, faire des incisions dans les chairs, et toutes les autres opérations à quoi notre humeur bouillante, aussi bien que la mauvaise constitution de notre climat, nous rend sujets.*
>
> *Le médecin de l'hôpital se tient à la porte, depuis huit heures jusqu'à midi, sur un petit échafaud portatif, de trente-cinq à quarante pouces de diamètre, et y donne ses avis et ses ordonnances gratis à qui vient le consulter. Les drogues et la nourriture des malades sont payées des deniers légués ; mais il y a toujours là si peu de malades, comme je l'ai dit, que ce qu'on se fait payer pour eux est autant d'argent volé. Les raisons sont premièrement, qu'on ne voit pas à beaucoup près en ces pays-là tant de sortes de maladies que dans les nôtres, ni de si longues et enracinées, à cause de la bonté de l'air ; secondement, qu'on n'a pas dans cet hôpital la charité qu'il serait à souhaiter* [...] *Il y a un autre hôpital à Ispahan, qui n'est pas plus grand, ni mieux entretenu que celui-ci, et c'est tout ce qui qu'il y en a*[23].

Chardin note aussi l'existence d'hôpitaux dans les autres villes principales de la Perse, sans cependant en offrir de descriptions plus détaillées : « Je n'en ai vu qu'un aussi dans les plus grandes villes de Perse, et il n'y en a point dans les autres[24] ».

Un autre témoignage, de la deuxième moitié du XVII^e^ siècle, est donné par Raphaël du Mans, prêtre français et père supérieur de la mission des Capucins d'Ispahan, où il vécut quarante ans avant de s'y éteindre en 1696. Raphaël du Mans écrivit un ouvrage intitulé *Estat de la Perse en 1660*, dans lequel il écrit que chaque ville de Perse possédait un ou deux établissements hospitaliers. A propos de l'hôpital d'Ispahan, Raphaël du Mans précise qu'il s'agissait d'un bâtiment peu fréquenté, à tel point qu'à l'époque où l'auteur l'avait visité, seuls y étaient hospitalisés un indien et

---

23 Chardin 1811, vol. 7, pp. 389–393.
24 Chardin 1811, vol. 7, p. 393.

un fou enchaîné. Aussi Raphaël du Mans note que la population appelait l'hôpital, la maison de la mort :

> Dar el Chepha, *hospitaux, qui dans une grande ville sera un ou 2, sont appellés par les gens mesme du pais* dar el mergue[25], *le lieu de la mort, non pas de la santé. Car jaçoit qu'il y aie quantité de chambres, toutes néantmoins comme les chambres pour les gens du Roy, c'est à dire les 4 murailles, sans aucun meuble. Quelque bien légué,* mal vekfe, *toute fois il ne se donne rien aux pauvres, qui mouroint plus tost de faim que pe[r]mettre que l'on les transportast là, le médecin et autres officiers mangeant tout le revenu. Dans celuy d'Hispan, faisant tout le tour, car il est comme un cloistre quarré, les chambres toutes à l'entour, la porte servant de fenestre comme dans les caravanserra, je ne vis là qu'un pauvre Indien moribond, couché à plat de la terre, et en une autre un pauvre fol attaché avec une chaisne*[26].

Comme nous l'avons vu, les sources et documents sur les hôpitaux en Perse, lors des XVI^e^ et XVIII^e^ siècles, sont assez limités, et notamment, les descriptions concernant l'activité de ces établissements à l'époque de l'épanouissement des sciences et des arts sous les Safavides. Cependant, on peut souligner quelques caractéristiques importantes résultant des descriptions disponibles. En premier lieu, il faut remarquer que des médecins éminents furent en service dans ces hôpitaux, et surtout sous Šāh Ṭahmāsp (r. 1524–1576) et Šāh ʿAbbās I^er^ (r. 1588–1629), ce qui fait penser qu'il s'agissait d'un travail capable d'attirer à cette époque des membres importants de l'élite médicale. Certains de ces établissements faisaient partie d'un ensemble de bâtiments, attenant parfois à une mosquée ou à un mausolée, ou à un caravansérail, comme dans le cas d'Ispahan, où un jardin occupait le centre de l'hôpital. Or il ne demeure rien aujourd'hui de ces bâtiments hospitaliers.

On ne connaît pas de nouveaux hôpitaux qui aient été créés à l'époque safavide après Šāh ʿAbbās I^er^, bien que ceux qui avaient été établis auparavant restèrent en général en activité. Les voyageurs européens qui visitèrent la Perse dès les années trente du XVII^e^ siècle, donnent souvent des descriptions négatives de ces établissements. Ces témoignages indiquent qu'après le règne de Šāh ʿAbbās I^er^, avec l'amorce du déclin de la dynastie, la situation des hôpitaux dut se dégrader considérablement. Cependant, on peut noter qu'en 1051/1641–42 encore, un médecin éminent tel ʿAlī Afżal Qāṭiʿ était en service à l'hôpital de Qazvin. Les récits des Européens indiquent en même temps que les hôpitaux des grandes villes du pays

---

[25] En persan *dār al-marg*.

[26] Richard 1995, vol. 2, p. 171.

étaient encore ouverts à la fin du XVII^e^ siècle. Enfin, on ne connaît presque rien de la situation de ces établissement au siècle suivant, durant la dernière période des Safavides puis sous les Afsharides (1736–1747) et les Zand (1750–1794).

## Bibliographie


Chardin, Jean, 1811, *Voyages du chevalier Chardin en Perse, et autres lieux de l'Orient*, L. Langles, éd., 10 vols. Paris, Le Normant (nouvelle édition).

Elgood, Cyril, 1970, *Safavid Medical Practice*. London, Luzac & Co.

Ḥasan Ḫān, Muḥammad Ṣanīʿ al-Dawla, 1363 h. š./1984–5, *Maṭlaʿ al-šams*, 3 vols. Téhéran (1e éd. 1301–03/1883–86).

Ḫvāndamīr, Ġiyāṯ al-Dīn ibn Humām al-Dīn al-Ḥusaynī, 1353 h. š./1974–5, *Ḥabīb al-siyar*, 4 vols. Téhéran.

Kaempfer, Engelbert, 1712, *Amoenitatum exoticarum politico-physico-medicarum fasciculi V : quibus continentur variæ relationes, observationes & descriptiones Rerum Persicarum & Ulterioris Asiæ, multá attentione, in peregrinationibus per universum Orientem, collectae / ab auctore Engelberto Kæmpfero*. Lemgoviæ : Typis & Impensis Henrici Wilhelmi Meyeri, Aulæ Lippiacæ Typographi.

Munšī, Iskandar Beg, 1350 h. š./1971–2, *Tārīḫ-i ʿālamārā-yi ʿAbbāsī*, 2 vols., Īraj Afšār, éd. Téhéran, Intišārāt-i Amīr Kabīr.

Qazvīnī, ʿAlī Afżal Qāṭiʿ, *Manāfiʿ-i Afżaliya*, ms. Téhéran, Bibliothèque Centrale de l'Université de Téhéran, pers. 13/d.

——, *Favāʾid-i Afżaliya*, ms. Téhéran, Bibliothèque Centrale de l'Université de Téhéran, pers. 3288.

Qummī, Qāżī Aḥmad, 1359–1363 h. š./1980–1984, *Ḫulāṣat al-tavārīḫ*, 2 vols., Téhéran, Intišārāt-i Dānišgāh-i Tihrān.

Richard, Francis, éd., 1995, *Raphaël du Mans : missionnaire en Perse au XVII^e^ s.*, 2 vols., Paris, Société d'Histoire de l'Orient - L'Harmattan.

Ṣafavī, Sām Mīrzā, 1314 h. š./1935, *Tuḥfa-yi Sāmī*, Vaḥīd Dastgirdī, éd. Téhéran.

Tadjbakhsh, Hasan, 1379 h. š./2000, *Tārīḫ-i bīmāristānhā-yi Īrān*. Téhéran, Pažūhišgāh-i ʿulūm-i insānī va muṭālaʿāt-i farhangī.

——, 2003, *History of Medicine and Veterinary Medicine in Iran*. Lyon, Fondation Mérieux.

Tavernier, Jean-Baptiste, 1976, *Les six voyages de Jean-Baptiste Tavernier, … qu'il a fait en Turquie, en Perse, et aux Indes, … Première partie, Où il n'est parlé que de la Turquie et de la Perse*. Paris, Hachette (reproduction de l'édition de Paris, G. Clouzier – C. Barbin, 1676).

# HOSPITALS IN SAFAVID AND QAJAR IRAN: AN ENQUIRY INTO THEIR NUMBER, GROWTH AND IMPORTANCE

Willem Floor

## Introduction: What Size Population Did Hospitals Serve?

The common wisdom is that the continuation of the institution of the Sasanian hospitals "was one of the most remarkable achievements in the Islamic East."[1] However remarkable the potential of the *dār al-šifā* was they did not deliver on their promise. For seen within the context of the size of the problem, neither the traditional *dār al-šifā* nor the nineteenth century modern European hospitals constituted an adequate response to the public health problem in Iran in view of their limited impact. To obtain a better understanding of the relative importance of hospitals I discuss their occurrence and activities in Iran. Given the scope of this publication, I have limited my remarks to the Safavid (1501–1722) and Qajar periods (1794–1925), but these remarks also apply to earlier periods. First, I raise the question as to the significance of hospitals given their number in relation to the size of the population. Second, I discuss the introduction and development of European hospitals and dispensaries and what conclusions one may draw from that experience.

Until recent times Iran had always been an agrarian subsistence economy. During the Safavid period its population probably was never higher than 9 million during the seventeenth century, a number likely to be lower in the sixteenth century due to the many wars that were fought. Most of the population (85–90%) was rural in nature, while the pastoral population was never more than one-third of the total population. There were about 70, mostly small provincial towns in Safavid Iran. Isfahan may have had 500,000 inhabitants, while Tabriz had more than 100,000, may be even more than 200,000, but Qazvin had many less inhabitants, even when it was the capital. The urban population, therefore, oscillated around 1 million during the Safavid period.[2] No population data are available on the eighteenth century, but, given the wars and oppression that characterized that period, it is likely

[1] Sajjādī 1990, pp. 257–259.
[2] Floor 2000, pp. 2–8.

that the urban population decreased. By 1900, Iran had an estimated population of about 9.8 million. The majority of that population was still rural and engaged in agriculture.[3] The urban population doubled between 1850 (9%) and 1910 (18%), with three towns having more than 100,000 inhabitants: Tehran with about 280,000, Tabriz with 200,000 and Isfahan with 100,000. Four other towns each had 50,000 inhabitants or more.[4]

What the above means is that between 1500 and 1925, even in the best of times, 85% of the population was rural, and only by 1910 did this figure drop to 82%. These figures imply that the vast majority of the population, therefore, had no access to hospitals at all. Because hospitals were only to be found in large cities, they thus did not serve most of the rural population (whether sedentary or nomadic), who hardly visited the large cities. That leaves still 1 to 1.8 million people in urban areas, where hospitals are located, but most of these never saw the inside of a hospital either, because of their small number, their limited staff and means as well as the nature of their function, but above all their lack of appeal to the public at large.

## How Many Hospitals Were There in Safavid Iran?

The number of traditional hospitals or *dār al-šifā* had never been large, despite their alleged importance during the period before the fourteenth century. It is, of course, likely that there were many more hospitals than the few indicated by the existing sources, but even if we assume a tenfold increase of the known ones their total number would probably still not exceed 100. Most scholars agree that the number of hospitals greatly decreased after the Ilkhanid period, although there is no evidence for that. This alleged decline took place despite the fact that Timur had given orders that there should be at least one hospital in every city in his realm.[5] There is no proof, however, that these actually were functioning let alone built.

The situation under the Safavids did not differ that much from the preceding centuries in terms of the nature of medical services offered to the public. However, there is no evidence that the number of *dār al-šifā* was less than in the preceding centuries. Allegedly one or two hospitals existed in every city, according to Du Mans. Unfortunately, we only have

---

[3] Floor 2003, p. 45.
[4] Gilbar 1976, pp. 147–149.
[5] Sajjādī 1990, pp. 257–259.

information about the existence of a few of these hospitals, but that seems to confirm Du Mans' observation. According to Tavernier, there were no hospitals in Iran as beautiful as the ones that existed in Europe.[6] Nevertheless, some of them were quite nice; at least that is what Chardin thought. He agreed with Tavernier that the one in Isfahan did not resemble anything like a European hospital. It was more like a two-storied convent around a garden, consisting of 80 rather nice, but small low rooms. This description is not unlike the one given by Du Mans.[7] The Isfahan hospital was situated near the *Qayṣariya*, behind the copper-smiths' bazaar that was also known as the *bāzār-i dār al-šifā*, because its caravanserai had been built as an endowment to ensure the payment of the hospital's staff's wages. The hospital was part of the traditional complex consisting of a madrasa and mosque with facilities for pilgrims such as a hospital, which buildings, therefore, were referred to as *madrasa-yi* and *masjid-i dār al-šifā*.[8] It is not superfluous to point out that usually the *dār al-šifā* mainly served pilgrims and other travelers (*ġurabā, zuvvār, mutaraddidīn*) who came to the Shrine or mosque-madrasa complex, but not necessarily the inhabitants of the town in which it was located. In this respect its function is roughly the same as that of a hospital in the meaning as used in Europe during medieval times, viz., an almshouse for the poor and pilgrims.

Isfahan was not the only town with a hospital, for there was also a hospital or *māristān* in Tabriz that had been built by Uzūn Ḥasan (r. 1453–1478), which was large, having many buildings, "and within it is even more beautifully ornamented than the mosque, having many large wards about ten yards long and four broad, each of them being fitted with a carpet to its measurement."[9] It still existed under the early Safavids. Some one hundred fifty years later, according to Chardin, there were even three clean and well-maintained hospitals in Tabriz.[10] In 1680, an additional *dār al-šifā* was built in Tabriz as part of the usual endowment complex consisting of a (founder's) tomb, a mosque, a madrasa and sundry buildings.[11] In Mashhad there probably was a *dār al-šifā* since the reign of Šāh Ṭahmāsp I (r. 1524–1576). At that time, assistance was most likely given to the sick, because the

---

[6] Tavenier 1930, p. 277; see also St. Joseph 1985, p. 133.

[7] Chardin 1811, vol. 7, pp. 389–390; Du Mans 1890, p. 219; Richard 1995, vol. 2, p. 171.

[8] Chardin 1811, vol. 7, p. 391; Jābarī-Anṣārī 1373, pp. 147, 287, 341; Gaube – Wirth 1978, pp. 284–285; Naṣrābādī 1361, p. 326; Munšī 1350, vol. 2, pp. 1070, 1110.

[9] Barbaro – Contarini 1873, part 2, p. 177; Tadjbakhsh 1379, pp. 162–164.

[10] Chardin 1811, vol. 2, p. 324.

[11] Werner 2000, p. 99 (*Ẓāhiriya awqāf*), of which no trace is left.

endowment deed of 1524 states that part of the Shrine's income had to be spent on the sick.[12] Šāh Ṭahmāsp I even appointed one of his court physicians ʿImād al-Dīn Maḥmūd, an opium addict, as physician of the shrine, who spent some time there treating the sick.[13] Elgood also mentions a hospital in Ardabil, which was attached to the shrine of Šayḫ Ṣafī al-Dīn, as well as one in Qazvin, called the 'royal hospital', to which ʿAlī Afżal Qāṭiʿ was attached as physician.[14]

There also were hospitals or dispensaries elsewhere in Iran such as in Yazd where there was a so-called 'house of health' or *ṣiḥḥat-ḫāna*.[15] In 1515, in Astarabad, Ḫvāja Muẓaffar ibn Ḫvāja Aḥmad Bitikčī Astarābādī endowed the *Dār al-šifā-yi Muẓaffariya*, which he had established previously, with new endowments. A third of the endowment was to be used, among other things, to pay for a professor (*mudarris*), students (*ṭalaba*), a tutor (*muʿīd*), a servant (*ḫādim*), and an orderly (*sāʿī*), and another third for the physician (*ṭabīb*) and the sick. The deed further noted that the professor had to be knowledgeable about medicine.[16] In Shiraz there was a *dār al-šifā*, which was founded by Šāh Šujāʿ Muẓaffarī in 1384 and functioned in the Timurid period, but there is no report that it was still used as such during the Safavid period.[17] According to an unpublished document, however, there still was a hospital attached to the mosque-madrasa complex in Safavid Shiraz located on the Maydān-i Šāh (see map 1 for its probable location).

This hospital perhaps still existed in the eighteenth century, for among the good works of Karīm Ḫān Zand are mentioned the order to keep the streets and the bazaar lanes clean as well as to fund the *dār al-šifā*, which had to make its services available free of charge to the poor and orphans.[18] In 1695, the existence of a *dār al-šifā* is mentioned in Damghan.[19] There had been, or perhaps there still was, a *dār al-šifā* in Ashraf, because Rabino lists among the mosques of that town one that was called *Masjid-i Dār*

---

12 Mu'taman 1348, p. 401.

13 Munšī 1350, vol. 1, p. 168; Savory 1978, vol. 1, p. 264. For other physicians employed at the Mashhad hospital see Elgood 1970, p. 29.

14 Elgood 1970 p. 29; Tadjbakhsh 1379, pp. 175–183.

15 Bāfqī 1340, vol. 3, p. 398. Elgood 1970, p. 29 refers to this hospital as Dār al-ʿIbādat or Place of Worship, which is wrong as his source, Munšī 1350, vol. 1, p. 168 only refers to the city of Yazd, which was known as Dār al-ʿIbādat.

16 Sutūda 1366, vol. 8, pp. 184–186.

17 Fasā'ī 1367, vol. 2, p. 943; Furṣat-i Šīrāzī 1312, p. 459; Musṭafavī 1343, p. 385 (part of the madrasa still exists).

18 Tavassoli – Naser 1371/1992, p. 68, quoting Nāṣir Bunyādī, *Madārik-i muntašir našuda-i ṭarḥ-i tārīḫ-i ijtimāʿī-i Šīrāz*, Tehran, 1358/1979; Āṣaf 1348, pp. 255–56.

19 Nasīrī 1373/1994, p. 115.

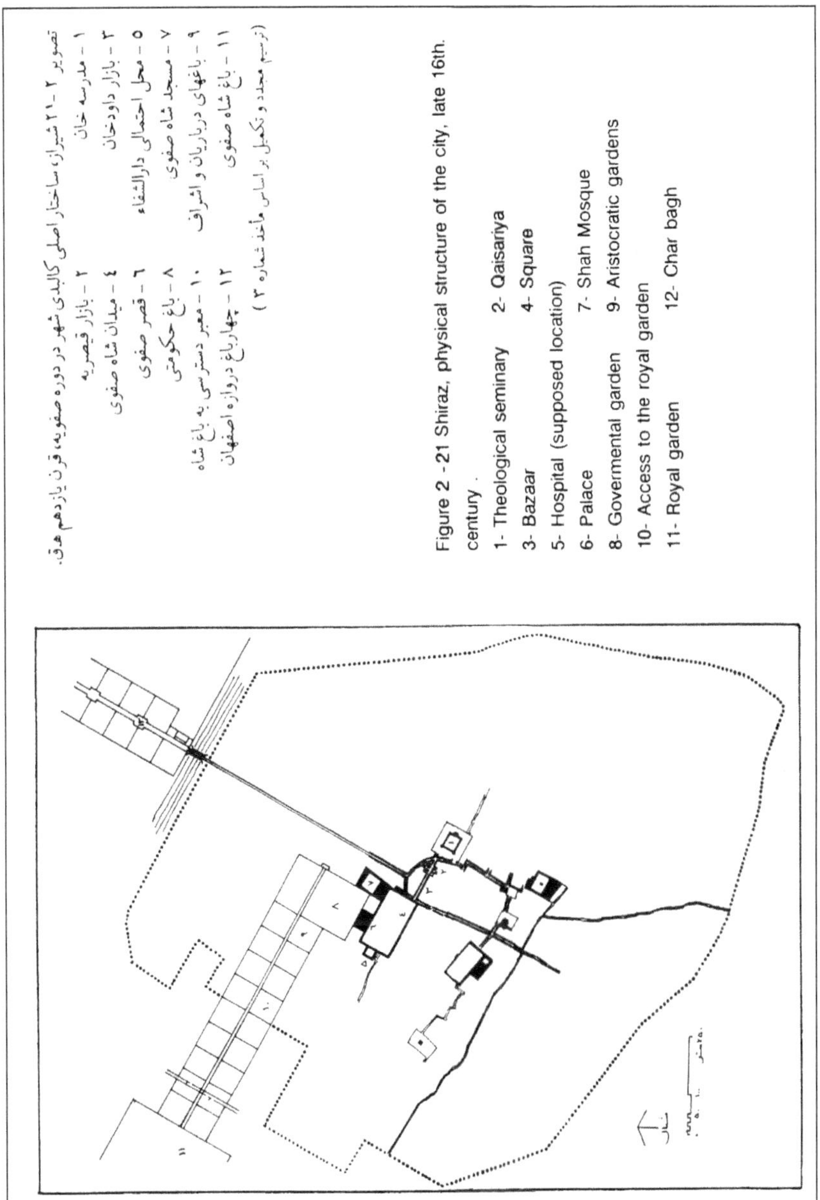


Map 1. Map of Shiraz indicating the supposed location of the hospital. From Tavassoli – Bonyadi, 1371/1992, *Urban Space Design*. Tehran, p. 68.

*al-šifā*. Such a mosque or a hospital is not mentioned in similar descriptions of Ashraf.[20] There was even a hospital in Ben Isfahan, a very large village near Isfahan.[21] There further existed a so-called charitable dispensary (*šarbat-ḫāna-yi ḫayrī*) which was managed by Ḥakīm Yār ʿAlī Tihrānī. He was known for his care of the poor and indigent, hence he was nicknamed *ḥakīm-i ḫayrī* or 'the welfare doctor.'[22] All these instances suggest that the information provided by Du Mans about the prevalence of hospitals is correct, thus belying the generally held opinion that after the fourteenth century there was a decline in the number of hospitals in Iran.

There seems to have been a court official, who is mentioned as functioning at the end of the Safavid period and who was known as the chief of the hospital (*tīmārčī-bāšī*).[23] It is not clear what precise function this official had. There was no hospital or dispensary in the royal palace grounds. Perhaps the official was in charge of the hospitals in Isfahan, of which one or two existed in Isfahan as well as in other large towns. It would not be the first time that a court physician was put in charge of the *dār al-šifā*. It happened to the one in Isfahan founded by ʿAbbās I, which was under the court physician for some time.[24] But it is more likely that he was in charge of the appointment of all physicians, who had to follow his instructions, just as the chief physician of the hospital (*sāʿūr-i bīmāristān*) in Ilkhanid times had been in charge of all physicians.[25]

Apart from these Iranian hospitals, there also was a European hospital, the first of its kind in Iran, which was built by the Portuguese on the island of Hormuz in 1516. It was run by Augustinian friars and provided, among other things, charitable services to the poor. Its impact, of course, was limited. First, because at that time the type of medicine practiced by European doctors did not differ that much from that of Iranian ones. Second, Iranian physicians were more knowledgeable as to the diseases in the Persian Gulf and Iran than the Portuguese monks, who, certainly initially, therefore learnt more from Iranian physicians than the other

---

20 Rabino 1928, p. 64; Sutūda 1366, vol. 5, pp. 615–16.

21 Jābarī-Anṣārī 1373, p. 323.

22 Munšī 1350, vol. 1, p. 169; Savory 1978, vol. 1, p. 265; Tadjbakhsh 1379, pp. 192–193; Tadjbakhsh also notes that there was a dispensary in the royal train, when the *šāh* was on the move, Ibid., p. 194.

23 Āṣaf 1348, p. 101. In medieval Khvarezm this official was known as *tīmārdār*. Jurjānī 2535, p. 644.

24 Du Mans 1890, p. 219; Richard 1995, vol. 2, p. 171; Munšī 1350, vol. 2, pp. 1070, 1110; Savory 1978, vol. 2, p. 1295; vol. 1, p. 536.

25 Naḫjavānī 1964, vol. 2, pp. 235–236.

way around. Third, the institute of a hospital per se was not unknown to Iranians; in fact there was one on the island prior to the arrival of the Portuguese. Also, the nature of the Portuguese hospital was not that different from that of a *dār al-šifā*, i.e., it was also a place to receive spiritual consolation and care and where one died, as indicated by the title of the manager of the Portuguese hospital (*provedor do esprital e defuntos*). Also, the capacity of the hospital was very limited (certainly in the first few years of its existence) and often the sick had to stay on the ships due to lack of room in the hospital. Its staff consisted of a physician, a surgeon, and a barber, while there also was a medical drug store (*botica*) in the fort.[26] All this suggests that the impact of this Portuguese institution on the medical situation in Iran, if any, was probably neutral.

The two hospitals in a hamlet near Bandar ʿAbbas reported by Fryer, were not hospitals, although he used that term and Elgood took his remarks at their face-value. What Fryer actually referred to was the use of the natural sulfur springs at Ghinaw, near Bandar Abbas by infirm people. The use of hot springs for medical and other purposes was already known since Antiquity,[27] and they were widely used in Iran where they abounded.

> Nakoda Biram, the Dutch Broker, and Tockserey, our Banyan, have Built to these natural Baths, each an handsome Hospital: That of the first is an open one, Built Square, Capped with Four round Tubilated Cupilo's about an huge one in the middle, with Two Rows of Pillars to support it. The latter has made his more close, upheld by Nine Pillars on the sides, and Four in the middle, with a stately Portico at the Entrance, and a close Cell behind, commodious to Sweat in, besides a Stone Repository for Rain Water; they being both neat and durable Works.[28]

From the above description it is quite clear that this was not a hospital, but an establishment to make use of the waters, of which there were many in Iran. Other travelers, who have written about this place, including Kaempfer (a physician), make no mention of a hospital at all, only of the beneficial qualities of the hot springs.[29] The Dutch who went there, not to get treated for illnesses, but to ease the pains of their aging bones, never referred to it as a hospital either. There was no physician attached to these hot springs, either by the Dutch or the English. But even if it had been a

26 Aubin 2000, pp. 401–403; Floor 2006, pp. 12, 27, 29, 54; Elgood 1951, p. 512.
27 On the merits of which Fryer 1909–15, vol. 2, pp. 330–335 expounds; see also the observation of Chardin regarding their use in Iran. Chardin 1811, vol. 5, p. 188.
28 Fryer 1909–15, vol. 2, pp. 329–330; Elgood 1951, p. 399.
29 Kaempfer 1968, p. 137; Hamilton 1930, vol. 1, pp. 60–61.

hospital it is clear that these baths were private establishments, inaccessible to those who had not been invited. Thus, their impact was very limited. The same remarks apply to the alleged hospital operated by the East India Company in Bandar ʿAbbas in 1727 and in the 1770s in Basra, which, more than likely, was just a room where the sick could receive drugs and consolation, and die or recuperate, as the case might be, not unlike the alleged 'hospital' or rather sick room that the Carmelites operated in the 1660s in Basra.[30] Even if these establishments had really been hospitals then their impact on the medical situation in Iran was negligible as their services were limited to a certain group of people only, i.e., Europeans and their Asian co-workers and there was no cross-fertilization with Iranian physicians.

## How Effective Were Hospitals in Safavid Iran?

In short, it is my contention that the number of hospitals was too small to have had a significant impact on the public health situation in Safavid Iran. Even assuming that the number of *dār al-šifā* was much larger than the number we know about, they could not have been very effective due to the limited number of doctors. Physicians, i.e., those who called themselves or were called *ḥakīm*, practiced medicine that was Galenic in nature. Not only was their number limited, but often, they were attached to the families of the rich and mighty, thus leaving little time for others. Those that still had the time and the inclination to serve patients in hospitals would not have been able to serve many. I am leaving aside here the question whether these *dār al-šifā* actually gave, or were able to provide, effective health care. The reality, therefore, was that the majority of the population, whether rural or urban, relied on home remedies and folk medicine that was mostly pre-Islamic in nature and did not flock to the *dār al-šifā*.[31]

The abovementioned analysis is borne out by the little we know about the actual functioning of Iranian hospitals in the Safavid period. For example, sick people did not come to the hospital in Isfahan to find healing, despite the fact that it had a staff that consisted of one doctor, a druggist, a mullah, a cook, a porter and a sweeper. There was no surgeon among them, "because surgery was not a specialty and moreover rather unknown in

[30] Elgood 1951, p. 341; Wright 2001, p. 122; Martin 1990, p. 427.
[31] See for an analysis of the situation in Qajar Iran, Floor 2004; Ibid., 1386/2007.

the east", according to Chardin. In the Isfahan hospital, the physician could be found at the hospital's door from 8 AM until noon, where he gave medical advice and prescriptions free-of-charge. Although the advice, drugs, and food were free, the few people who actually came there for treatment paid for the service and drugs. This was partly due to the fact that the hospital was badly endowed. It had 2,000 *écus* or 666 *tūmān*s in rents to feed the sick, but these rents had been based on a source of income which was difficult to collect. Du Mans, Chardin and Ange de St. Joseph all agree that hardly anybody came to the *dār al-šifā* to find treatment. The only people they saw were some mad men who were chained to the wall or a poor moribund Indian. According to Chardin, as little as 1,800 *écus* or 600 *tūmāns*[32] had been allocated for its medical staff, which may explain that not only was medical care limited in scope if not absent, but that the hospital's funds were stolen, or as Du Mans formulates it, the physicians and other staff "ate" all the allocated funds. This despite the fact that ʿAbbas I had assigned a rather reliable source of income for the 1,800 *écus*, viz., the income of the adjacent caravanserai of the copper-smiths, which the *šāh* had built at the same time as the hospital. As a result, the hospital thus was not really charitable, while, moreover, the sick and mad men were badly treated and died as a result in the hospital. Poor people, travelers and strangers, only came there to die, hence this and other *dār al-šifā* were known in popular parlance as the "house of death", *dār al-marg* or *dār al-mawt*.[33] In Tabriz the situation was not much different. Chardin noted that hardly anybody stayed in its three *dār al-šifā*. However, food was given twice per day to those who came there. Hence the three hospitals were popularly known as Ach-tacon (*āš-maqām*) in Tabriz, i.e., the place where food (in this case soup or *āš*) was distributed.[34]

The endowment deed of the shrine in Mashhad of 1747 suggests that its *dār al-šifā* was still functioning and assisting patients, although there is no way of knowing whether the money was really spent in accordance with

---

32 Chardin qualifies this amount as being inadequate (*l'hôpital est fort pauvrement fondé*), but in fact it was an enormous amount, certainly if one takes into account the total amount of funds as well as the level of wages paid to the staff of the Shrine hospital at Mashhad (see Table 1) and that the average annual wages of an army officer were six *tūmāns* at that time.

33 Du Mans 1890, p. 219; Richard 1995, vol. 2, p. 171 (*dār al-marg*); Chardin 1811, vol. 7, pp. 389–393; St. Joseph 1985, pp. 132–133 (*dār al-mawt*). A contemporary Persian text states that in Isfahan "the *dār al-šifā* is [built] in the form of a caravanserai; in it are sick people and madmen." Gaube – Wirth 1978, pp. 284–285.

34 Chardin 1811, vol. 2, p. 324.

the terms of the deed, as suggested by the reality in Isfahan. The deed states that in the past 94 *tūmān*s had been fixed for the expenses of the *dār al-šifā* annually, but now in view of the increased number of sick and poor it had been decided to add to that annual amount from the endowment funds as follows:

Table 1: Wages and Other Expenditures of the *Dār al-šifā* of Mashhad in 1747

| Wages | Cash | In kind |
|---|---|---|
| Physician | 20 *tūmāns* | 20 *ḫarvār* of wheat |
| Two overseers (*nāẓer*) | 12.5 *tūmāns* | 27 *ḫarvār* of wheat |
| Surgeon with the cost for ointments | 8 *tūmāns* | 2 *ḫarvār* of wheat |
| Orderly, porter, etc. | – | 20 *ḫarvār* of wheat |
| Expenses for food, medicines, etc. | 200 *tūmāns* | – |
| Total | 240.5 *tūmāns* | 69 *ḫarvar* of wheat |

Source: Mu'taman 1348, p. 402.

Given the fact that Iran before 1850, like all other countries, suffered from a lack of sanitation and in the case of Iran remained so well into the 1950s, the need for effective preventive health care is evident. However, there were neither enough hospitals nor enough physicians to provide the necessary medical care. But even those hospitals that existed did not address the need for health care and as a result Iran remained a public health nightmare. The contribution of *dār al-šifā* in Iran to the public health situation, therefore, was irrelevant and thus, we also need to re-assess our appreciation of the objective value of this institution in medieval Iranian society. This is further underlined by the limited impact that modern European dispensaries and hospitals had on the public health situation in Qajar Iran, despite much better clinical and diagnostic knowledge and much more effective treatment methods and medicines. This is mainly due to the fact that the real public health challenge in Iran, as in all countries all over the world, was and is the lack of sanitation and of personal hygiene. The answer to that problem of providing limited curative care, however effective that may have been in individual cases, could not and did not address the sanitation and hygiene problem. As a result, people remained sick or repeatedly fell sick, because of the continued existence of endemic and contagious diseases.

## The Situation in Qajar Iran

In what follows I will give an overview of what is known about dispensaries (*darmān-ḫāna*) and hospitals (*bīmāristān* or *marīż-ḫāna*) in various Iranian cities between 1850 and 1925. This inventory, which starts with the capital Tehran and thereafter alphabetically lists the cities about which we have data, also serves, where data are available, to gauge the impact hospitals and dispensaries had and what the major problems were that they had to overcome to have some measure of success. This section is completed with a discussion of the implications of these data.

### Tehran

Tehran, the capital city of Iran since 1796, had a population of more than 220,000 (even 300,000 according to some) in 1920. Until 1852, when it had a population of about 100,000, Tehran had no real hospital. There was a *dār al-šifā*, which had been built by Fatḥ ʿAlī Šāh (r. 1797–1834). As was usual for this type of institution it was attached to a religious school and mosque, where sometimes a few sick people stayed and were fed. It still existed under Muḥammad Šāh (r. 1834–1848), but fell into disuse. It was then turned into a madrasa, although the students did not receive stipends. It does not seem to have had any active medical function anymore under Nāṣir al-Dīn Šāh (r. 1848–1896).[35]

In 1850, at the instructions of Amīr Kabir construction was begun of a state hospital (*marīż-ḫāna-yi dawlatī*), which was the first modern hospital built in Iran.[36] The new hospital, which was situated outside Tehran, was opened in January 1852. It also had a pharmacy and could house 400 patients. The first director was Mīrzā Muḥammad Walī *ḥakīm-bāšī*, and Dr. Kazulani, chief-doctor of the army, was responsible for medical

---

35 ʿAyn al-Salṭana 1376, vol. 1, p. 306; Sipihr 1377, vol. 3, p. 1183; Tadjbakhsh 1379, p. 217. It was located opposite the Masjid-i Šāh, part of it was situated in the Ḫiyābān-i Buzurgmihr. Šahrī 1368, vol. 5, p. 700, n. 3. When the street was broadened the *dār al-šifā* was destroyed and a plaque was erected to commemorate its location, which was later occupied by a branch of the *Bānk-i Bāzārgānī*. Muʿtamadī 1381, pp. 104, 197, 629.

36 Ebrahimnejad 2000, p. 171, mentions an anonymous Persian manuscript (*Risāla dar ḫuṣūṣ-i ta'sīs-i marīż-ḫāna*), written in the early 1850s, that proposed, amongst other things, the establishment of a military hospital. It seems likely that this text was written at the suggestion of the Amīr Kabīr, in which case it must have been written in 1849, because construction work of his hospital had started already in 1850. For an English translation of this text see Ebrahimnejad 2004.

treatment. The doctors with three students were busy everyday till noon, and the patients were satisfied with the service offered and left the hospital in good health, according to the government newspaper. From January 1852 till January 1853, 2,238 patients were treated in the hospital, who suffered from difficult diseases.[37]

It would seem that this hospital was inadequate, for in 1857 Nasir al-Dīn Šāh ordered the establishment of another hospital in Tehran.[38] It was built outside Tehran at the instigation of Dr. Polak, the Austrian medical advisor and teacher, who had seen that sick soldiers were kept in dark cellar-like barracks, where they died like flies. Whether Polak referred to the first hospital that Amīr Kabīr had built in 1852, or whatever happened to that first hospital, is not known. Polak does not even explicitly refer to this first hospital, although he had worked in it. Polak's original design was a roomy and light building, that formed a square with a spacious courtyard, in the middle of which was the inevitable pond. Around the building he had planned that bushes and trees were to be planted, while a wall would surround the entire site. The rooms were three and a half feet high above the ground. The design was completely changed by the chief general during his absence, but Polak was able to get most of his way. Once the hospital had been built in 1857, the next battle began; how to get funds for its operation. The army doctors had an allocation for a large establishment, but spent most of it on themselves. Even the most necessary drugs, such as quinine, they did not buy. The doctors shared the hospital's operational budget with the army's officers and were not interested in changing this arrangement. Polak's students, whom he had entrusted with the management of food, clothing, instruments, and drugs, diverted the money for their own use. Instead of showing how a proper hospital might function, Polak received a demonstration of how Iran functioned. Nevertheless, it was not a wasted effort, because the students still learnt the concepts of hospital management, saw many patients, and learnt how much you could do for the soldiers with limited means. Hundreds of patients were

---

[37] I'timād al-Salṭana 1306, pp. 62, 73; Government of Iran 1373, vol. 1, p. 611 (nr. 102, 8 *rabīʿ al-ṯānī* 1269/19 January, 1853) states that 1,238 patients were treated, but vol. 1, pp. 618–619 (nr. 103, 10 *rabīʿ al-ṯānī*, 1369/21 January, 1853) gives the higher number. On Dr. Kazulani, about whom I have not been able to find other particulars, see Ibid., vol. 1, pp. 34, 64, 260, 303 (his death) and Ādamiyat 1348, p. 327 who stated that he was the brother of Kazulani the chief painter (*naqqāš-bāšī*), about whom I have found no further information.

[38] I'timād al-Salṭana 1300, vol. 3, pp. 218, 255; Polak 1859, p. 140.

treated at the hospital, and despite their initial mistrust of the hospital, the sick gradually begged for admission.

Because Polak was appointed the *šāh*'s personal physician he could no longer manage the hospital and its management was transferred to an Iranian doctor. When Polak came back later, he was shocked to see the conditions in which the patients were kept. It was like a scene from medical hell. "Patients with typhus and dysentery literally danced in their own feces and vomit." Also, all trees and bushes that he had financed with his own money had disappeared.[39] By 1860, it no longer deserved to be called a hospital, according to Häntzsche, a German physician who had worked for many years in northern Iran.[40] Polak also insisted on appointing a number of physicians as sanitary inspectors of army barracks. It was their task to ensure that preventive measures were taken to maintain proper hygienic conditions in the barracks, and to acquaint new recruits with preventive medical rules. To provide them with guidelines he had written instructions in Persian.[41]

In 1868, a new hospital was built for the army. The old one was now dedicated for civilian use and was placed under the management of a German physician who taught at the Dār al-funūn. The hospital remained under German management until World War I. The old hospital became known as the Marīż-ḫāna-yi dawlatī.[42] A director and sub-director managed it. The staff consisted of three doctors, a manager (*mubāšir*), a chemist (*davāsāz*), two supervisors (*nāẓir*), one cook (*tabbāḫ*), one receiver, six nurses (*parastār*), one bathhouse attendant, one barber, and five washer-men.[43] The new military hospital may have been the same described as the Dār al-šifā-yi jadīd-i Nāṣirī-i tūpḫāna which had a staff of 15, consisting of two physicians, one surgeon, one chemist, one supervisor (*nāẓir*), four nurses (*parastār*); two cooks/washer-men, and four guards.[44] Whether the same or not, the new army hospital was a small building with only a few rooms with about 20 beds. It was ominously nicknamed 'the cemetery of the living,' reminiscent of the nickname of the *dār al-šifā* in Safavid times

39 Polak 1859, p. 140; Ibid., 1865, vol. 1, 307–311. According to Elgood 1951, p. 512, the hospital was first put under the management of Drs. Polak and Schlimmer.

40 Häntzsche 1869, p. 442.

41 Polak 1859, p. 140.

42 Elgood 1951, p. 512. Wright 2001, p. 126 reports that the hospital was established with German help in 1869, but he does not provide any reference for that statement and this assistance is nowhere mentioned in publications dealing with German-Persian relations.

43 I'timād al-Salṭana 1306, p. 405.

44 I'timād al-Salṭana 1306, pp. 349, 361. The chief army surgeon was Muḥammad Niẓām al-Ḥukamā Ṭabīb, Sipihr 1368, pp. 97–98.

(see above). There were no sick patients in it, for nobody came there, which explains its nickname. After the opening of the hospital its staff had left, because there was no money allocated for its operation, at least none was made available to the hospital. The idea behind its creation was that the medical students at the Dār al-funūn would receive part of their practical training at the hospital. However, after the death of the European professor, who only gave one course there, the project was abandoned. According to Mme. Serena, the *šāh* had charged his uncle ʿAlī Qulī Mīrzā Iʿtiżād al-Salṭana to manage the hospital, which is contradicted by Nafīsī. Iʿtiżād al-Salṭana used the funds for his own private use and let the hospital slowly deteriorate.[45]

There also was a military dispensary in Tehran, "exactly opposite the entrance to the [Golestan] Palace," where soldiers went to be treated for minor injuries.[46] Afżal al-Mulk reported that Mīrzā Muḥammad Nāẓim al-Aṭibbā, the chief army surgeon, was credited with having established effective army dispensaries (*davā-ḫānahā*) for which he had been awarded a diamond ring.[47]

In addition to the new army hospital built in 1868, another civilian one had been built in 1874 or thereabouts. The new hospital was built after Nāṣir al-Dīn Šāh returned from his first tour to Europe. Ḥājj Mīrzā Ḥusayn Ḫan Mušīr al-Dawla Sipahsālār-i Aʿẓam, the grand vizier, took steps to build a hospital in Tehran like the ones he had seen in Europe to which end he assigned one section of the Madrasa-yi Nāṣirī, later known as Madrasa-yi Sipahsālār, to be used as a hospital. He put ʿAlī Akbar Ḫān, a recent graduate from the Dār al-funūn, in charge of the construction of the Marīż-ḫāna-yi dawlatī, who managed the hospital until 1880. It is of interest to note that the hospital was still part of the traditional triad: mosque, madrasa, and hospital.[48]

---

45 Serena 1883, pp. 143–144; Nafīsī 1325, p. 57; Curzon 1892, vol. 1, p. 606. For the introduction of modern European medical science in Iran in the nineteenth century see Floor 2004; Ibid., 1386/2007.

46 Collins 1925, p. 221.

47 Afżal al-Mulk 1361, p. 139. Prior to that time there had been surgeons attached to the army, who managed field dispensaries. Tadjbakhsh 1379, pp. 214–216.

48 Elgood 1951, pp. 511–512, where he confuses it with Polak's military hospital; his description on Ibid., p. 454f is correct; Nafīsī 1325, pp. 56–57; Ibid,. 1329–31, p. 19; Iʿtimād al-Salṭana 1306, p. 83. The new hospital director later became Mīrzā Muḥammad Duktur Muʿtamad al-Aṭibbā, who also taught Western medicine at the Dār al-funūn. The hospital fell under the jurisdiction of the Minister of Science, Hospitals and Arts (*Vazīr-i ʿUlūm va Dār al-šifā va al-Funūn*), see Afżal al-Mulk 1361, p. 5. The *šāh* and his minister were not the

The need for hospitals was something to which many among the Iranian elite were receptive. In February 1886, for example, Āṣaf al-Dawla wrote that he intended to build a hospital in Tehran. The land had already been bought and land preparation had started. However, there is no further mention of this hospital in Āṣaf al-Dawla's published documents. He further proposed to establish dispensaries in Sarakhs and Sistan and argued that such facilities should be established all over Iran.[49] Iqbāl al-Salṭana, another member of the elite, had built a hospital in Tehran, which ʿAyn al-Salṭana visited in May 1889. He commented that it was very clean and proper.[50] But it would seem that this hospital did not remain operational. The 1317/1899 census of Tehran recorded the existence of only two unnamed hospitals, both in the Dawla quarter.[51] The census probably referred to the army hospital built in 1868 and the new civil hospital built in 1874.

In 1904, at the suggestion of Ḥajj Sayyāḥ a small hospital was established in Tehran to respond to the need for medical assistance created by the 1904 cholera epidemic. In collaboration with Mr. Naus, the Treasurer-General, and Muḥtār al-Salṭana, the chief of sanitation (*muḥtasib*) of Tehran, a building was rented and Faylasūf al-Salṭana Mīrzā ʿAbd al-Karīm was hired as its medical director, at a salary of 250 *tūmān*s per month. They also organized a system whereby sick people were transported to the hospital by droshky, all free of charge. Those that died were taken by the same service to the washers of the dead. The hackneys were paid one *tūmān* per patient. Dr. Morel, a French physician, assisted in the operation, in particular in managing the women's hospital that had been set up. Some wealthy individuals such as Mušīr al-Dawla provided further financial assistance.[52]

Šahrī does not even list this hospital, which, therefore, must have been a temporary solution (using a rented building) to an immediate and pressing problem, i.e., the 1904 cholera epidemic.[53] In fact, Šahrī states that

only Iranians who were impressed with European hospitals so was Šūštarī 1363, p. 262, as is clear from his description of the sights of London.

49 Āṣaf al-Dawla 1377, vol. 1, p. 220.

50 ʿAyn al-Salṭana 1376, vol. 1, p. 208.

51 Saʿdvandiyān – Ittiḥādiya 1368, pp. 353, 359, 451. For the location of the Dawlatī hospital, west of the Maydān-i Tūpḫāna, see the map in Moghtader 1992, p. 47, figure 2.

52 Sayyāḥ 1347, pp. 536–540.

53 This supposition is confirmed by Wishard 1908, pp. 219–220 who mentions that during the 1904 epidemic his general hospital was converted into a cholera hospital; furthermore, "a house was taken as a refuge hospital on the west side of the city [Sayyāḥ's hospital], and also a place was opened in Shiran [Shemiran?]. These three centres of work,

around 1920, there were only two Iranian hospitals in Tehran, the State or Imperial Hospital (then called Aḥmadī, but later again Dawlatī and ultimately Sīnā) and the Najmiya Hospital, in addition to the American and Russian hospital.[54] The Najmiya Hospital was founded by Dr. Muṣaddiq's mother Princess Malik Tāj Fīrūz Najm al-Salṭana as a charity hospital in 1928, and located in the Ḫiyābān-i Ḥāfiż.[55] According to Mrs. de Warzée, in 1912 there was only one Iranian hospital, viz., the State or Imperial Hospital, which was managed by Dr. Ilberg. He was assisted by another German physician (Dr. Beck), one Iranian physician, a chemist and a number of well-trained male nurses. The hospital had at least 60 beds, including rooms for better class Persians and Europeans, and two operating rooms. The poor received free consultations, medicines, bandages, and vaccinations. Mrs. de Warzée also mentions that a military hospital was to be built.[56] She mentions a second Iranian hospital, most likely the Vazīrī hospital (see below), but it did not function as such in 1912.

> A Persian sinner who had misdirected public funds repented of his sins at the eleventh hour and just before his death gave a large sum of money to build a hospital. He was told that by doing so he would gain Paradise. A great building was erected outside Teheran towards the mountains, but, unluckily, the money was not only insufficient to run the hospital, but also to complete the building, and until now it has stood unfinished and useless. It is to be turned into barracks for the new Persian gendarmerie.[57]

American missionaries had opened their medical dispensary in 1881 in Tehran (Dr. N. Torrence, in 1890 joined by Dr. Mary J. Smith, the first female physician in Iran) and established the Ferry Hospital there in 1893, which also served as a teaching hospital. They added a women's ward to it in 1897. A separate women's hospital was built and equipped in 1907 with

together with a dispensary in the Jewish quarter of the town, were kept in operation day and night for nearly a month, when the epidemic ceased." On this epidemic see Burrell 1988, pp. 258–270.

54 Šahrī 1368, vol. 1, p. 294.

55 Rustā'ī 1382, vol. 1, pp. 532–539 (includes the text of the *vaqf-nāma*); Tadjbakhsh 1379, pp. 242–243.

56 De Warzée 1913, pp. 171–172. Wishard 1908, p. 234 reports on this subject that recently, the German government had opened a free general hospital in Tehran, which does not seem to be correct. She probably mistook German management of the Imperial hospital (see below) as this being a German hospital, which it was not. For example, Litten 1925, p. 404 only mentions the management of the Imperial hospital by Dr. Becker, and no other German involvement with the hospital.

57 De Warzée 1913, p. 172.

the funds donated by a wealthy Iranian lady.[58] The establishment of the first hospital building had not been without difficulties. The Americans had already bought a piece of land in 1887, but the *šāh* demanded that (i) no women be admitted, (ii) the call for prayer to be given by one of the future hospital's staff; these were unacceptable conditions for the American missionaries. When Dr. Wishard arrived in Tehran in 1893 he was able to have the *šāh* agree to drop these conditions and as a result the hospital was built.[59] The hospital's dispensary was open every morning, except Sunday, from 9 a.m., and closed when the last patient had been treated. On good days some 100 people visited the dispensary.[60] The American Hospital for Men and Women was not always open for business such as in 1912 when the male ward had been closed for almost one year, because there was no male physician. The male ward had been closed again from 1916 or 1917 until early 1919 for the same reason, when with the arrival of Dr. Post it was reopened. The female ward, however, had remained open all this time and was led by Dr. Mary Smith, who intermittently was assisted by an American trained nurse. Both of them taught Iranian nurses through on-the-job training; "they were made responsible for the care of the women patients in the hospital, the preparation of the surgical dressings, sterilizing and the getting ready of the surgery and the instruments for operations." In 1918, moreover, two additional dispensaries had been opened in the south of Tehran, although this seems to have been a temporary measure in response to provide relief to victims of the famine and influenza, typhus, and cholera epidemic.[61] Dr. Mary Griscom, who worked there as of 1919, reported that

---

[58] Wilson 1896, pp. 259–260; ʿAyn al-Salṭana 1376, vol. 1, pp. 377, 865; Kumīsyūn 1343, vol. 2, pp. 1449–1451; Elgood 1951, pp. 511–512, 534; Wishard 1908, pp. 12, 99; Muʿtamadī 1381, pp. 632–633; Richter 1910, p. 322.

[59] Waterfield 1973, p. 135; Muʿtamadī 1381, pp. 632–633.

[60] Wishard 1908, p. 232.

[61] De Warzée 1913, p. 171; *One Hundred Seventeenth Annual Report of the Home Missions of the Presbyterian Church of the U.S.A.*, 1919, p. 259; *The Eighty-third Annual Report of the Board of Foreign Missions of the Presbyterian Church in the U.S.A.*, 1920, p. 310; Griscom 1921, p. 239. Hence there were two dispensaries (male and female) at the same hospital. *The Eighty-fourth Annual Report of the Board of Foreign Missions of the Presbyterian Church in the U.S.A.*, 1921, p. 326. The female ward of the hospital had been closed for three months in 1918, while the main dispensary had been open irregularly due to the quasi-disappearance of droshkies from the streets, while walking was not possible. However, emergency cases on those days were taken care of by Drs. Petros and Saʿīd Ḫān, who lived nearby. *One Hundred Seventeenth Annual Report of the Home Missions of the Presbyterian Church of the U.S.A.*, 1919, p. 260.

> At the dispensary I saw from fifteen to thirty patients, two or three times a week. Poor Armenians, beggars, members of Persian ministers' families and relatives of the Shah all rubbed elbows in the waiting-room. The majority of them had eye-diseases demanding operation. Persian ladies of high degree never expected to be seen ahead of the others. They took it as a matter of course that they were to be examined in their turn.[62]

In 1919, the nurses training class completed its first three-year term and graduated its first class of Iranian nurses.[63] The Russian hospital, which was supported by the Russian Red Cross, practically only served Russians and was managed by the Russian Legation's doctor. According to Wishard, it was opened in 1907. There also was "an infirmary in the Russian (sic) Cossack Brigade buildings, where the brigade and their families are attended. There are over a thousand consultations monthly in this infirmary and the dispensary is free."[64] French nuns (*Filles de la charité*) also had a small hospital-dispensary in Tehran.[65] Finally, there was the dispensary of the British Legation, which had "consulting-rooms for men and women, and an operating room attached to the English Legation doctor's house; it is financed by the English government and the consultations are free."[66]

By 1924, there were four civil and two army Iranian hospitals in Tehran. The largest and oldest was the Imperial or State Hospital (*marīż-ḫāna-yi dawlatī*), built in 1874 (see above) with a nominal capacity of 50 beds, although this number could be increased if funds were available. Most patients treated were those with acute malaria. During the summer many patients were treated in the garden under the trees. The staff consisted of a

---

[62] Griscom 1921, p. 239. By 1920 Dr. McDowell was also working in the hospital. *The Eighty-fourth Annual Report of the Board of Foreign Missions of the Presbyterian Church in the U.S.A.*, 1921, p. 328. In 1918 there were four dispensaries in Tehran that treated 11,561 patients. *One Hundred Seventeenth Annual Report of the Home Missions of the Presbyterian Church of the U.S.A.*, 1919, p. 256 (with picture of Dr. Mary Smith in an operating room). In 1921 it was noted that 80% of the patients of both the hospital and dispensary were from outside of Tehran, mostly from its nearby districts. Patients also included pilgrims coming from or going to Mashhad and Karbala. *The Eighty-fifth Annual Report of the Board of Foreign Missions of the Presbyterian Church in the U.S.A.*, 1922, p. 364.

[63] *The Eighty-third Annual Report of the Board of Foreign Missions of the Presbyterian Church in the U.S.A.*, 1920, p. 310.

[64] De Warzée 1913, pp. 171–172; Grothe 1911, p. 131; Wishard 1908, p. 234.

[65] Hassendorfer 1954, p. 61; Wishard 1908, p. 234.

[66] De Warzée 1913, p. 172; Wishard 1908, p. 234. There also was a hospital in Rey built by Ḥājjī Sayyid Rižā Fīrūzābādī, possibly around 1925. It was built on a land of 62,000 sq.m. and was situated on the old Šahr-i Rey road, above the ʿAbd Allāh Imāmzāda. He later build a mosque and an orphanage next to the hospital. Initially his salary as member of parliament was used to meet the operational cost of the hospital, Tadjbakhsh 1379, pp. 243–244.

medical director, a surgeon, an assistant surgeon, a physician, an assistant physician, a surgeon aide and a physician aide, who dealt with patients who came for consultations. The nursing staff consisted of one trained nurse, two assistant nurses and 6 orderlies. The hospital had treated 499 hospitalized patients (450 men; 32 women; 17 children) during March 1923–March 1924. During the same period 6,450 outpatients were treated. Apart from tracking incoming and outgoing patients no database was kept.[67] Until November 1915, two German embassy physicians (Dr. Ilberg and Dr. Becker) managed the Imperial Hospital. After their departure, Iranian physicians ran the hospital. In 1917, the Russians used the hospital, its staff and equipment rather roughly, so that by 1918 the hospital could only receive 30 patients.

The British government offered to assist with the management of the hospital and improve it, to which the Iranian government agreed. As a result, between 1919–23, the British government helped to reorganize the government hospital at Tehran with 90 beds, and also supplied staff (Dr. A. R. Neligan, the physician of the British legation, and Dr. I. Scott, head of the medical staff of the Indo-European Telegraph Department, IETD), as well as medical stores and equipment, as did the Anglo-Persian Oil Company (APOC). Dr. Luqman al-Dawla was the director of the hospital and was assisted by three Iranian physicians, Drs. Lisān Šams Lisān al-Ḥukamā, Mīrzā Muḥammad Ḫān ʿAlāʾī, and Mūsā Ḫān as well as by Drs. Neligan and Scott. As a result of the British involvement the hospital soon became known as 'the English hospital.' Because the Iranian government did not provide any real support for the operation of the hospital, the unpaid and neglected Iranian staff blamed the British for their problems. The British doctors, however, were but advisers and had no decision-making authority. British involvement, therefore, became an embarrassment (especially as the political climate had become very anti-British), and this was the reason Great Britain withdrew its assistance in 1923. It asked the Anglo-Persian Oil Company to take charge of the hospital. The Company accepted to do so, provided there would be a continued role of the British with the hospital, which the government of Iran refused. The APOC dropped this condition and assumed charge of the hospital, but made it clear that it could halt its subsidy at any time without notice.

---

67 Gilmour 1924, p. 26.

It also accepted joint management of the hospital by APOC and Iranian physicians.[68]

The Vazīrī Hospital had been made possible by Mīrzā ʿĪsā Tafrašī Vazīr (d. 1892), one of Nāṣir al-Dīn Šāh's ministers, who had bequeathed one-third of his wealth for the construction and operation of a small hospital as well as of a mosque, in which he was buried. The combination of a mosque, hospital and the founder's tomb is clearly modeled after that of the traditional *dār al-šifā*. The construction started in 1898 under the supervision of the cleric Ḥājj Šayḫ Hādī Najmābādī, who had been made *mutavallī* or administrator of the Vazīrī endowment. The hospital was completed in 1900. It had two physicians, Dr. Abū Tūrāb for the medical department and Dr. Wolf (a German) who was in charge of the surgical section. After the death of Najmābādī the hospital's work was hampered because the foundations that Najmābādī had created questioned the hospital's finances. The hospital was then managed by Yūsuf Buzurgmihr (ʿĀlam al-Salṭana).[69] As a result, the hospital never functioned properly, which was why the state took over its management in 1918. The hospital had 30 beds for both medical and surgical cases. The director of the hospital was the chief medical officer at the same time. He also taught at the Medical School, as did the hospital's surgeon. Three final year students functioned as their assistants. There were eight nurses, two of which were female. During 1923–1924 the hospital admitted 344 patients and treated 1,104 outpatients. In 1926, the hospital was transferred to the Ministry of Health.[70]

Third, the Women's Hospital, a small one with 20 beds, had become fully operational only in 1918. The proposal for the hospital had been submitted by Dr. Amīr Aʿlam on 5 May 1915. The government adopted the idea on 20 July 1915 and a government-owned building was assigned as the premises for the hospital. Two French midwives were supposed to have been hired to train Iranian midwives, but the outbreak of the Great War made that impossible. Instead the services of Mme Fraskina, who had been trained as a midwife in Europe and was working as such in Tehran, were engaged. When the hospital was officially opened much money was collected, but it was not

---

[68] Elgood 1951, pp. 546–554 (with details on the state of the building and staff, and how it developed later). Litten 1925, pp. 6, 242; Wright 2001, p. 127.

[69] Hemmati n.d., p. 161; Bāmdād 1347, vol. 2, pp. 514–515 (with biography); Tadjbakhsh 1379, pp. 240–242.

[70] Gilmour 1924, pp. 26–27; Hemmati n.d., p. 161 (which relates how the hospital fared thereafter).

enough to make the hospital functional. In 1916 there was no money to buy 50 beds and other equipment, but the Iranian government allocated 3,600 *tumans* to pay for the staff. As a result the hospital functioned as a genealogical outpatients' dispensary, which, between March 1916 and 1924, was managed by Dr. ʿAlī Riżā Bahrāmī Muhaddab al-Salṭana. In September 1918, the then Minister of Endowments (*Awqāf*) tried to raise funds to properly equip the building and turn it into a real hospital. He was only able to acquire funds to buy six beds, where from September 1918 until March 1919 about sixty women gave birth. During that period Mme. Fraskina trained 10 Iranian women to become mid-wives. After the end of Great War funds became available to establish an internal medicine and surgical (obstetrics) department in the Women's Hospital, which was led by Dr. Saʿīd Malik Luqmān al-Mamālik. Mme Fraskina was replaced by a French female physician Dr. Dermes, who remained there until 1934.[71] Thereafter, the hospital served as training center for the Medical School for Women, while women continued to be admitted to give birth. During 1923–24, some 107 patients were admitted, 20 of whom suffered from malaria. Some 1,342 outpatients were treated, of whom 192 suffered from malaria. In 1921, the Medical School for Women had 13 students, who all belonged to the elite families; instruction was in French. They received a training of three years that was focused on women's diseases and obstetrics. On graduating the student received a diploma. They were not physicians, but more broadly trained than mid-wives.[72]

Fourth, the so-called Fārābī Hospital was situated in a garden, which the government of Iran acquired in 1921. From 1921 until 1940, with many interruptions it was the municipal hospital, a.k.a. Hospital Nr. 2, and was later made available to the medical faculty of the University of Tehran.[73] Gilmour does not mention the Fārābī hospital, but it was probably the same as what he called the Municipal Hospital, which by 1924 existed already for a number of years. It had 72 beds (30 medical; 32 surgical; 10 isolation), one surgeon, four physicians, one ophthalmologist, one director of the laboratory, three medical interns, twelve male nurses, six female nurses and two pharmacists. Its dispensary treated patients from all over Iran. In 1923 the hospital admitted 818 inpatients, while it treated some 50–80 outpatients daily. Like in the Imperial hospital many outpatients were treated in the open-air, some in tents, and others in the shade of

71 Hemmati n.d., pp. 163–164.
72 Gilmour 1924, p. 27.
73 Hemmati n.d., p. 165.

the trees in the hospital garden. Although malaria was one of the major diseases none of the beds had a mosquito-net. The monthly budget for the hospital was 575 *tūmāns*, of which 250 served to pay the staff.[74]

In addition there were two army hospitals in Tehran which exclusively treated army personnel. One, situated outside Tehran and known as the Aḥmadiya Military Hospital, was housed in old barracks and had 150 beds although its capacity could be increased to 250 beds, and was led by Russians (administrator, surgeon and chief doctor) in 1924. The barracks had been transformed into a hospital by Dr. Amīr Ḫān and opened its doors for business in 1914. The other army hospital was in the center of Tehran and had a capacity of 50 beds, but was being extended to receive 100 inpatients. It had an important dispensary attached to it; the service was good and the patients were well looked after, but there was no regular disinfection of the clothing and bedding. Also, each regiment had a regimental physician as well as a dispensary, and thus the army had a better medical organization than civil society.[75]

Finally, for completeness' sake, the existence of the mental hospital or *dār al-majānīn* has to be mentioned. Until 1905 there was no facility in Tehran to receive and treat psychiatric patients. However, in that year, after complaints to the police about mad people going about naked in the streets, the Minister of Police, Saʿīd al-Salṭana sent them to the Imperial Hospital. In consultation with Drs. Luf [?] and Abū Turāb a psychiatric ward was constructed there at the minister's expense. This seems to have consisted of four to five small rooms closed with an iron door in an isolated part of the Imperial Hospital. Because psychiatric cases were the responsibility of the police it was at the initiative of general Westdahl, the Swedish chief of police of Tehran (1922–24) that a separate and larger mental institution was built in Akbarbad. The building had four rooms above ground and four below ground. In one of the rooms below ground there were four dark narrow cells to hold agitated patients. Treatment of the patients was harsh. There was one orderly per 50 patients. The orderlies, who were bullies, used violence to keep order, while the food that patients received was bad and insufficient. In short, the patients suffered not only from their illness, but also from poor treatment, hunger and bad food. According to Šahrī, referring to a later period, apart from the real

---

74 Gilmour 1924, pp. 57–58.

75 Gilmour 1924, pp. 30–31; Rustāʾī 1382, vol. 2, p. 125. For a picture and description of the first army hospital see Šahrī 1368, vol. 1, p. 295. The Aḥmadiya was situated in the Ḫiyābān-i Sipah and the other hospital (later known as Pahlavī) in Yūsufābād, Rustāʾī 1382, vol. 1, p. 179.

mental cases, most of the inmates of the mental hospital were there for political, financial or other non-medical reasons.[76]

## ABADAN

Since 1914, the British APOC maintained its own medical service for its staff, although it also extended its gratis services (including dental treatment) to the local population who did not have any relationship with the Company. The Abadan hospital, one of the most modern in the Middle-East, was one of the three hospitals the APOC operated (see also Ahvaz and Masjed-Soleyman), as well as 12 separate dispensaries, nine in the Oil Fields, one at Mohammerah, one at Bawardah, and one at the refinery.

The Abadan hospital had a capacity of about 100 beds (36 for administrative staff and 60 for workmen plus special private wards), an outpatient department, a dispensary, a dental surgery, an operation room, a pathological laboratory, a disinfection station and X-ray equipment. In 1926, the hospital at Abadan treated more than 180,000 patients, or some 500 per day. At that time, its population was about 30,000 and growing. The APOC employed a senior medical officer, two resident medical officers, a visiting medical officer, a consulting surgeon, a pathologist, and an ophthalmologist. These were assisted by 26 local nurses under a European matron and assisted by eight European nurses.[77]

Table 2: Number of Patients Treated and of Activities Undertaken in Abadan APOC hospital (1926)

| Activity | Number |
|---|---:|
| Hospital inpatients | 2,228 |
| Outpatients (a) new cases | 40,129 |
| (b) attendances | 137,169 |
| Major operations | 214 |
| Minor operations | 1,815 |
| Pathological examinations | 4,733 |
| Dental cases | 892 |
| X-ray photographs | 99 |

Source: Williamson 1927, p. 130.

76 *Rūznāma-yi sulṭānī va Īrān* 1380, year 58, nr. 11, p. 2 (10 *jumāda al-ṯānī* 1323/12 August 1905), p. 346; Šahrī 1368, vol. 1, pp. 436–437; Rustā'ī 1382, vol. 1, pp. 488, 522–524 (with more details about its lay-out and use of the various available spaces). For a photograph of the asylum see Afšār 1371, p. 349.

77 Williamson 1927, pp. 128–132; Gilmour 1924, p. 39.

## Ahvaz

In 1914 or thereabouts, Ahvaz had an estimated population of 12,000 and no modern medical institutions.[78] In 1906, a dispensary was opened under the aegis of the British consulate, where in 1908 average daily attendance was 85[79] From 6 May until 17 December 1908 the dispensary was closed, because the hospital assistant, Fażl Ilāhī, had to accompany the consul on mission. This gave rise to unease and apprehension on part of the population, and "the community deputied some of their leading members to beg that the Hospital Assistant should be left in Nasiri [Ahvaz] and painted in gloomy colours the fate which otherwise would befall them."[80] The British government transformed the dispensary into a Civil Hospital, although the exact date this took place is not known. The first mention of the Civil Hospital dates to 1918, when it is reported that Sub-Assistant ʿAṭā Muḥammad was attached to it.[81] A year after The Civil Hospital had grown from a charitable dipensary to a 30-bed hospital. The British hoped to extend the activities to Shustar and Dezful and stressed the political value of the hospital:

> Except for the pay of the Civil Surgeon, and a Sub-Assistant Surgeon, it is self-supporting and it is hoped to arrange for its activities to extend to Dizful and Shushtar in the future. The cost of drugs, however, a large item of expenditure, which has up till quite lately been bore by the Iraq revenues, will no doubt seriously hamper the work of the hospital if further local support is not forthcoming.
>
> Patients of all classes from Bakhtiari, Kughilu and Luristan attend, and its undoubted political value cannot be under-estimated.
>
> The Civil Surgeon is also responsible for the organisation of the Municipality and is thus able to control the sanitation of the town, the cleanliness of which compares very favourably with any other in the East.[82]

In 1921 it was reported that the Civil Hospital treated 2,236 outpatients and 221 inpatients; and carried out 14 major and 175 minor operations. This was a good result since in that same year the civil surgeon died and there was no replacement for him. The consul, therefore, proposed to

---

78 *Administration Report on the Persian Gulf Political Residency for the year 1919 in Government of India* (henceforth *Administration Report*), p. 10.

79 *Administration Report* 1906–1907, p. 24; *Administration Report* 1907–1908, p. 29.

80 *Administration Report* 1908, p. 21. In 1909, the dispensary was again closed for some time (24 May till 26 November), but the hospital assistant provided medical assistance while on tour. Eye diseases, malaria and worms were the most common diseases met, *Administration Report* 1909, p. 52; *Administration Report* 1910, p. 63.

81 *Administration Report* 1918, p. 43.

82 *Administration Report* 1919, pp. 44–45.

Table 3: Attendance and Operation at Ahvaz Civil Hospital (1918–1920)

| | 1916 | 1917 | 1918 | 1919 | 1920 |
|---|---|---|---|---|---|
| Inpatients | – | – | 662 | 670 | 452 |
| Outpatients | 5,627 | 6,661 | 5,104 | 6,383 | 3,235 |
| Major operations | 1 | 8 | 29 | 55 | 60 |
| Minor operations | 171 | 296 | 189 | 358 | 420 |

Source: *Administration Report* 1916, p. 59; Ibid., 1917, p. 40; Ibid., 1918, p. 45–46; Ibid., 1919, p. 48; Ibid., 1920, pp. 44–45.

abolish the hospital and revive the old charitable dispensary.[83] As a result, the Civil Hospital was closed in March 1922. Probably due to lack of funds, the charitable dispensary also closed in November 1922. Efforts were then made to open a town dispensary funded by public donations.[84] This does not seem to have met with success as nothing more is heard about the matter. Perhaps the effort was abandoned, because in 1921 it was made public that the APOC would establish a new hospital at Ahvaz, staffed with one medical officer and two nurses. This hospital indeed was operational in 1922.[85] It was set up with similar equipment, staff and capacity as the APOC hospitals in Abadan and Masjed-Soleyman (q.v.).[86]

## Arak

In 1914 the British Church Missionary Society (CMS) allegedly founded a hospital in Arak or Soltanabad, a town of some 20,000 inhabitants.[87] However, it does not seem to have been started or, if it did, not to have lasted very long for there is no mention at all to be found of this hospital or of activities by the CMS in the local histories of Arak.[88] Moreover, in various CMS tracts (Linton, Rice, etc.) no mention is made of any activity in Arak, while they list their medical facilities in Isfahan, Yazd, Kerman and Shiraz. However, in 1926, the Adventists, a Protestant denomination, opened a dispensary in Soltanabad led by the Iranian Dr. Arzu, who shortly thereafter established a 15-bed hospital. In the early 1930s, the dispensary treated

83 *Administration Report* 1921, p. 43.
84 *Administration Report* 1922, p. 43.
85 *Administration Report* 1921, p. 43; Williamson 1927, p. 124.
86 Williamson 1927, p. 124.
87 Elgood 1951, p. 535.
88 Tabrīzī 1966–1967, pp. 362–460; Dihgān 1950.

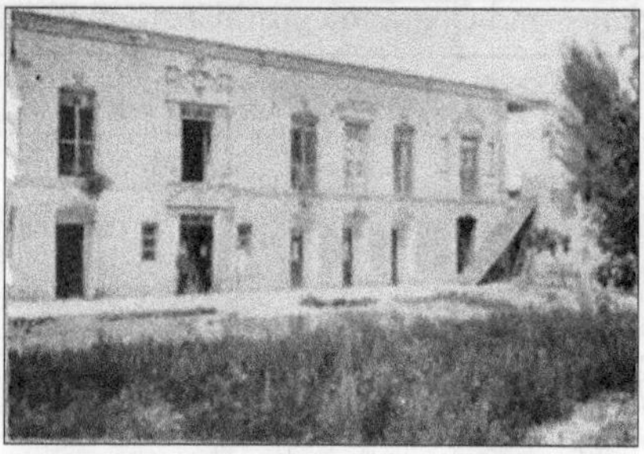

Figure 1a. The Adventist dispensary and hospital at Soltanabad. From Rühling, 1934, *Quer durch Persien*. Hamburg, p. 80.

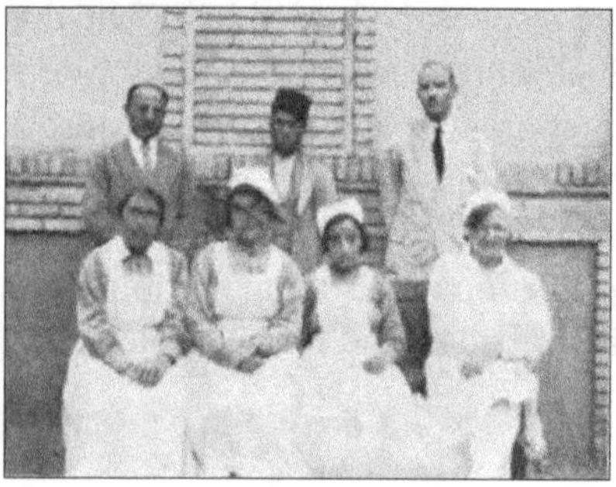

Figure 1b. The staff of the Adventist dispensary and hospital at Soltanabad. From Rühling, 1934, *Quer durch Persien*. Hamburg, p. 80.

4,000 patients per year or 12,000 treatments. The inpatients had to pay a fixed amount per day per bed, which barely covered fifty percent of the variable operating cost of the hospital.[89]

## Ashuradeh

There was a small hospital of 14 beds established by the Russian government on the island of Ashuradeh in 1848 to treat its Russian naval as well as consular staff in the Caspian littoral, although the date of its

[89] The average daily pay of a worker in Iran was 60 *pfennig*, while the cost per bed was 100 *pfennig*, which was a great burden for patients, Rühling 1934, pp. 82–85. Already in 1913 there was a call to US physicians to fill a vacancy in Soltanabad. Muirhead 1913, p. 205.

establishment may have been earlier.[90] In 1844 there were no buildings on the island. Holmes described it at that time as follows : "The only habitations are two large sail-cloth tents, occupied by the sick. [...] They were much exposed in these tents, and a building of wood was in the course of construction as an hospital".[91] Twenty years later Melgunof reported that there were some wooden buildings on the island, amongst which he mentioned "the hospital, a house for both physicians (one for the Russian, the other for the Persian)".[92] The hospital is not mentioned in a description of the island around 1900.[93]

## Bandar ʿAbbas

Given the fact that Bandar ʿAbbas had 20,000 inhabitants by 1914, almost as many as Bushire,[94] and no medical facilities or even an Iranian physician,[95] it was no surprise that the British consul submitted that "A charitable dispensary was sadly required at Bunder Abbas owing to the large numbers of the very poor. One was opened under the charge of the Quarantine Medical officer in March 1906 and does an immense amount of good in reliving suffering, apart from the political influence which such institutions always bring in their train in Persia."[96] Although the dispensary was well received and was a great benefit to the population the consul opined, "At the same time, the advisability of placing the equipment for a charitable dispensary in the hands of a subordinate who is not precluded from taking fees and engaging in private practice, is thought to be open to question, while the fact that in this case, the individual is the Quarantine Medical Officer and as such a the servant of the Persian Sanitary Administration, has the effect of concealing the source of benevolence from those visiting the dispensary

90 Elgood 1951, p. 512; Teymūrī 1363, pp. 269–271, who also reports that Russia in addition obtained a concession for the establishment of a hospital in Astarabad. In 1848, the Russians had first asked for such a concession at Gaz, the port of Astarabad, while in 1850 they were again denied to build a hospital there despite a renewed request, although later (with more success) they asked for permission to build a hospital at Astarabad, see Kazembeyki 2003, pp. 55–57, 124. However, the Russians did not build a hospital in Astarabad, at least no published source mentions it.

91 Holmes 1845, p. 250.

92 Melgunof 1868, p. 75.

93 Adamec 1981, vol. 2, p. 32.

94 *Administration Report* 1919, p. 10.

95 Sadīd al-Salṭana 1342, p. 169.

96 *Administration Report* 1905–06, p. 59.

Table 4: The Number of New Patients Treated and of Operations Performed in the Bandar ʿAbbas Dispensary (1908–25)

| Year | New patients | Operations |
|---|---|---|
| 1908 | 1,894 | – |
| 1910 | 2,855 | – |
| 1911 | 2,345 | – |
| 1912 | 2,879 | – |
| 1913 | 2,092 | – |
| 1916 | 3,122 | – |
| 1917 | 3,388 | – |
| 1918 | 3,889 | – |
| 1919 | 3,673 | – |
| 1920 | 4,279 | 92 |
| 1921 | 4,215 | 182 |
| 1922 | 4,526 | 195 |
| 1923 | 4,425 | – |
| 1924 | 4,419 | – |
| 1925 | 5,848 | 258 |

Source: *Administration Report* 1908, p. 63; Ibid., 1899–1900; Ibid., 1912, p. 47; Ibid., 1913, p. 48; Ibid., 1917, p. 13; Ibid., 1918, p. 16; Ibid., 1919, p. 19; Ibid., 1920, p. 18; Ibid., 1921, p. 19; Ibid., 1922, p. 19–20; Ibid., 1923, p. 35; Ibid., 1924, p. 27; Ibid., 1925, p. 36.

and thus there results no political influence."[97] The consul, therefore, argued that the dispensary should be moved from the Quarantine station to the new consulate that was to be ready in 1909. "The charitable dispensary is indeed a boon to the poor who swarm in Bunder Abbas and now that free treatment has become a regular feature, the shifting of the local from the Quarantine Medical Officer's house to the Consulate will bring yet more prominently before the public that their well-being is closely identified with the British flag".[98] Attendance remained steadily increasing thereafter, while the opening of the new charitable dispensary in 1920 provided a considerable additional boost to attendance.[99]

The major diseases treated at the dispensary were malaria, eye and skin diseases, which three accounted for 52.5% of total admissions in 1908.[100] Vaccinations were also given.[101] The British consul believed that the dis-

97 *Administration Report* 1906–07, p. 50. However, Sadīd al-Salṭana 1342, p. 169 was quite aware that the British government, not the Quarantine Service, provided the medical services to the public.

98 *Administration Report* 1908, p. 63.

99 *Administration Report* 1920, p. 18.

100 *Administration Report* 1908, p. 63; for further data see *Administration Report* 1921, p. 19; *Administration Report* 1922, p. 19; *Administration Report* 1923, p. 35.

101 *Administration Report* 1907–08, p. 74.

pensary created good-will, if not political influence, and he was right. For, although a British operated and funded institution, it met an enormous need. It was the only medical institution in the town and in the region and its services were free and therefore it also received local support from the most influential persons in Bandar Abbas. For example, in 1924, "The floor of the operation room was repaired and the expense met by Haji Sheikh Ahmed Galledary, a local merchant. A well was built in the compound of the dispensary which supplied a great need, the expense in this case being met by Haji Mukhtar Divani another local merchant. The latter is erecting at his own expense ten small cubicles for the purpose of accommodating poor persons coming in from distant villages for treatment at the dispensary. When completed the cubicles will be of great convenience to the poor."[102] Similarly, the next year, "The roof was replastered paid by Haji Mukhtar Divani, while Haji Sheikh Ahmed Galledary paid for the cost of extra drugs and dressings of Rs 520."[103]

## Bushire

Bushire, with 24,000 inhabitants,[104] had a much higher attendance at its dispensary that those in Bandar Abbas or Lengeh with a similar population size. This may have been due to the fact that as of the 1870, if not earlier, the British had what they classified as a second-class dispensary at Bushire. It was a great success, not only as it was the only modern medical facility in town, but its services were also gratis.[105] As a result the number of patients increased steadily (see Table 5). The statistics showed that the largest daily attendance took place during the height of the hottest weather, i.e., June, July, and August.[106] Many of the patients were and continued to be women as well as children, whose numbers were also on the rise as indicated by the data available (see Table 6).[107]

---

102 *Administration Report* 1924, p. 27.

103 *Administration Report* 1925, p. 36.

104 *Administration Report* 1919, p. 10.

105 "It is the only place for free treatment in Bushire", *Administration Report* 1914, p. 12. A dispensary was already kept at Bushire since 1873 under the control of the Civil Surgeon for the relief of the poor. "This boon is much prized by the natives, and if there was an arrangement for treatment of indoor patients, the results would be still more satisfactory than at present." *Administration Report* 1873–74, p. 7.

106 *Administration Report* 1907–08, p. 19.

107 *Administration Report* 1914, p. 12; *Administration Report* 1913, p. 34.

Table 5: The Number of Out- and Inpatients and of Operations in the Bushire Dispensary-Hospital (1898–1925)

| Year | Total | Outpatients | Inpatients | Operations inpatients | Operations total |
|---|---|---|---|---|---|
| 1898–99 | 6,418 | 6,418 | – | – | 395 |
| 1899–1900 | 5,026 | 5,026 | – | – | 315 |
| 1900–01 | 8,050 | 8,050 | – | – | 525 |
| 1907–08 | 13,383 | 13,254 | 129 | 69 | 540 |
| 1908 | 8,821 | 8,734 | 87 | – | 476 |
| 1909 | 16,581 | 16,422 | 59 | – | 589 |
| 1910 | 13,094 | 13,045 | 49 | – | 389 |
| 1911 | 13,470 | 13,397 | 73 | – | 599 |
| 1912 | 13,747 | 13,716 | 31 | – | 589 |
| 1913 | 15,153 | 15,009 | 146 | – | 552 |
| 1914 | 13,295 | 13,190 | 105 | – | 636 |
| 1915 | 14,667 | 14,537 | 140 | – | n.a. |
| 1916 | 15,575 | 15,520 | 55 | – | 639 |
| 1918 | 14,759 | 14,696 | 63 | 63 | 583 |
| 1919 | 12,764 | 12,711 | 53 | n.a. | n.a. |
| 1920 | 12,374 | 12,302 | 72 | 69 | 709 |
| 1921 | 11,453 | 11,365 | 88 | – | 614 |
| 1922 | 13,571 | 13,461 | 110 | – | 945 |
| 1923 | 10,912 | 10,766 | 146 | 148 | 664 |
| 1924 | 18,854 | 18,747 | 105 | 94 | 1,169 |
| 1925 | 42,177 | 42,030 | 147 | 119 | 1,649 |

Source: *Administration Report* 1898–99, p. 15; Ibid., 1899–1900, p. 11; Ibid., 1900–1901, p. 11; Ibid., 1907–08, p. 19; Ibid., 1908, p. 12; Ibid., 1909, p. 17; Ibid., 1910, p. 20; Ibid., 1912, p. 43; Ibid., 1913, p. 34; Ibid., 1914, p. 12; Ibid., 1915, p. 10; Ibid., 1916, p. 10; Ibid., 1918, p. 8; Ibid., 1919, p. 10; Ibid., 1920, p. 7; Ibid., 1921, p. 9; Ibid., 1922, p. 9; Ibid., 1923, p. 14; Ibid., 1924, p. 8; Ibid., 1925, p. 10.

Table 6: Number of Male, Female and Child Patients Visiting the Bushire Dispensary (1899–1901)

| Year | Total | Daily attendance | Men | Women | Children |
|---|---|---|---|---|---|
| 1898–99 | 6,418 | 58.5 | 2,849 | 1,959 | 1,610 |
| 1899–1900 | 5,026 | 27.7 | 2,266 | 1,652 | 1,108 |
| 1900–01 | 8,050 | 43.7 | 3,465 | 3,470 | 2,115 |

Source: *Administration Report* 1898–99, p. 15; Ibid., 1899–1900, p. 11; Ibid., 1900–1901, p. 9.

The dispensary is referred to as a hospital for the first time in 1907,[108] and usually thereafter as hospital-dispensary and as of 1922 as the Bushire Civil Hospital or Bushire Residency Dispensary and Charitable Hospital.[109] The qualification of hospital was determined by the fact that as of 1907 inpatients were treated and what was qualified as major operation (e.g. lithotomy, removal of urethral calculus) could be and were performed. Minor operations were mainly the extraction of the teeth, evacuation of abscess and removal of wax.[110]

The most important diseases treated included: malaria, skin diseases, eye diseases, worms, and diseases of the respiratory system.[111] However, the physicians commented that there were "no statistics that would be of value are available to show the extent of the ravages of the diseases."[112] Most of the cost was represented by the salaries of the European medical staff. Medicines were both imported from Europe and bought in the local bazaar.[113] The most modern methods and treatments were introduced as soon as these became available. For example, with some pride, the Political Agent reported the "Successful treatment of leprosy cases by means of the new Nastine treatment inaugurated by Professor Deycke Pasha."[114]

The Bushire facility had so much success that in 1908 it was reported that "The hospital has been open the whole twelve months under report. Owing to the gradually increasing attendance the rooms hitherto occupied by the dispensary in the Residency building having become too small for requirements, and the congregation of patients in the Residency court-yard a source of considerable inconvenience, the government of India was pleased to sanction the renting of a capacious house next door to the town Residency and the hospital and dispensary were moved in."[115] The move made in 1912 to other premises was in hindsight not a good one, for although the building was well situated it "was poorly adapted for taking-in patients," which made the work for the medical staff difficult.[116] "The provision for a decent hospital for Bushire is much to be desired and had been mooted

108 *Administration Report* 1907–08, p. 19.
109 *Administration Report* 1922, p. 9; *Administration Report* 1925, p. 10.
110 *Administration Report* 1898–99, pp. 15–20.
111 *Administration Report* 1900–01, pp. 9–13; *Administration Report* 1914, p. 12; *Administration Report* 1913, p. 34.
112 *Report 1920–21. The Persian Gulf Trade Reports 1905–1940. Bushire* (henceforth *Report 1920–21*), p. 2.
113 *Administration Report* 1899–1900, p. 15.
114 *Administration Report* 1908, p. 12.
115 *Administration Report* 1907–08, p. 19.
116 *Administration Report* 1913, p. 34; *Report* 1921–22, p. 1.

by a few leading members of the community, but it seems desirable it take the form of a development of the existing Residency Dispensary rather than that the latter should suffer or be eclipsed in any way by an independently conducted institution."[117] One of the main problems of the new location was that the building was owned by a Persian, who did not maintain it and therefore, the medical staff considered that they needed better housing soon.

> A small fund, accumulated by contributions of some of the chief habitants of Bushire, has for some time been destined by them to go towards the provision of a good hospital, and until recently it appeared as if the intention was that the new hospital should be run by Persians. A counter-proposal with some considerable authority to back it is to effect that funds raised locally to assist in the building of a new hospital on a site to be granted free by its proprietor. The hope has been expressed that the Government of India would be good enough to permit the Staff of the Residency Dispensary to run the new Hospital intended to replace it, and that further the Government of India might possibly assist in the expense of building the hospital. There is little doubt that it will be a considerable time before the local efforts, if united, will suffice to build and maintain a good hospital.[118]

According to Wright, a new hospital was established in 1916 with financial help from local merchants,[119] which is incorrect. Indeed such a plan for a hospital and a free dispensary had been initiated many years ago, but its realization was delayed by the Great War. It was only by the end of 1920 that "work had started by the residency mason and under the supervision of the British Executive Engineer for the Gulf Ports,"[120] and the first storey was almost complete by September 1921.[121] It was expected that in 1922, the dispensary would move to better place; therefore, "the old place is demolished and is being reconstructed on a better and more sanitary basis."[122] In 1922 it was reported that "The work on the new Charitable Hospital, built by public subscription, was practically complete by the end of the year. The equipment still remains to be purchased. It is hoped that it may be opened during the next year,"[123] which indeed it was.

117 *Administration Report* 1913, p. 34.
118 *Administration Report* 1914, p. 12.
119 Wright 2001, p. 127.
120 *Report 1920–21*, p. 1.
121 *Report 1920–21*, p. ii.
122 *Administration Report* 1920, p. 7.
123 *Administration Report* 1922, p. 9.

> The new hospital was occupied in April 1923. Its design is a compromise between what is needed for a hospital on the one hand and local Persian ideas of architecture coupled with insufficiency of funds on the other. As a result, when occupied, it lacked electric light, a water-supply, cookhouses, quarters for staff, and a sanitary and drainage system. Electric light has been installed, two engines purchased and, thanks to the Anglo-Persian Oil Company, a free supply of kerosene oil and petrol for power. A proper drain has been made into the sea, latrines constructed and a water-tank on the roof for finishing purposes supplied by an automatic electric pump from a well, is in course of erection. A large 'Ab-ambar' has been constructed to be connected by a semi-rotary hand pump to another tank on the roof for the supply of water to the operation theatre and dispensary. But until the quarters of the staff have been built the hospital can only be considered to be an 'outdoor' dispensary.[124]

The facilities were still insufficient to receive inpatients. The Hospital, therefore, continued to operate as dispensary, because much equipment was still lacking as was a chief medical officer.[125] By the end of 1925, shortages were overcome and the Bushire Residency Dispensary and Charitable Hospital was fully operational. Nevertheless, there were still problems, because the great demand on outpatients hampered the extension of inpatient work.[126] The new hospital was staffed by a British physician and administered by a committee composed of two Iranians and two Englishmen.[127] Apart from the dispensary maintained by the Indian government, there was no government medical aid of any kind. The residency surgeon and his staff therefore performed practically the whole of the medical work of Bushire.[128]

In 1929 some significant changes took place as to the status of the Charitable Hospital. On 9 February the Residency Dispensary was removed from the hospital to the Residency compound. This dispensary only treated Residency staff and their families, employees and families of the Imperial Bank of Persia, and the employees of the three European firms, to wit: the Mesopotamia Persia Corporation, Messrs. Ziegler & Company and Messrs. A. and T. J. Malcolm. This move was due to the fact that in September 1928 the head of the finance department (*ra'is-i maliya*), who was acting

[124] *Administration Report* 1923, p. 14. It was nevertheless, considered to be "quite an improvement on the present building where the residency surgeon carried on his work under adverse conditions." *Report* 1921–22, p. 1.

[125] *Administration Report* 1924, p. 8.

[126] *Administration Report* 1925, p. 10.

[127] Elgood 1951, p. 548.

[128] *Report 1920–21*, pp. 1–2.

governor of Bushire at that time, informed the Residency Surgeon that the Charitable Hospital had to be handed over to the Iranian authorities. To put some pressure behind this 'suggestion' shortly thereafter the Customs Department withdrew its financial contribution to the hospital. It further instructed its employees to henceforth go to a dispensary that had been opened within the Customs Department and which was operated by Iranian physicians. Soon thereafter the Post Office and the Finance Department likewise withdrew their financial contribution and their sick. The collection of the so-called *šāhī* voluntary fee, which represented 50 per cent. of the Hospital's income, for some time had systematically been underperforming and it was not paid at all during the last quarter of 1928. It was clear to the British authorities that all these measures were aimed to bankrupt the hospital and thus embarrass the British. As a result, the British government decided to sever its relationship with the Charitable Hospital on 9 February 1929, a relationship that has lasted some 60 years. The medical responsibility was immediately transferred to Dr. Bahrāmī, the Iranian chief quarantine medical officer, who, assisted by Dr. 'Alī Ḫān carried out the medical work. The British government divided all medical supplies and surgical equipment in half, one of which was moved to the Residency dispensary. As a result the operating room equipment was incomplete and serious cases could not be dealt with. During a visit made in January 1930 at the request of the governor of Bushire, the Residency Surgeon noted that "the Hospital was not conspiciously clean and that Dr. 'Alī Ḫān's learning was not of a very high order, in fact not even of mediocre standards."[129]

## Enzeli

In the summer of 1897 a group of Russian physicians arrived in Enzeli and established a dispensary, according to a report in the newspaper *Ḥabl al-Matīn*. They made use of a kind of prefabricated house, which allegedly was made of cardboard (*muqavā-yi qārdūn*) and that could be disassembled and re-assembled. The Russian physicians provided medical care free-of-charge to the poor and gave their patients quinine as well as a kind of greasy oil (*rawġan-i zamāt*). They also carried out operations and therefore had many patients. Wealthy patients had to pay for the medical service and

---

[129] *Administration Report* 1929, p. 8.

were given a prescription made out to the new pharmacy in Enzeli.[130] It is unknown for how long this group of Russian physicians remained in Enzeli and if they had anything to do with the establishment of a hospital there, which was established in 1905 or thereabouts. At that time, the town had some 8,000 inhabitants.

In 1908 people in Enzeli complained about the shortages at the hospital, which means that it must have been established prior to that date. There certainly was a hospital in 1907 as the newspaper *Ḥabl al-Matīn* published data on its income and expenditures. In 1911 the hospital still existed, because a newspaper article mentions that a victim of an attack was treated at the hospital. In 1924, the by then municipal hospital had 15 beds, 10 for men and five for women. It had further a dispensary and pharmacy. Despite its limited capacity (one physician, two Russian nurses and one male nurse) Gilmour had the impression that the hospital was rendering excellent services. From March 1923 until March 1924 the hospital treated 375 inpatients, most of them suffering from malaria, and 3,000 outpatients. The hospital was still functional in 1926. By that time, there also was a hospital for women, which continued to exist in the years there after. Apparently it was a two-storey building with a few rooms, located just behind the municipality.[131]

## Golpaygan

When in 1915 all British subjects were ordered to leave Iran many returned to Great Britain. J. R. Garland, a young clergyman, who in 1915 worked in Isfahan, went to Ahvaz and when in 1916 the situation in Iran had become less volatile he returned to Isfahan. He then opened among other things a dispensary at Golpaygan, a town of some 15,000 inhabitants. His work was supervised by Mīrzā Yūsuf Ḥakīm and Mīrzā Ayūb Ḥakīm. It is not known to me how long this dispensary lasted, but probably only for a short period given the demand on medical manpower to deal with the famine of 1917–18 followed by the outbreaks of influenza, cholera and typhus in Iran.[132]

130 Ṭavīlī 1371, vol. 2, pp. 210–211 quoting *Ḥabl al-Matīn*, nr. 8, Calcutta, 2 *ša'bān* 1315/27 December 1897, p. 90 and nr. 36, 15 *rabī' al-avval* 1318/24 July 1899. Andreeva 2007, p. 193.

131 Ṭavīlī 1371, vol. 2, pp. 218–220, 223–224, quoting *Ḥabl al-Matīn*, nr. 225, Tehran, 5 *muḥarram* 1326/8 February 1908; Ẓahīr al-Dawla 1351, p. 319; Gilmour 1924, p. 29. However, in 1909, the *Diplomatic and Consular Reports* (henceforth *DCR*) 4828, pp. 11, 14 under the heading "Public Health" makes no mention of a hospital in either Rasht or Astarabad.

132 Waterfield 1973, p. 121. Išrāqī 1383, p. 886 does not mention this dispensary when he deals with the subject of health in Golpaygan.

## Hamadan

Around 1907, Hamadan had a population of about 60,000 for whom hardly any medical assistance was available. As of 1882, American missionaries had Dr. E. W. Alexander operating in Hamadan, who was succeeded by Dr. G. Holmes in 1893, who operated a small hospital-cum-dispensary. He was joined in 1891 by Dr. Jessie C. Wilson, and later in 1900 by Dr. Blanche Wilson Stead. In 1903, Dr. Arthur Funk established the Lily Reid Holt Memorial Hospital for Men in Hamadan, which was expanded in 1916. This was probably the Whipple Memorial Hospital for Women, which is mentioned in 1921, but clearly existed before that time, while both hospitals shared one dispensary. In the early days he had no skilled assistants or nurses, although he performed ten to twelve operations per day. According to Morton, it was "a three-story, up-to-date hospital, which he [Dr. Funk] designed and supervised in every detail so that he was in fact architect, contractor, and builder."[133] In 1917–18, the hospital suffered greatly because of the hostilities. The Russian Red Cross had taken occupation of the hospital for men, so all patients had to be treated in the women's hospital. When the Russian Red Cross left the hospital was like a pigsty and had to be thoroughly cleaned. Because all the bedding had been destroyed or lost, new mattresses, quilts, pillows, sheets, etc. had to be made, but when the hospital was about to be cleaned "unrestrained Russian soldiers" occupied the hospital for six weeks, causing damage to the building estimated at 200 *tūmāns*. Shortly thereafter British troops who were better behaved, arrived. They asked for permission to be housed in the hospital, and it was given. Meanwhile, the work at the dispensary continued, but at a lower attendance than before, because Dr. Funk had been called to Soltanabad and Tehran.[134] In 1920, the hospital was closed because Dr. Funk was on furlough as of March 1920, but the dispensary was operated by his assistant, Dr. Khachatur. Most of the patients were women. However, because the British military still occupied the Hospital for Men a reduced number of patients had to be received in the Hospital for Women. Despite these setbacks the four medical trainees all graduated on Dr. Funk's departure and were given their MD certificate.

[133] Morton 1940, pp. 262, 268 (training of Iranian staff); Wilson 1896, pp. 260, 374; 'Ayn al-Salṭana 1376, vol. 1, pp. 377, 865; Kumīsiyūn 1343, vol. 2, pp. 1449–1451; Elgood 1951, pp. 511–512, 534; Ẓahīr al-Dawla 1351, p. 133; Waterfield 1973, pp. 136–137. Dr. Holmes became later personal physician to the *šāh*; *The Eighty-fourth Annual Report of the Board of Foreign Missions of the Presbyterian Church in the U.S.A.*, 1921, p. 329; Dr. Holmes also had trained many Jewish merchants in the principles of modern medicine. *DCR* 3189, p. 40.

[134] *One Hundred Seventeenth Annual Report of the Home Missions of the Presbyterian Church of the U.S.A.*, 1919, p. 263.

The government of Iran issued them all a license to practice as physicians.[135] In 1921 Dr. Khachatur continued the dispensary, while Mrs. Zoeckler regularly assisted with examinations and the treatment of special cases. As the Women's Hospital had not been used for some time one of the dispensary rooms was turned in a hospital ward for men, while the hospital was being readied to receive women. With the arrival of Dr. Dodd (from Urmiyeh) and Ms Wells (from Tabriz) as well as three Iranian nurses (from Urmiyeh) the Hamadan hospital had never known such medical efficiency. Meanwhile in 1921 Dr. Funk returned, but the Hospital for Women still required major repairs due to its use by the Russian military as well as having been used as an orphanage for Assyrian children. However, he intended to receive female inpatients again as soon as the repairs were completed.[136]

Also, there was a 12-bed municipal hospital in Hamadan, housed in part of the Municipality building. It had been established around 1920, which was financed by a tax on transportation, and although it was a bare-bones operation it provided better treatment to patients than they would have received at home. However, there was no surgical service, even of the most elementary kind.[137]

## Isfahan

Isfahan was a city with 60,000 inhabitants, where, as of 1883, a dispensary with waiting rooms for either sex was operating in Jolfa-Isfahan, which had been established in 1880 and had been managed since then by Dr. E. F. Hoernle of the British Church Missionary Society. "Another room had been set apart as a hospital where the more serious cases are treated surgically."[138] Mary Bird of the CMS opened a dispensary for Muslim women in the Isfahan bazaar in 1891, which, despite the opposition by the ulama, who forcibly shut it down no fewer than five times during 1894–97, remained open due to popular support from her patients.[139] In

135 *The Eighty-fourth Annual Report of the Board of Foreign Missions of the Presbyterian Church in the U.S.A.*, 1921, p. 332; *The Eighty-third Annual Report of the Board of Foreign Missions of the Presbyterian Church in the U.S.A.*, 1920, p. 313.

136 *The Eighty-fifth Annual Report of the Board of Foreign Missions of the Presbyterian Church in the U.S.A.*, 1922, pp. 366–67.

137 Gilmour 1924, p. 29. It is sad that Hamadānī 1382, p. 176 does not even mention these earlier hospitals, thus relegating the endeavors of these physicians, both Americans and Iranians, to the dustbin of history.

138 Wills 1893, p. 164; Elgood 1951, p. 534; Waterfield 1973, p. 150.

139 For the story of the clerical opposition see Rice 1916, pp. 70–77; Waterfield 1973, pp. 155–156.

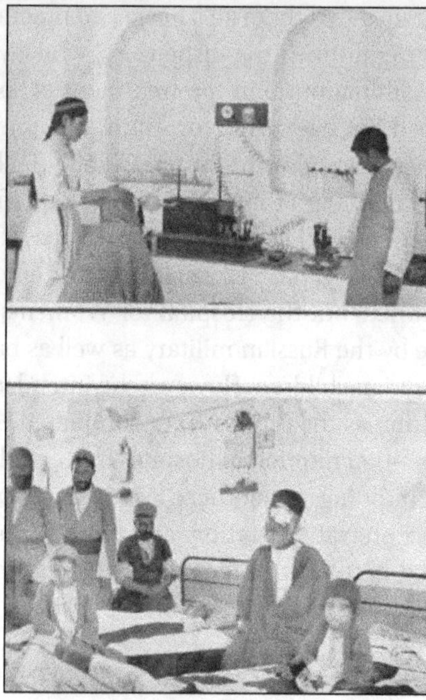

Figures 2a and 2b. The Jolfa CMS hospital at Isfahan. From Hume-Griffith, 1909, *Behind the Veil in Persia and Turkish Arabia*. Philadelphia, p. 148.

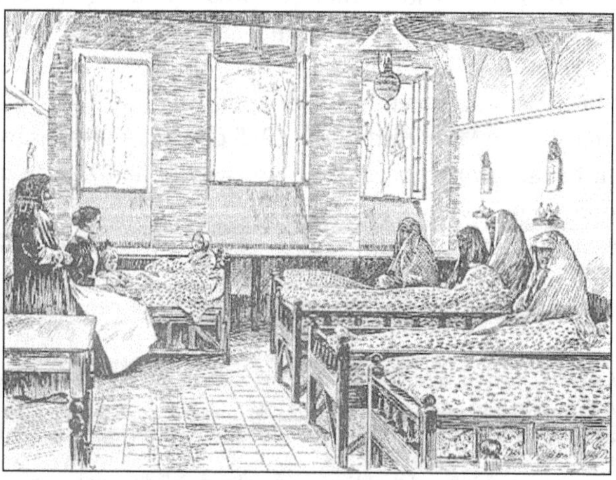

Figure 3. A ward of the Jolfa CMS hospital at Isfahan. From Stileman, 1902, *The Subjects of the Shah*. London, p. 38.

1894, Dr. Donald Carr took over medical operations, and in 1896 the CMS opened a hospital with dispensary in Jolfa-Isfahan and made great progress in improving its facilities. In 1901 Dr. Carr observed:

> When he came he found the hospital in a very bad state of repair, more like a caravanserai than a hospital, with only three wards accommodating six men and seven women. In 1901 there was an entire wing for women and beds for twenty-three men. In 1894 there was no nursing staff, each patient being looked after by a friend or relative. In 1901 nursing care had been revolutionised by the Canadian sister, Helen McKin. In 1894 there was a minimum of hygiene and cleanliness and the patients remained in their own clothes, which were often torn and filthy. In 1901 they had clean linen and clean hospital garments and there was a high standard of antisepsis in the hospital. Between 500 and 600 patients passed through the hospital during the year 1900, with an average stay of fourteen days.[140]

In 1902 a clinic was opened in Isfahan itself, and in 1904 a hospital was built helped by a land gift from a local rich merchant. Subsequently a women's hospital was founded and placed under the supervision of Dr. Emmelina Stuart.[141] In 1915 the hospital was closed, because British subjects were ordered to leave, but they returned in 1916 after the Russians had occupied the city in May of that year.[142]

## Kerman

In September 1897, the governor of Kerman, Bahjat al-Mulk, opened a hospital for the poor inside the citadel of Kerman, which had 20 beds as well as a nursing staff. The medical director was Ḥājj Maḥmūd H̯ān Kirmānī.[143] Whether this hospital lasted beyond the governor's time in office is not known. A fact is that when in 1902 the CMS operation established a small hospital, with a male and a female section, it certainly satisfied a great need in the town of 50,000 inhabitants. In 1913 a bigger hospital was completed, mostly with funds and land gifts from the local Kermani community. In the 1920s the hospital was further enlarged and modernized.[144]

---

140 Waterfield 1973, p. 158.

141 Wright 2001, pp. 118, 122. The British therefore noted that "there are two British hospitals in the city." Adamec 1981, vol. 1, p. 251. It was in this hospital the late Queen Suraya was born in 1936.

142 Waterfield 1973, p. 162; Rice 1916, p. 189.

143 Sipihr 1368, pp. 169–170.

144 A Friend of Iran 1940, pp. 27, 34, 54–56, 58–59, 63; Rice 1916, pp. 133–134; Wright 2001, pp. 188, 121. For a description of the modern equipment the Isfahan hospital had acquired by around 1920 see Stuart n.d., pp. 17–19.

Table 7: Number of Patients Seen, Operations Performed in Kerman and House Calls Made (1910–1925)

| Type/Year | 1910 | 1912 | 1913 | 1919 | 1920 | 1921 | 1925 |
|---|---|---|---|---|---|---|---|
| Total | | | | | | | |
| Male | | 8,442 | | | | | |
| Female | | 12,647 | | | | | |
| New patients | | | 4,981 | | | | |
| Male | 2,933 | 2,040 | – | 1,466 | 1,502 | 217 | – |
| Female | 2,705 | 2,669 | – | 1,615 | 2,094 | 2,078 | – |
| Repeat patients | | | 12,042 | | | | |
| Male | 7,080 | 6,025 | – | 4,394 | 3,109 | 1,035 | – |
| Female | 9,038 | 9,555 | – | 3,267 | 8,203 | 6,535 | – |
| Outpatients | | | 4,982 | | | | |
| Male | 2,311 | – | – | – | – | – | – |
| Female | 1,417 | – | – | – | – | – | – |
| Inpatients | | | 469 | | | | 581 |
| Male | 224 | 208 | – | 169 | 155 | 30 | – |
| Female | 214 | 166 | – | 155 | 148 | 111 | – |
| Operations | 204 | | | | | | |
| Major | – | 175 Men | 377 | 287 | 144 Men | 80 | 522 |
| Minor | – | 157 Female | not recorded | – | | – | – |
| Urban house calls | – | – | 1,537 | 2,427 | 803 | 2,103 | 2,150 |
| Rural visits | – | – | 475 | 505 | – | – | 70 |

Source: *Administration Report* 1910, p. 33; Ibid., 1912, p. 56; Ibid., 1913, p. 70; Ibid., 1919, p. 31; Ibid., 1920, p. 30; Ibid., 1921, p. 29; Ibid., 1925, p. 39 (581 inpatients compared with 565 last year [1924] and 447 the year before [1923]; 522 operations as compared with 540 in 1924.).

Table 7 shows that the Kerman hospital-dispensary was well attended even during the years for which no data are available, such as in 1914.[145] In 1915, the CMS hospital-dispensary, which was doing well, unexpectedly suffered a major setback due to the local 'coup-d'etat' by the Democrats, which led to a temporary departure of staff.[146] In 1916, the Kerman hospital-dispensary was not operational, because the Democrats did not allow the return of superfluous British citizens, a description that they also applied to CMS medical

145 *Administration Report* 1914, p. 25.

146 *Administration Report* 1915, p. 23. The hospital was also visited by German soldiers. Waterfield 1973, p. 162.

staff.[147] In 1917, the political situation became favorable again and the CMS staff returned to Kerman. However, CMS Kerman had to start almost anew as most of its medical equipment had been looted by the Democrats during the staff's absence.[148] As of 1918, attendance grew, as expected. A positive development was the acquisition of a car in 1925, which made rural visits more efficient. "Visiting rural patients on mule or horse back in the past required 27 days, now the same trip lasted only 42 hours."[149]

Starting anew had also its advantages, for the old buildings was cramped and inadequate, and thus plans to have a new building were initiated. In 1919 it was reported that "building work has been continued on the new site, where the men's new outpatient department, one new ward block for 28 men's beds, the new kitchen and store rooms, and part of the new Doctor's house have been put up."[150] In 1925, the new hospital was nearing completion. "The compound is about eight acres in size and the most modern types of building have been erected."[151]

In Kerman, as of 1910, the CMS has a female doctor, Dr. Westlake and two nurses (Ms Parry and Ms Carrick), who together with Dr. and Mrs. Dodson formed the medical team. Sometimes, they received occasional assistance from the Isfahan-based Drs. Donald Carr and C. Merrill Schaffter for a few months, during the leave of absence of Dr. Dodson.[152] By 1919, the Kerman CMS staff consisted of Dr and Mrs. Dodson, 7 male and 4 female Iranian assistants.[153]

In addition to the CMS, and the so-called *Mursalīn* (i.e., Missionaries), hospital, there were two other medical establishments in Kerman. In 1912, the IETD's dispensary was operating in Kerman, but it is unknown from and until when. The dispensary was managed by assistant surgeon Mr. Steinhoff.[154]

---

147 *Administration Report* 1916, p. 42.
148 *Administration Report* 1917, p. 26.
149 *Administration Report* 1925, p. 39.
150 *Administration Report* 1919, p. 31; Cash 1930, p. 40.
151 *Administration Report* 1925, p. 39.
152 *Administration Report* 1910, p. 33; *Administration Report* 1912, p. 56; *Administration Report* 1913, p. 70.
153 *Administration Report* 1919, p. 31.
154 *Administration Report* 1912, p. 56.

Table 8: Performance of the Indo-European Telegraph Department Dispensary at Kerman (1912)

| | Male | Female |
|---|---|---|
| Fresh cases | 620 | 316 |
| Repeated visits | not known | not known |
| Operations | 97 | 15 and 25 minor ones |

Source: *Administration Report* 1912, p. 56.

Finally, there was the so-called Nūriya Hospital, which was a *vaqf* or endowed medical institution, which had been established in 1924. In that same year, Dr Mūsā Ḫān, an Iranian physician with French qualifications and English experience, had come to Kerman to take charge of this hospital as well as to act as ex-officio Health Officer for the town. After a few months he resigned and left Kerman "as he was unable to obtain either his pay or medicines from the Mutawalli."[155] In 1925, he was succeeded by Dr. Arīsṭū Ḫān.[156]

## Kermanshah

At the turn of the twentieth century, Kermanshah had a population of over 60,000 inhabitants and no mention is made of any medical institution in the detailed study of the city by Rabino.[157] In 1904, ʿAbd al-Ḥusayn Mīrzā Farmānfarmā, when governor of Kermanshah, opened a newly built hospital in the town. However, when Farmānfarmā was dismissed one year later the hospital was neglected and became dilapidated. When Farīd al-Mulk visited it in 1905 it had no patients, although its doctor was present. He told the new governor that Farmānfarmā had given 70 *tūmāns* per month, which was insufficient for the operating expenses of the hospital, excluding the salary of the doctor and the cost of charcoal were 100 *tūmāns* per month.[158]

This medical gap was filled by American missionaries. In 1905, Dr. B. W. Stead and Mrs. Stead (who was a physician a.k.a. Dr. Blanche Wilson) initiated medical services in Kermanshah. In 1907, Mrs. Stead enlarged her dispensary with a few rooms and henceforth also received

155 *Administration Report* 1924, p. 36.

156 Rustāʾī 1382, vol. 2, p. 45.

157 *DCR* 590, p. 13.

158 Sulṭānī 1370, vol. 1, pp. 533–534; Farīd al-Mulk Hamadānī 1345, pp. 64–65, 228, 238, 223.

inpatients. They established a general clinic there in 1912 and a small hospital in 1922, because the old dispensary had suffered during the Great War. In fact, during 1917–18 the dispensary had to be closed due to the hostilities and the lack of medical supplies.[159] In 1919 Mrs. Stead was able to open the dispensary, but she also provided medical care to outpatients. Meanwhile, some of her work was taken care of by the British Medical Corps, although as of March the latter received orders not to treat civilians anymore.[160] When the British army left Kermanshah in April 1921, it offered huts for sale to the American missionaries. The 21 huts, 12 of which 80 feet long, were nicely located on a hill outside the city. Moreover, they were located at a distance from one another such that this made the establishment of a cottage-hospital possible. The Americans bought them for 3350 *tūmāns*, much below market value, but they had to break down the "ideal hospital" as they had neither the staff to guard them nor a doctor to work there, while looting of building materials had already occurred. On Dr. Stead's return in March 1920 she opened the dispensary in her sewing room, where she received 30 patients every day. Dr. Stead-Wilson died 21 February 1922 in Kermanshah, aged 52 years.[161]

The British also opened a charitable dispensary and Civil Hospital, at an unknown date, probably in 1906 or 1907, which in 1908 was transferred from the consulate to more commodious quarters in town, consisting of: surgeon's office, hospital assistant's office, dispensing room, two dressing rooms (two small waiting rooms, one for male and one for female patients), an operating room, one small ward for emergency cases and hospital assistant's quarters. It was open for 174 days in that year, because for the remainder of the time, the medical staff accompanied the consul on tour. In 1908 it treated 20,981 patients of which 8,000 were males, 10,762 females and 5,942 children. At the Civil Hospital a total of 308 in-house patients were treated, of which 284 were men and 24 women. As in other cities malaria was a main problem, tuberculosis was also frequently encountered, while syphilis

159 'Ayn al-Salṭana 1376, vol. 1, pp. 377, 865; Kumīsiyūn 1343, vol. 2, p. 1451; Elgood 1951, pp. 511–512, 534; Waterfield 1973, pp. 139–140; *One Hundred Seventeenth Annual Report of the Home Missions of the Presbyterian Church of the U.S.A.*, 1919, p. 266. In 1921 the dispensary was closed due to the absence of Mrs. Stead. *The Eighty-fourth Annual Report of the Board of Foreign Missions of the Presbyterian Church in the U.S.A.*, 1921, p. 335.

160 *The Eighty-third Annual Report of the Board of Foreign Missions of the Presbyterian Church in the U.S.A.*, 1920, p. 318.

161 *The Eighty-fifth Annual Report of the Board of Foreign Missions of the Presbyterian Church in the U.S.A.*, 1922, pp. 68, 368–369.

Table 9: Number of Visits to the Charitable Dispensary of Lengeh (1912–1925)

| Year | Total | Men | Women | Boys | Girls |
|---|---|---|---|---|---|
| 1912 | 947 | – | – | – | – |
| 1913 | 1,846 | – | – | – | – |
| 1914 | 2,072 | – | – | – | – |
| 1916 | 2,587 | – | – | – | – |
| 1917 | 2,023 | – | – | – | – |
| 1918 | 2,630 | – | – | – | – |
| 1919 | 2,318 | – | – | – | – |
| 1921 | 1,521 | – | – | – | – |
| 1922 | 1,630 | – | – | – | – |
| 1923 | 2,203 | – | – | – | – |
| 1925 | 2,095 | 1,284 | 476 | 190 | 145 |

Source: *Administration Report* 1914, p. 16; Ibid., 1915, p. 15; Ibid., 1916, p. 15; Ibid., 1917, p. 14; Ibid., 1918, p. 14; Ibid., 1919, p. 14; Ibid., 1923, p. 36; Ibid., 1925, p. 37.

and eye diseases were very common. The dispensary performed also simple operations.[162]

## Lengeh

The British opened a charitable dispensary in Lengeh, although the date is not known. Although similar in population size[163] as Bushire and Bandar Abbas and having the same kind of diseases, attendance at the dispensary was lower in Lengeh.[164] This did not mean it was unpopular, for patients came from the outlying districts with the caravans as well as from the islands to receive treatment. Although women patients remained in the minority, by 1925 it was noted that a "better class women now attend the dispensary."[165]

162 The more important operations included "removal of sequestrum of palatal process of upper jaw; excision of rodent ulcers in the inner angle of the eye, fistula *in ano*, lateral lithomy", *Administration Report* 1908, pp. 49–54.

163 Lengeh had a population of some 20,000 in 1919. *Administration Report* 1919, p. 10. The doctor's house "is a very large straddling edifice very much out of repair. The Persian clearly has an aversion to repairing." Cursetjee 1918, p. 72.

164 The prevailing major diseases were malaria, eye diseases and of digestive organs, *Administration Report* 1913, p. 43; Ibid. 1914, p. 16; Ibid. 1923, p. 36.

165 *Administration Report* 1923, p. 36; Ibid. 1925, p. 37. In nearby Basidu, on the island of Qeshm the British army had a small military base since 1823, which included a small hospital. This hospital remained functional until the 1883 when the base was abandoned. The derelict hospital building was still there in 1925. There is no evidence that the services of

## Malayer

In 1920, the first hospital was built in Malayer, a town of 8,000 people, from funds made available from the large endowment left by Prince Sayf al-Dawla, a member of the Qajar family. It had ten beds and was still in use in the 1960s.[166] Prior to that time, American missionaries had already established a school in Dowlatabad as Malayer was known at the time and provided irregular medical care from Hamadan. But with the departure of Mr. and Mrs. Zoeckler in November 1918 their medical work was discontinued.[167]

## Mashhad

As a major pilgrimage city, part of the population of Mashhad was fluctuating, sometimes doubling in size from 50,000. Before the 1890s, there was no real hospital, although there was a *dār al-šifā* at the shrine of Imam Riżā at Mashhad, which seems to have been established by Nādir Šāh.[168] Prior to 1862, when Eastwick visited Mashhad, this hospital was either renovated, or as he reported a new one had been built. Eastwick wrote that he visited "the new hospital, built by the Mashir [the Mashhad shrine's manager] for eighty sick persons. It is in a fine large garden, and the Mashir told me he intended to endow it with funds."[169] When Nāṣir al-Dīn Šāh visited Mashhad, the *dār al-šifā* was situated opposite the Gawhar Šād Mosque, which he did not consider an appropriate location. This place later became known as the *Sarā-yi Nāṣirī*. The Šāh instructed the chief-manager (*mutavallī-bāšī*), ʿAżud al-Mulk, to build a new hospital some 500 meters farther away from the shrine, on the south side of the Bālā-yi Ḫiyābān. In 1880, ʿAlī Akbar Ḫān, who had overseen the construction of the State Hospital in Tehran, moved to Mashhad. Mušīr al-Dawla was the chief-administrator of the shrine complex and, at the latter's request ʿAlī

this hospital were available to the population of Basidu. For a description of the military hospital of Basidu in 1856 see Shepherd 1857, pp. 71, 73, 75–76, 97. See also *Administration Report* 1882–83, p. 6; Wilson 1928, p. 212.

166 Zahereddini 1966, p. 38; Gilmour 1924, pp. 29–30; Momeni 1976, pp. 46, 49.

167 *One Hundred Seventeenth Annual Report of the Home Missions of the Presbyterian Church of the U.S.A.*, 1919, p. 263.

168 Iʿtimād al-Salṭana 1294–97, vol. 1, p. 552; Ibid., 1301–03, vol. 2, p. 235; Āṣaf al-Dawla 1377, vol. 1, pp. 20 (*marīż-ḫāna*), 39 (*dār al-šifā*); Rustāʾī 1382, vol. 2, p. 512. For the situation prior to 1500, see Tadjbakhsh 1379, p. 184.

169 Eastwick 1976, vol. 2, p. 213.

Akbar Ḫān constructed the Rażavī Hospital (*Dār al-šifā-yi Rażavī*) in one of the shrine's gardens, which was mainly financed through donations and partly from the shrine's foundation funds. It had separate male and female wards, while the rooms for people with contagious diseases were separated from the other wards. Because the hospital was not completed during Mušīr al-Dawla's tenure his son, Muḥammad Ṣādiq Ḫān completed the building with funds his father had endowed for that purpose.[170] The new building apparently replaced the old *dār al-šifā*, as it was reported that it was the only medical facility in the city.[171] This makes perfect sense as it was also reported that when Mušīr al-Dawla arrived in Mashhad in 1277/1861, mention was made of the former *dār al-šifā*, which was situated adjacent to the Friday Mosque and had fallen into disuse. However, it seems that the old building was renovated and new buildings added to it.[172] This was further borne out by a report in 1924, in which Gilmour reported that there were two old dilapidated shrine hospitals in Mashhad (see below).

Table 10: Funds Paid to the Staff of the *Dār al-šifā* of Mashhad (ca. 1870)

| Name and function | Remuneration (in *tūmāns*) |
|---|---|
| Ḥājj Mullā Ḥusayn *Nāẓir* (overseer) of the hospital | 15 |
| Ḥājj Mullā Ḥusayn *Nāẓir* of food and medicines | 5 |
| Mīrzā Muḥammad *Ṭabīb* (physician) | 17.5 |
| Mīrzā Bāqir *Mušrif* (inspector) | 7 |
| Aqā Muḥammad Isma'īl | 10 |
| Mīrzā Abū al-Qāsim | 5 |
| Mullā 'Abd al-Raḥmān | 5 |
| Orderlies: male 6; female: 2 | 14 (males: 8 + 5 *qirāns*; females: 5 + 5 *qirāns*) |
| Mullā Karīm, the druggist | 9 |

Source: 'Attārdī 1371, pp. 501–502.

170 Elgood 1951, pp. 511–512; Nafīsī 1325, pp. 56–57; I'timād al-Salṭana 1301–03, vol. 2, pp. 237, 268; 'Attārdī 1371, pp. 498–501; Tadjbakhsh 1379, pp. 247–248. According to Muḥammad Ḥasan Ḫān, Malik al-Ḥukamā, who was the public health officer (*ḥāfiẓ al-siḥḥa*) of Mashhad at that time, Nāṣir al-Dīn Šāh took this decision after he had submitted a paper to the *šāh* outlining 32 defects of the *dār al-šifā*. Prior to that decision he had already modernized its surgery and pharmacy. For details see Rustā'ī 1382, vol. 2, pp. 512–513.

171 Ḥakīm al-Mamālik 1356, p. 259; Nafīsī 1329–31, p. 20; Hemmati n.d., p. 101. In 1881 it was reported that some mad people were brought to the *dār al-šifā* for treatment. *Rūznāma-yi Īrān* 1375, p. 1868 (9 *šavvāl* 1298/4 September 1881).

172 I'timād al-Salṭana 1301–03, vol. 2, pp. 237, 268; Mu'taman 1348, p. 403.

As is clear from Table 10, the *dār al-šifā* of the Shrine was under a general manager, who also doubled as the overseer of food and medicines. The hospital only employed one physician, whose prescriptions for drugs were supplied by the druggist. The latter did not receive much money, thus suggesting that there was no great demand for his services. It is of no surprise to find that the hospital employed both male and female orderlies as there was both a male and female ward. The other persons listed presumably had administrative and/or religious functions.

Not much is known about the quality of medical service offered by the Rażavī Hospital. From one description it is clear that much of the *dār al-šifā*'s work was devoted to "the preparation of food and medicines, so that the sufferers, the sick and ill from among the strangers, travelers, and pilgrims of the holy land with the help of the staff of that institution: the physician, the overseer, the eye-doctor, the surgeon, the orderly, the nurse, Koran reciter, and assistant may find healing for their illnesses and diseases in that place and after having taken the food and medicine may become healthy."[173] Around 1905 the Shrine hospital had "a staff of about five or six native physicians. The hospital is nearly always full, and some kinds of surgical operations are undertaken, but not often with satisfactory results. This hospital is used mostly by pilgrims."[174] In 1900 Yate wrote that men, who had been sentenced to be subjected to corporal punishments by a court of law, "with the maimed feet and hands duly turned up for treatment at the British Consulate dispensary. I have never heard of any one going to the Persian hospital in the shrine under such circumstances, though that was the place that ought to have been open to all."[175] Dr. Hoffman noticed that conditions had much deteriorated at the Shrine hospital. He stated that when he arrived in Mashhad in 1913, "it was a place where men went only to die; hardly a pane of glass in the whole place, wooden bedsteads without sheets or pillow cases, a dirt floor, and no stove."[176]

In 1885, in addition to the Rażavī Hospital there was a clean and well-provisioned dispensary, established by Mīrzā Mullā Ḥusayn Ḥakīm-Bāšī-i Niẓām-i Ḫurāsān, which reportedly took good care of the troops in Mashhad.[177] Whether this dispensary continued to operate is not known.

173 'Attārdī 1371, p. 498.
174 Adamec 1981, vol. 2, p. 486.
175 Yate 1900, p. 336.
176 Morton 1940, p. 253.
177 Āṣaf al-Dawla 1377, vol. 1, p. 176.

There was yet another Iranian hospital in Mashhad. During his life, Ḥājj Muḥammad Ḥasan Mīrzā Muntaṣir al-Mulk had deeded a number of villages to his fourth wife, Iḥtirām al-Salṭana, on condition that she used those properties to build a hospital in Mashhad. In 1918 she used the funds from the sale of part of that property to buy a piece of land of 3,500 sq. cubits situated on the Ḫiyābān-i Darvāza-yi Jinnat and constructed there the Muntaṣiriya Hospital. She endowed the hospital with the remainder of the property. She remained the endowment manager until she died, when the management was transferred to the Shrine.[178] The hospital was not explicitly mentioned by Gilmour when he made his inventory of medical institutions in Iran and therefore, it is likely that it was included in his observation that the two endowed hospitals of Mashhad (that of the Shrine and this one) had suffered great neglect.

The impact of the Rażavī Hospital clearly was insufficient, for there was a growing demand, also from pilgrims, for the other hospital services available at Mashhad. First, there was the small British consular hospital with 12 beds, 6 for men and 6 for women.[179] It had one British doctor and one Indian hospital assistant, who treated about 6,000 patients per year around 1900. In the doctor's absence the hospital assistant ran the dispensary.[180] Until the arrival of the American missionaries,

> The British Consulate-General hospital is the only one in the city which is equipped for the reception and scientific treatment of in-patients, and for the undertaking of serious surgical work. It has recently been largely repaired, renovated and altered; also a good deal of modern equipment has been added, an operating room fitted out and an ophthalmoscopic 'dark room'. The average daily attendance of out-patients throughout the year is 112. During the year 1904–05, before the renovations and re-equipment were completed, 41 major operations and a large number of minor operations were performed. Eye operations have hitherto formed the large proportion of the major operations. About 36,000 patients are seen annually.[181]

All patients received treatment and drugs free-of-charge, while the poor were fed at the British hospital's expense. Wealthy, presumably paying, patients received house-calls. The hospital's services, therefore, were

---

[178] Mu'taman 1348, p. 414 (with a picture of the hospital); 'Attārdī 1371, pp. 509–510.

[179] Gilmour 1924, pp. 29–30; Grothe 1911, p. 131. Although the *dār al-šifā* of Mashhad had ceased to operate it continued to receive endowments, such as in 1334/1915–16 and 1338/1919–20, thus lack of funds cannot have been the reason for its negligence and the discontinuation of its operations. Sutūda 1366, vol. 7, pp. 561–562; vol. 8, pp. 257–258.

[180] Yate 1900, p. 336; Wright 2001, p. 126.

[181] Adamec 1981, vol. 2, p. 487.

becoming popular by 1905; it even received patients from as far as Herat. In February 1905, therefore, the government of India, allocated a sum of 5,000 Rupees for the re-equipment of the hospital, and later additional funds were made available to completely repair and renovate the hospital buildings.[182]

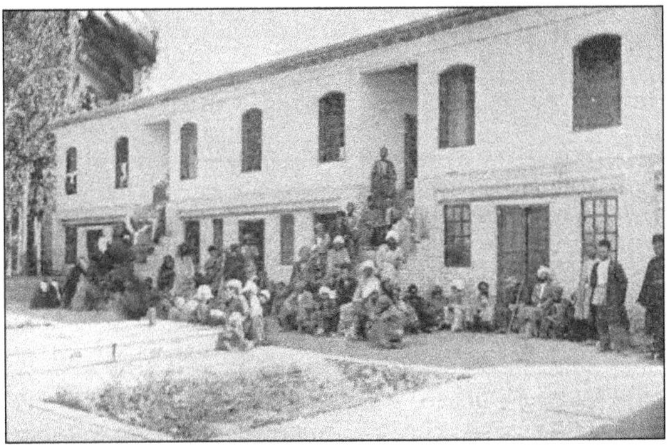

Figure 4. The British charitable dispensary at Mashhad. From Yate, 1900, *Khurasan and Seistan*. London, p. 336.

Table 11: Number of Patients Treated in the British Hospital at Mashad in 1904–05

| | Male | Female | Children | Total | Remarks |
|---|---|---|---|---|---|
| Outpatients (new and old) | 21,814 | 11,387 | 2,561 | 35,762 | |
| Outpatients (new only) | 7,926 | 3,082 | 1,195 | 12,203 | |
| Inpatients (new and old) | 33 | 12 | . 7 | 52 | From April 1 to November 11,1904, surgical inpatients only were registered. From November 12, 1904 to March 31,1905 both medical and surgical are included |

182 Sykes 1905, p. 22.

Table 11 (*cont.*)

| | Male | Female | Children | Total | Remarks |
|---|---|---|---|---|---|
| Major operations | 27 | 10 | 4 | 41 | Cataract, 28; bone, 2; liver abscess, 2; amputation, 2; litholapaxy, 1; lithotom, 3; supra-pubic lithomy, 1; other operations, 2 |
| Total (excluding operations) | 29,773 | 14,481 | 3,763 | 48,017 | |

Note: The average daily attendance of outpatients (new and old) was 114.25. The average daily attendance of new outpatients was 39.00.
Source: Sykes 1905, p. 22.

Even that service was not enough to satisfy demand, and the American missionary Dr. Joseph Cook started his medical work in Mashhad in 1913 (later joined by Dr. Rolla E. Hoffman), in a rented dispensary. The hospital, which had only a few beds, as well as its lone American physician was locally known as *Yangī Dunyā*, i.e., the 'New World.' "The villagers would sometimes say that they had gone to America when they had visited the hospital!"[183] In 1917 the hospital was changed into a soup kitchen to provide relief to thousands of hungry poor and re-opened on 11 October 1917. In the summer of 1919 the hospital remained closed, while in December the landlord canceled the rent contract giving one month's notice. Fortunately, a much better building was found, one that was ideally located, very well built and with access to clean water piped in iron tubes from the only pumping station of Mashhad. At the same time, the dispensary was open for business five days per week, although it was problematic to obtain medical supplies. The hospital now also drew many patients from across the border. In 1920, the medical staff was reinforced by the arrival of Dr. Hartman Lichtwardt. The latter operated the women's ward and dispensary together with Ḫānum Šarīfa, who acted as his interpreter, while Dr. Hoffman took the men's ward and dispensary. They held dispensary 3 days a week, while in 1921 the small hospital was extended by renting a house next door. Financially the hospital concluded a good contract with the Imperial Bank of Persia to treat all its employees. Patients continued to be a mix of local people and those from outlying

183 Donaldson 1972, pp. 108, 113; Elgood 1951, pp. 511–512, 534; Funk 1920, p. 153. According to Miller 1989, p. 50 Dr. and Mrs. Cook spent only a few months in Mashhad to see whether there was potential for medical mission work and Dr. Hoffman only came in 1916.

districts, including many pilgrims and Russian refugees. Dr. Hoffman also visited Nishapur where he provided medical assistance. Around 1923–24 a new hospital with some residences was opened (or re-opened), which was operated by Dr. Rolla Hoffman and Dr. Hartman Lichtwardt, who had arrived in December 1919.[184]

Again, there was a small hospital or charitable dispensary led by the Russian consular physician. It had "a daily attendance of about 40 to 50 outpatients in the summer; in the winter it is less."[185] When the Russian consular physician had finished his duties at the Russian dispensary "he proceeds to the [Russian] Bank dispensary, where he sees all the male patients. The female patients are seen by a Russian lady doctor, the wife of one of the bank employees. The average attendance here in the summer is about 70, and less in winter. The dispensary was established as a 'draw' for the Russian Banque d'Escompte de Perse."[186] These two dispensaries stopped functioning after 1917. Foreign medical establishments were the only source of medical service as of 1914 "there were only a few half-trained Persian doctors in the entire province of Khorasan" and no other hospital.[187]

In short, by 1914 there were four hospital/dispensaries operating in Mashhad: (i) the British Consulate-General dispensary/hospital; (ii) the Russian Consulate-General dispensary; (iii) the Russian Bank dispensary; and (iv) the American missionary hospital/dispensary. The two Mashhad Iranian hospitals (the Shrine's *dār al-šifā* with 70 beds and the Muntaṣiriya with 20 beds) had been totally neglected and had ceased to operate, allegedly due to lack of funds, probably after 1910. However, four years later the two Russian

184 Waterfield 1973, p. 139; Miller 1989, pp. 56–57 (Nishapur); *One Hundred Seventeenth Annual Report of the Home Missions of the Presbyterian Church of the U.S.A.*, 1919, p. 269; *The Eighty-third Annual Report of the Board of Foreign Missions of the Presbyterian Church in the U.S.A.*, 1920, pp. 319–321; *The Eighty-fourth Annual Report of the Board of Foreign Missions of the Presbyterian Church in the U.S.A.*, 1921, p. 337; Miller gives the date of the opening (or re-opening) of the hospital as 1924, Miller 1989, pp. 55, 98. According to Miller the hospital was closed for six months in 1921, because the missionaries fled to Zabol, due to the threat of an invasion by Soviet troops, thus, it is possible that the hospital was opened earlier than 1924 Miller 1989, pp. 60–62; see also *The Eighty-fourth Annual Report of the Board of Foreign Missions of the Presbyterian Church in the U.S.A.*, 1921, p. 337, which states that the absence was during the last 8 months of 1919; *The Eighty-fifth Annual Report of the Board of Foreign Missions of the Presbyterian Church in the U.S.A.*, 1922, pp. 371–372.

185 Adamec 1981, vol. 2, p. 486; Grothe 1911, p. 131.

186 Adamec 1981, vol. 2, p. 486.

187 Donaldson 1972, p. 108. Although there were many Russian troops in Mashhad apparently there was no Russian military hospital, or the military medical service was considered to be inadequate, as Russian soldiers came for treatment to the American hospital. Ibid., p. 112.

hospitals had closed down. In 1919, the President of the Sanitary Council made a pilgrimage to Mashhad and at the time took steps to re-open the two run-down and neglected Iranian hospitals as well as to organize a public health service for the province of Khorasan.[188] However, prodded by the success of the Christian hospital the Shrine authorities had already decided to improve their hospital in 1917, although the visit by the health official in 1919 may have spurred them to continue the competition of who offered the best medical services in Mashhad. Dr. Hoffman of the American missionary hospital reported about this chain of events as follows:

> But in 1917 there was a reform; it [the Shrine hospital] was rebuilt; a new doctor was secured, and the workers put on white gowns; a new operating suite was built, and surgery was begun on a small scale. Again, when we secured a larger and better hospital building in 1919, the Shrine hospital was moved into a larger and better house and more doctors were added to its staff. And when, again, in 1924, the Mission hospital advanced a decided step forward, through securing its own land and erecting a good building, along with many other reforms, the Sacred Shrine authorities soon began planning a really modern hospital building, which was begun three years later, a very elaborate series of buildings, costing around one million dollars![189]

In addition to these hospitals there was a leprosaria, which had been established one km outside Mashhad in 1884 or 1885 in the old castle of Miḥrāb Ḫān. Prior to that time lepers had lived among the people and congregated near the shrine to beg. Given the contagious nature of the disease it was therefore decided to concentrate them outside the city. They were taken care of by the Shrine.[190]

## Masjed-Soleyman

In 1914, the APOC established one of the most modern hospital in the Middle East, in the Fields (near Maydān-i Naft), as it was known for a

188 Gilmour 1924, pp. 29–30. Although the *dār al-šifā* of Mashhad had ceased to operate, apart from its existing endowments, the hospital continued to receive new endowments, such as in 1334/1915–16 and 1338/1919–20, therefore, lack of funds cannot have been the reason for its negligence and the discontinuation of its operations. Sutūda 1366, vol. 7, pp. 561–562; vol. 8, pp. 257–258.

189 Morton 1940, p. 254. Dr. Hoffman considered this competition a good thing as it was his policy to slowly give up one sphere of activity after another to Iranian hospitals, because finally the Mission hospital "seeks to eliminate itself."

190 Mu'taman 1348, p. 411. There were two other leprosarias in Iran, see Floor 2004, pp. 36–37.

Table 12: Number of Patients Treated and of Activities Undertaken in the Fields APOC Hospital (1926)

| Activity | Number |
|---|---|
| Hospital inpatients | 1,666 |
| Outpatients (a) new cases | 38,270 |
| (b) attendances | 88,913 |
| Major operations | 290 |
| Minor operations | 1,378 |
| Pathological examinations | 6,039 |
| Dental cases | 607 |
| X-ray photographs | 483 |

Source: Williamson 1927, pp. 127–128.

long time, which later developed into the town of Masjed-Soleyman. This was part of a comprehensive hospital construction and health development program led by Dr. Young. The Fields Hospital had a capacity of 88 beds (administrative staff 27; workmen 57 + 2 beds for European ladies and another ward for 2 beds for clerks' wives), a dispensary, two operating rooms (one for septic, the other for aseptic cases), a laboratory, and a radiology unit. The number of patients treated in the Fields numbered more than 128,000 in 1926.

In the Fields, the APOC employed a senior medical officer, two resident medical officers, a visiting medical officer, a consulting surgeon, a pathologist, and an ophthalmologist. These were assisted by 26 local nurses under a European matron with by eight European nurses.[191]

## Mohammerah

Mohammerah had an estimated population of 25,000 after the Great War[192] and no medical institutions until the establishment of a charitable dispensary by the British government. It is unclear when this took place, but most likely it must have been around 1908. In 1911, 242 patients were treated monthly.[193] The dispensary clearly satisfied a felt need as the growing number of visits indicates (See Table 13).

---

191 Isolation hospitals for quarantine purposes were also maintained by APOC. Williamson 1927, pp. 123–128; Šahnī 1374, pp. 320–321; Gilmour 1924, p. 39.

192 *Administration Report* 1919, p. 10.

193 The annual dispensary cost were 150 Rupees plus free medicines, *Administration Report* 1909, p. 38; *Administration Report* 1911, p. 67. For a discussion of the most common

Table 13: Number of Outpatients Treated at the Mohammerah Dispensary (1911–1925)

| Year | Outdoor patients |
|---|---|
| 1911 | 2,209 |
| 1912 | 3,395 |
| 1913 | 4,275 |
| 1921 | >5,500 |
| 1924 | >4,000 |
| 1925 | 3,800 |

Source: *Administration Report* 1913, p. 86; Ibid., 1921, p. 38; Ibid., 1924, p. 49; Ibid., 1925, p. 60. For the years between 1913 and 1924 the British reports only mention that the dispensary was "well attended." Ibid., 1914, p. 36; Ibid., 1916, p. 53; Ibid., 1918, p. 42; Ibid., 1919, p. 43; Ibid., 1920, p. 40; Ibid., 1923, p. 62.

Table 14: The Common Diseases Treated in the Mohammerah Dispensary (1911–1913)

| Disease/year | 1911 | 1912 | 1913 |
|---|---|---|---|
| All diseases | 2,909 | 3,395 | 4,275 |
| Malarial fever | 213 | 312 | 415 |
| Eye diseases | 430 | 491 | 618 |
| Skin diseases | 182 | 265 | 280 |
| Digestive system | 272 | 487 | 683 |
| Venereal | 212 | 220 | 307 |
| Total named diseases | 1,309 (45%) | 1,775 (52%) | 2,303 (54%) |

Source: *Administration Report* 1913, p. 86; see also Ibid., 1912, p. 65 ("Eye diseases are exceedingly common. 66 minor operations were performed.").

Given the rising demand for medical services, the establishment of a hospital had been proposed. This plan was put in jeopardy in 1913 when the medical officer left. The British consul commented, this "has been very unfortunate since not the least of the methods which we should employ to mark our predominance and to extend our influence is by the erection of a Hospital. It is to be trusted that His Majesty's Government will realise the importance of this point." He further noted that despite this set-back, the plans for a hospital were being submitted.[194] The enthusiasm for the hospital was tempered by the outbreak of WWI, for "Owing to the disturbed

diseases and their frequency as well as of the lack of hygiene in the town, see *Administration Report* 1912, p. 65.

194 *Administration Report* 1913, p. 86.

state of the country no progress was made with the proposal to build a hospital. The dispensary maintained by the Government continued to do good work staffed by Quarantine Medical officer."[195] In 1916, it is reported that the "Charitable Dispensary in the town continued to be well attended." This may have been partly due to an outbreak of cholera and plague during that year.[196] There also were British and Indian Convalescent Depots at Mohammerah since 1916. The Imperial Bank of Persia offered its accountant's house as a hospital, which the medical authorities accepted. As a result, this building began to be used as hospital on 1 July 1917 under the charge of Assistant Surgeon K. S. Dick, who was replaced by Civil Surgeon Captain T. H. Bishop, IMS on 11 September.[197] In 1918, the charitable dispensary continued to be well attended. There was an oubreak of the plague as well of the Spanish influenza from the beginning of October until the end of November, which resulted in a considerable loss of life among the population.[198] In 1924, the Charitable Dispensary treated over 4,000 outpatients, amongst which 40 cases of plague and 26 cases of cholera.[199] In 1925, it treated about 3,800 outpatients.[200] There is no further information available on this dispensary, but its function seems to have been taken over by the dispensary established by the APOC in Mohammerah.[201]

Ḥajj Ra'is al-Tujjār, C.I.E. (Commander Indian Empire), a leading merchant, had started to build a 20-bed hospital in Mohammerah in 1921 for the use of the local population, with adequate accomodation for the European and clerical staff of local firms in case of an emergency. Šayḫ Ḫazʿal (d. 1936), the ruler of Mohammerah, decided to make an endowment (*vaqf*) to the hospital "on a scale adequate for its needs." The hospital, which was named in his honor Aqdasiya, was formally opened by Sardār-i Aqdas (Šayḫ Ḫazʿal) on 8 January 1923. The APOC donated the entire equipment of the hospital.[202]

---

195 *Administration Report* 1914, p. 36.

196 Ass. Surgeon C.H. Lincoln was the quarantine officer, *Administration Report* 1916, p. 53.

197 *Administration Report* 1917, pp. 36, 37; *Administration Report* 1916, p. 52. The British convalescent depot was closed as per 1 December 1918, but the Indian one was continued. *Administration Report* 1918, p. 41. It was closed and moved to Basra in April 1919, *Administration Report* 1919, p. 43.

198 *Administration Report* 1918, p. 42. Captain Kirk, RAMC relieved Captain Bishop, IMS as civil surgeon, until November when Major Napier, IMS was appointed. Both also acted as assistant political officers. Ibid. p. 39. The dispensary continued to be well attended in 1919; in June-August some cases of the plague occurred. *Administration Report* 1919, p. 43; *Administration Report* 1920, p. 40; *Administration Report* 1922, p. 40.

199 *Administration Report* 1924, p. 49.

200 *Administration Report* 1925, p. 60.

201 Williamson 1927, p. 129.

202 *Administration Report* 1923, pp. 60–61, 62; Gilmour 1924, p. 30.

## Qazvin

In Qazvin, a town of some 40,000 inhabitants, the first hospital was established by the Russian Road Company, which maintained a small hospital for its staff. In 1923, when its assets had been transferred to the government of Iran, the Tehran municipality wanted to transfer all its equipment to Tehran, against which the population of Qazvin protested. Nevertheless, despite assurances to the contrary the transfer took place.[203] The Russian government had established an additional hospital in Qazvin at the beginning of World War I, when the Russian army transformed the Sipahdār mansion in Qazvin into a hospital. The Russian Orthodox Sisters of Compassion managed it till 1918 when the Russians left and handed it over to the British.[204] It would appear that the British had established a military hospital in Qazvin as well, which, by early 1919, was empty.[205] Also, there was an American missionary dispensary in Qazvin, established in 1905. It was situated in the center of the town, near the post-house and hotel. However, as of April 1918 it has been 'temporarily' closed due to lack of staff, but it was still closed in 1922.[206]

In 1917, at the initiative of Ḥājj Muḥammad 'Alī Amīnī the Amīnī Hospital (Marīż-ḫāna-yi Amīnī) had been built in Qazvin. It had 25–30 beds and a dispensary. For the operational cost Ḥājj Muḥammad Amīnī had endowed some villages to the hospital. It continued to function till 1927 when the endowment funds were insufficient to keep it operational and reconstruction had to be funded by the State.[207]

## Qom

As one would expect, there was a *dār al-šifā* attached to the shrine of Fāṭima in Qom, a town of about 30,000 inhabitants, which was visited

203 Varjāvand 1377, vol. 2, p. 1822.

204 Taymūrī 1363, pp. 269–271; Elgood 1951, p. 512; Varjāvand 1377, vol. 3, pp. 1818, 1822.

205 Griscom 1921, p. 239.

206 Wishard 1908, p. 80; Grothe 1911, p. 131; Funk 1920, p. 142; Richter 1910, p. 322; *One Hundred Seventeenth Annual Report of the Home Missions of the Presbyterian Church of the U.S.A.*, 1919, p. 260; *The Eighty-third Annual Report of the Board of Foreign Missions of the Presbyterian Church in the U.S.A.*, 1920, p. 314; Speer – Russell 1922, p. 348.

207 Varjāvand 1377, vol. 3, p. 1820. On the Marīż-ḫāna-yi Amīnī see Omid Rezai's article in this volume.

by Muẓaffar al-Dīn Šāh in 1903.[208] This may have been the same as the one built, or perhaps renewed, by Fatḥ ʿAlī Šāh (r. 1797–1834) north of the madrasa Fayżiya, for the use of travelers and the pilgrims of the shrine. The *šāh* had assigned the income of a village for the annual wages of a physician and surgeon, who had to treat ailing pilgrims and travelers. It is not known when, but later the hospital was transformed into a madrasa and dormitory for theological students, which, of course, was called *madrasa-yi dār al-šifā*.[209] At least in 1849, a hospital still existed at the shrine at Qom, when Abbott visited the shrine city and reported that: "A small annual allowance was formerly made from the revenues of the country for the maintenance of this establishment." Abbott continues, "but at present, beyond the accommodation afforded by the bare apartments, there is no provision for distress and sickness."[210] According to oral reports, there also existed a joint-stock hopital (*bīmāristān-i sihāmiya*) in Qom, probably as of the early 1920s, which had been established at the urgings of Āyat Allāh Šayḫ ʿAbd al-Karīm Ḥāʾirī.[211]

## Rasht

In 1902, Dr. and Mrs. Schuler had begun medical work in Rasht, a town of 25,000 inhabitants. Before that time the town was provided with medical services from Tehran. Permanent medical work began with the arrival of Dr. J. D. Frame in 1904; his dispensary was right in the center of the city.[212] In 1905, Prince Abū al-Fażl Mīrzā ʿAżud al-Sulṭān, the governor of Rasht (1321–23/1903–06), built a hospital in Rasht for which he had donated £1,800 from his own private funds. According to an article in a British journal, "The hospital is situated in a well-chosen and healthy locality. It contains seven wards, each to accommodate ten to fifteen patients. It has [a] consulting-room, [an] operating-room, and all appliances of a modern

208 *Rūznāma-yi sulṭānī va Īrān* 1380, p. 156 (11 *ramażān* 1321/1 December 1901).

209 Ṭabāṭabāʾī 2535, vol. 1, pp. 28–30; vol. 2, p. 140; Hidāyat 1339, vol. 10, p. 106. Whether in the same building or in a new one, but there still seems to have been a *dār al-šifā* in Qom at a later date. Rustāʾī 1382, vol. 2, p. 199.

210 Abbott 1855, p. 9.

211 Tadjbakhsh 1379, pp. 245–246.

212 ʿAyn al-Salṭana 1376, vol. 1, pp. 377, 865; Kumīsiyūn 1343, vol. 2, pp. 1449–1451; Elgood 1951, pp. 511–512, 534; Wishard 1908, p. 76; Waterfield 1973, p. 139; Richter 1910, p. 322.

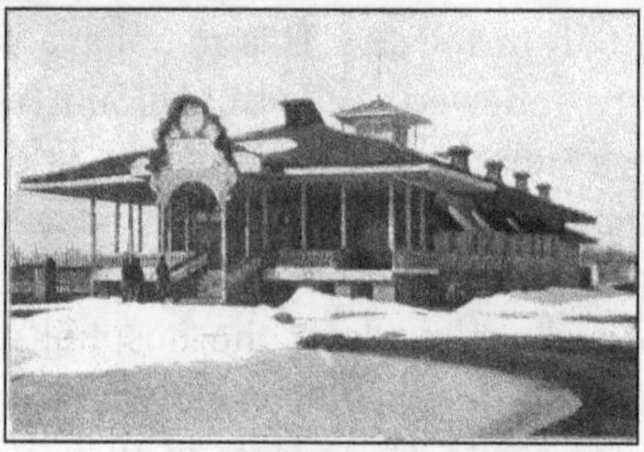

Figure 5. The hospital at Rasht. From "Royal philanthropy in Persia: A prince and his hospital", 1905, *The Graphic*, 7 October, p. 458.

hospital. The furniture for the place was brought from Russia."[213] ʿAżud al-Sulṭān wanted Dr. Frame to manage the hospital, but he did not like the arrangement and soon thereafter (most likely when the prince was no longer governor) started his own hospital. That hospital functioned until 1914 when work was discontinued until October 1918, when it was re-opened. However, it was in a different building than Dr. Frame had secured earlier. He did not have the means to open a proper hospital as yet and therefore, together with a few other physicians resident in Rasht he asked "about 100 gentlemen in the city to consider what could be done. Only a few responded." Due to this discouraging result, Dr. Frame had to close his dispensary in 1919, because he lacked funds. He then opened hospital with a capacity for 90 patients, which he had been able to do with dedicated funds that he received to that end from the American-Persian Commission. However, it was not a permanent solution, for he needed 2,000 *tūmāns* per year to maintain a 20-bed hospital. During the short Soviet occupation of Rasht in 1920 the Bolsheviks occupied the hospital. Dr. Frame allegedly built (or renovated?) a 31-bed hospital there in 1923, presumably in the Čirāġ-i Barq lane.[214]

213 "Royal philanthropy in Persia: a prince and his hospital", 1905, p. 458. Given the laudatory nature of the article it has all the trappings of an article commissioned by and ghost-written for the prince. There is no other report on the prince's hospital and it is not known to me to what other use it was put.

214 ʿAyn al-Salṭana 1376, vol. 1, pp. 377, 865; Kumīsiyūn 1343, vol. 2, pp. 1449–1451; Elgood 1951, pp. 511–512, 534; Wishard 1908, p. 76; Waterfield 1973, p. 139; Richter 1910, p. 322; *One Hundred Seventeenth Annual Report of the Home Missions of the Presbyterian Church of the U.S.A.*, 1919, p. 264; *The Eighty-third Annual Report of the Board of Foreign Missions of the Presbyterian Church in the U.S.A.*, 1920, pp. 314–316. As of 1921 Dr. Frame was assisted as matron nurse by a graduate from the girls' school; the assistant matron was a girl of 17. *The Eighty-fourth Annual Report of the Board of Foreign Missions of the Presbyterian Church in the U.S.A.*, 1921, p. 333.

## Sabzavar

In 1919 or thereabouts, at the initiative of Dr. Ġanī, a small hospital was constructed in Sabzavar, a town of some 15,000 people, which was financed by the local community.[215] No other information is available on its further development.

## Semnan

In or around 1885, the governor of Semnan, Anūšīrvān Mīrzā established a hospital (*marīż-ḫāna*) in that town, which had a population of some 20,000. It probably fell into disuse after the end of his governorship in early 1888, for in July 1901 the inhabitants of Semnan raised money and established a *dār al-šifā* with a pharmacy and engaged two physicians and one surgeon to provide gratis treatment and medicines for the poor and pilgrims. The total cost amounted to 700 *tūmāns*.[216] It is not known how long this institution lasted; it is not mentioned in local histories.

## Shiraz

The CMS hospital in Shiraz, which had a population of 30,000, was the last of its medical establishments. There had already been a CMS dispensary in Shiraz from 1900 until 1909, when it was closed due to a lack of staff.[217] Medical CMS work started again in 1922 when Dr. Carr, a missionary physician from Isfahan, opened a dispensary in Shiraz with the help of Dr. Emmeline Stuart and Alice Verinder, a British nurse, and a few local Christian nurses. They worked under difficult circumstances (cramped and crowded quarters, drugs in short supply), sometimes seeing 250 patients per morning. Initially a building in a garden had been rented, but in 1924 with a donation of land by Ḥājj Muḥammad Ḥusayn Namāzī a maternity hospital was built. It was subsequently converted into a large general

---

215 Ġanī 1367, vol. 1, pp. 190–191.

216 I'timād al-Salṭana 1306, p. 79; *Rūznāma-yi Īrān* 1378, p. 4020 (nr. 998, 12 *rabī' al-ṯānī* 1319/29 July 1901).

217 Grothe 1911, p. 131; Cash 1930, p. 54. Although Grothe called it a hospital, this was not the case, because Richter 1910, p. 330 explicitly states that it was intended to build a hospital, but it had not yet been completed, when he wrote his book.

hospital with financial assistance of the IETD. The hospital had male and female wards, a midwifery department plus an outpatient department.[218]

### Tabriz

According to Aubin, in about 1875 the American Presbyterian Missionary Society (APMS) established a 15-bed hospital with dispensary in Tabriz, which initially mainly served the Armenian population. However, other sources leave no doubt that missionary activity was started in 1873 (which Aubin misinterpreted to also mean missionary medical work), while it was only as of 1881 that Dr. G. W. Holmes began his medical work in Tabriz, and Dr. Mary Bradford, from 1888. Dr. Holmes was replaced in 1892 by Dr. William Vanneman who served there for the next 40 years. By 1896, there were two dispensaries (although Waterfield writes that it was a hospital as of 1893), one for men and one for women, with a separate receiving rooms for them. It was only in 1913 that Dr. Lamme established a hospital in Tabriz, which at that time had a population of 300,000.[219] In 1915 the APMS pioneered the formal training of a few nurses. Subsequently, in 1916 a three-year nursing school was established in Tabriz,[220] whose operation was interrupted by the departure of the American staff for Hamadan in June 1918 prior to the Turkish attack and occupation of Tabriz, during which period the Turks looted the American hospital. At that time, the staff of the Tabriz hospital consisted of Dr. Charles W. Lamme, who was the head of the so-called Colton Memorial hospital until May 1918, assisted by Dr. Edmund Dodd and Dr. Ms. Mary R. Fleming, who was in charge of the female section, known as the Whipple Memorial hospital. In reality these two were wings of the same hospital. Other medical staff included

[218] Elgood 1951, pp. 534–535; Waterfield 1973, p. 166; "Current Topics" 1924, p. 182; Williams 1994, pp. 60–61. The move in 1922 had been facilitated by the fact that the IETD had asked the CMS to take over the medical care of its employees, on generous terms, when its own physician retired. Waterfield 1973, pp. 165–166. According to Cash 1930, p. 54, describing the situation in 1928, "the hospital itself is a private house converted for the purpose. Every available corner of space has been utilized, but the congestion is terrible. However, a beginning has been made and the staff are bravely tackling the problems of extension." This means that the new hospital must have been built after 1928.

[219] Aubin 1908, p. 45; Wilson 1896, p. 259; Kumīsiyūn 1343, vol. 2, pp. 1449–1450; Waterfield 1973, p. 137. There also was a physician of the Russian road company working in Tabriz. Grothe 1911, p. 131.

[220] Salsali 1991, p. 190. It was operating again in 1920, if not earlier. *The Eighty-fourth Annual Report of the Board of Foreign Missions of the Presbyterian Church in the U.S.A.*, 1921, p. 344.

Dr. W. S. Vanneman and Ms. E. Jean Wells, a nurse. At that time they had all left Tabriz for Hamadan.[221] The APMS's work in Tabriz would only restart in 1919, when the looted hospital had to be restored under the leadership of Dr. E. M. Dodd, initially at a capacity of 20 beds. Bedding and other supplies were fortunately available in the bazaar, while the lack of instruments hampered the hospital in its work. The training class for nurses was also resumed.[222] The hospital was again closed when the missionaries fled Tabriz in November 1920, but they reopened it again in July 1921, after a thorough cleaning and repairs. Without the help of the Iranian army, which sold supplies to the hospital, it could not have been opened. As a result, a 30-bed hospital, with room for five babies, functioned again. The dispensary was open five days per week. Ms Wells was training four Iranian young women to become nurses, while three young Armenian young men worked as nurses in the men's ward. However, the lack of a female doctor was sorely felt, as Iranian women did not allow themselves to be examined by a male physician, even in their greatest need.[223]

There was a municipal hospital in Tabriz, which had been closed down, but by 1924 had been reopened. It had 30 beds, but no other details are available about its operations.[224] The American Adventists opened a dispensary in Tabriz in early 1925, which remained open till 1928. It was led by the Englishman Dr. H. E. Hargreaves.[225]

## Torbat-e Heydarieh

There were two small hospitals in Torbat-e Heydarieh, a town of 5,000 inhabitants. One established by the British, which was managed by the consular physician, the other by the Russians, who likewise had opened a small hospital under the Russian consular doctor. It is not known when these hospitals were established and how long these politically motivated

---

221 New York Times, "Outrage by Turks may presage war," 18 June 1918. The names of the hospitals are those of the families that made their construction financially possible; *One Hundred Seventeenth Annual Report of the Home Missions of the Presbyterian Church of the U.S.A.*, 1919, p. 276.

222 Speer 1920, p. 69; *The Eighty-third Annual Report of the Board of Foreign Missions of the Presbyterian Church in the U.S.A.*, 1920, p. 321–22; *The Eighty-fourth Annual Report of the Board of Foreign Missions of the Presbyterian Church in the U.S.A.*, 1921, p. 346.

223 *The Eighty-fifth Annual Report of the Board of Foreign Missions of the Presbyterian Church in the U.S.A.*, 1922, pp. 377–378.

224 Gilmour 1924, p. 29.

225 Sajjādī 1990, p. 261; Rühling 1934, p. 82.

establishments lasted.[226] The Russian hospital was the first to be established. The British Consul reported in January 1904 that the British hospital was not yet in proper working order, but patients were already lining up for its services in great numbers. "A large proportion seem to be patients who have tried the Russian cure and are now anxious to see if the English treatment is more successful. Special attention is paid to such cases, as, if they are treated successfully, it will at once raise the prestige of English methods."[227]

## Urmiyeh

Following the establishment of dispensary by Dr. A. Grant in 1835, the American missionaries continued to provide medical assistance at Urmiyeh. After Grant's death in 1844, the medical missionary work was assumed by several physicians, including Drs. T. L. van Orden (1866–73), Ms K. Cochran (1871–75), and G. W. Holmes (1874–77). In 1878, the latter was succeeded by Dr. Joseph Cochran, who constructed the so-called Westminster Hospital in 1883, where he also taught medicine. The 100-bed hospital was built in one year on a 15 hectare piece of land. There was a morgue and dissection room in the basement, while the upper floor had patient wards, two operating rooms, a pharmacy, and ten small isolation rooms. Because he worked alone at that time and needed more medical staff Dr. Cochran established a medical training school, a first for Iran. To that end he built a wooden building, which contained lecture rooms and a laboratory. This building still exists. Although he had to train the Iranian physicians himself, Dr. Cochran's clinical and teaching task was eased when Dr. Emma T. Miller arrived in 1892. General courses consisted of English and Persian, medical law and ethics. Basic medical sciences covered were physiology, anatomy, biochemistry and physics, and clinical sciences were pathology, contagious diseases and gynecology, while they also had to be knowledgeable in pharmacology. Students were required to attend the medical college for 9–10 months per year; however, the college was open the whole year round. Students would study several hours and

---

226 The British Consulate had one medical officer, while the Russian Consulate had two doctors, one of whom was stationed at Kariz. The main work of the Russian physicians was the enforcement of quarantine regulations. Grothe 1911, p. 131; Adamec 1981, vol. 2, pp. 653–654; Bricteux 1912, p. 192.

227 Tchalenko 2006, p. 47, see also pp. 54–55.

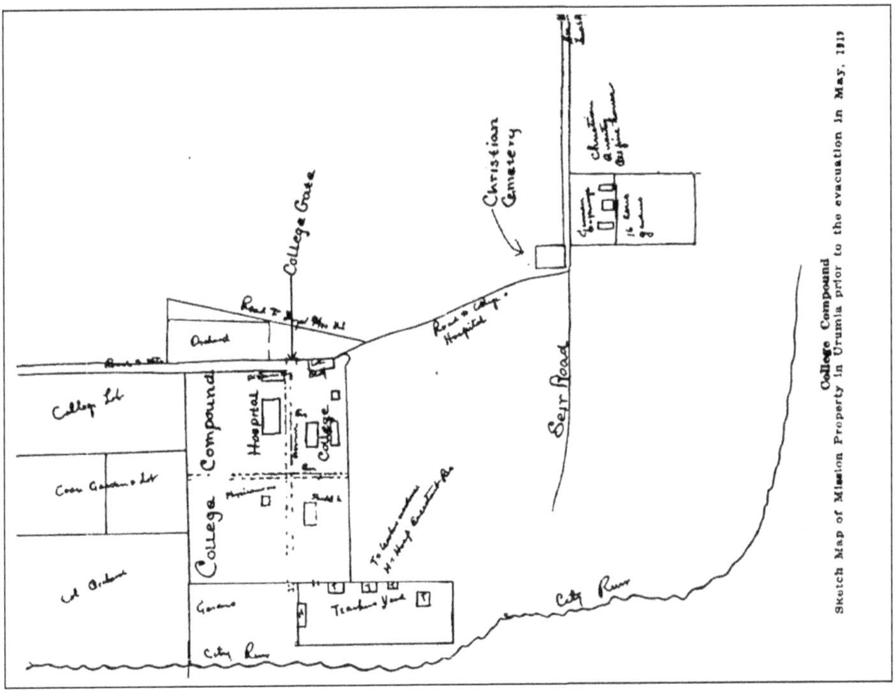


Map 2. A map of Urmiyeh indicating the location of the American missionary hospital. From *The Eighty-Third Annual Report of the Board of Foreign Missions of the Presbyterian Church in the U.S.A.*, New York, 1920, p. 328.

spend the rest of their time working in the hospital. The medical training school of Urmiyeh was active until 1905, when Dr. Cochran died. A total of 26 medical students had graduated at that time. The hospital included a female ward, the so-called Howard Annex (as of 1890), on one side of the hospital, and on the other side the dispensary, with rooms for medical students and assistants. Later, the so-called Lyman Memorial, a new operating room with a four-bed ward was added. Within the compound there also were residencies for the physicians. Its main building was 75 × 30 feet, two stories high, and accommodated up to 30 patients.[228] The hospital had an average of 300 inpatients, and performed operations, including those

---

228 Wilson 1896, pp. 74, 259; Kumīsiyūn 1343, vol. 2, p. 1449; *The Eighty-third Annual Report of the Board of Foreign Missions of the Presbyterian Church in the U.S.A.*, 1920, p. 237. On the training of Iranian physicians see Daniel 1901, pp. 207–209. For some time the Anglican mission also had a medical missionary in Urmiyeh in the 1890s, but he returned after a while. Richter 1910, pp. 310, 313.

on the eyes. In 1896 it had trained twelve Iranian physicians. The addition of a new operating room after 1906 made abdominal surgery possible, while 28 more beds were added to the hospital's capacity, both additions were made possible by the memorial to Dr. Cochran.[229] In 1904 the medical staff treated 12,754 patients of all creeds and ethnic groups.[230]

In 1910, when Urmiyeh had a population of some 20,000, there was a small Russian hospital, of which nothing else is known. It was not mentioned by Aubin who left an account of foreign activities in Urmiyeh in 1907, which suggest that it was established after that date.[231] After the occupation of Urmiyeh by Russian troops early in World War I, the Russian Consul Nikitine arranged for a sanitary team to visit and help to combat the cholera epidemic of 1915. The leader of that team, Dr. A. Kach, also set up a temporary hospital there. It was the only one sponsored by the Orthodox mission. It was discontinued when the Russian troops left in 1918.[232] After the war, the hospital could not be used, because it had been destroyed during the hostilities and medical services were carried out in two provisional buildings.

In the fall of 1917, a French military hospital to assist the Russians was established in Urmiyeh. This was abandoned by the staff in April 1918 and with them also left the French nuns who had been engaged in medical work. As a result the American Presbyterian Hospital was the only one in the town, for the Russian military hospital also had been abandoned with the withdrawal of the Russian troops.[233] Again, the American missionaries had left and their work had been wiped out by the war, while due to the prevailing insecurity in the area the missionaries did not return until after Riżā Ḫān had re-established central government control.[234]

---

229 Speer 1911, chapter 16; Wilson 1896, pp. 267, 275; *The Eighty-third Annual Report of the Board of Foreign Missions of the Presbyterian Church in the U.S.A.*, 1920, p. 237; http://www.ams.ac.ir/AIM/0252/0252127.htm.

230 Speer 1911, pp. 166, 270, 328–329.

231 Grothe 1911, p. 131.

232 Tamaddun 1350, pp. 243–244. Elsewhere in Iran, Russian military physicians and nurses also treated the local Iran population. Andreeva 2007, p. 191.

233 Shedd 1922, pp. 212, 246, 258, 273; Muʿtamid al-Vizāra 1379, pp. xxv, 9, 18–27, 74–75, 89–93, 99, 156; Coan 1939, 252, 260, 283; Hellot 1996; Ibid., 2002, pp. 340, 348; for an account of the French medical team in Urmiyeh by a participant see Zavie 1927.

234 Speer 1920, p. 69; *The Eighty-third Annual Report of the Board of Foreign Missions of the Presbyterian Church in the U.S.A.*, 1920, p. 327; *The Eighty-fourth Annual Report of the Board of Foreign Missions of the Presbyterian Church in the U.S.A.*, 1921, p. 340; *The Eighty-fifth Annual Report of the Board of Foreign Missions of the Presbyterian Church in the U.S.A.*, 1922, p. 374.

## YAZD

In 1892, Dr. and Mrs. White began medical missionary work in Yazd, a town of some 50,000 inhabitants. They first had a dispensary in the open air in a garden and then rented a house. The Whites were later joined by Dr. Urania Latham, who later married Napier Malcolm, and were assisted by Armenian orderlies. In 1899, the CMS opened a new maternity hospital in Yazd. In 1900, the Yazd CMS hospital treated 35,600 patients, some of who even came from Baluchistan and Afghanistan to seek treatment.[235] The buildings for the hospital were donated by a Zoroastrian merchant, Gūdarz Mihrbān, in the form of a caravanserai "and its property including a house that adjoined it. The structure of this erstwhile halting-place for caravans lent itself in a remarkable manner to the uses to which it was now to be put: the central court that was once filled with camels, asses, and pack-mules was turned into a pretty garden; and the old-time lodgings of the camel-drivers and muleteers were transformed into chambers

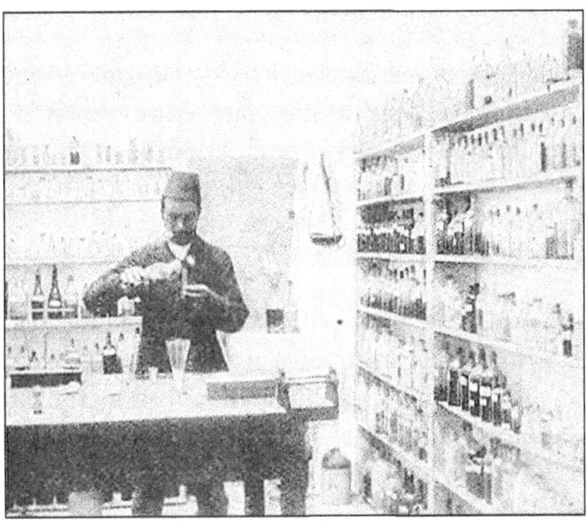

Figure 6. The CMS hospital of Yazd. From Stileman, 1902, *The Subjects of the Shah.* London, p. 74.

235 Stileman 1902, pp. 74–75; Wright 2001, pp. 188, 121; Afšār 1354, vol. 2, p. 803 (text of foundation plaque); Bricteux 1912, p. 235.

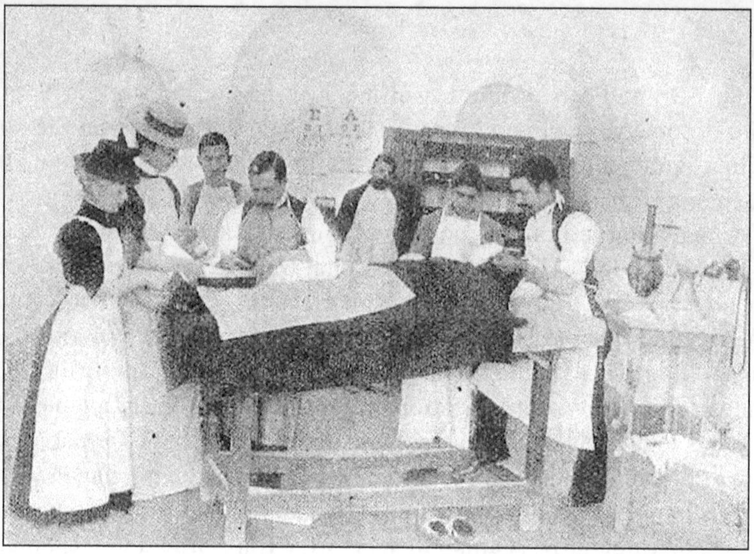

Figure 7. An operation at the CMS hospital of Yazd. From Stileman, 1902, *The Subjects of the Shah*. London, p. 75.

and wards for the Good Samaritan work."[236] In 1915 the hospital was closed when British subjects had to leave Iran, but it was reopened in 1916, when the political situation became less problematic.[237]

## Zabol

In 1921 when the American missionaries stationed in Mashhad fled the city, because it was feared that a Soviet invasion would take place, they went to Zabol and "cleaned up a dirty old building and turned it into a hospital," where every day they treated a large number of people. The missionaries

[236] Jackson 1909, p. 377; Stileman 1902, p. 74; Hume-Griffith 1909, p. 164. According to Richter 1910, p. 331, "for the erection of this [new] hospital (1907), Parsees in Yezd gave £200, and Muhammadans also made contributions." The hospital was later called Gūdarz hospital, to which later the Laal maternity hospital and nursing school were annexed.

[237] Waterfield 1973, p. 162. On the situation of the hospital of Yazd in 1928 see Cash 1930, p. 57.

stayed only for about six months, for when the Soviet threat proved to be unfounded they returned to Mashhad.[238]

## Conclusions

From the above it is clear that there did not exist a system of public health facilities such as hospitals or dispensaries in Iran prior to the 1850's. The few *dār al-šifā* that were to be found in a small number of cities did not really function as institutions that provided medical services. These traditional institutions mainly served poor and sick pilgrims and travelers; local inhabitants of the towns where these *dār al-šifā* were located usually looked for medical care elsewhere and preferred to die at home. The majority of the population, which was rural, also had no access to these hospitals even if they had wanted to. In case of illness they, therefore, relied on folk medicine that was available in a large variety of manifestations and probably was as effective as Galenic medicine that its practitioners offered at these hospitals. Moreover, physicians trained in Galenic medicine served urban areas, but their number was inadequate even for the cities in which they lived and they mainly served the rich. Formal sustained medical assistance to the poor (95% of the population), therefore, only became available to some extent, both geographically and numerically, through physicians who were attached to foreign Legations, foreign agencies (Indo-European Telegraph Department, Russian Red Cross, etc.), or missionaries (American and British). In addition, there were a few physicians attached to the royal court and some to provincial governors, who also had other paying private patients.[239] It was in particular the missionary physicians with their hospitals and dispensaries and the British charitable dispensaries in the Persian Gulf, who introduced the general population to quality medical care after 1880. They did so despite the many difficulties they had to overcome in their daily work, be they political, financial, social, staffing, linguistic, or the odd famine and/or epidemic outbreak.

---

238 The old building was that of the former Russian consulate, Miller 1989, pp. 60–64. According to *The Eighty-fourth Annual Report of the Board of Foreign Missions of the Presbyterian Church in the U.S.A.*, 1921, p. 337, these events took place in the second half of 1919.

239 I'timād al-Salṭana 1306, p. 390. By the end of the nineteenth century and the beginning of the twentieth century there were, e.g., the following French physicians: Dr. Coppin (Muẓaffar al-Dīn Mīrzā), Dr. Sorel (Ẓill al-Sulṭān), Dr. Broussière (Customs Service in the Persian Gulf), Dr. Bongrand (Nā'ib al-Salṭana) Dr. Roth (Šams al-Salṭana, Fars) and Dr. Ferte ('Ażud al-Sulṭān, Gilan), see Hassendorfer 1954, p. 61.

The first, although short-lived, European medical dispensary was established in Tehran by Dr. Salvatori, the physician of the French diplomatic Gardane mission in 1807–09.[240] It was the American Presbyterian Mission that established the first permanent dispensary in 1835 in Urmiyeh.[241] However, it was only towards the end of the nineteenth century that other dispensaries and hospitals were opened, often attached to foreign Legations and Consulates or by missionaries in Tehran, Bushire, Isfahan, Mashhad, Kerman, Urmiyeh and other towns. Also, a number of Iranian state, municipal, and private hospitals were established, as has been detailed above.

European doctors in Tehran not attached to missionary organizations only treated patients that could pay, with the exception of the British and Russian Legation doctors, who treated the poor free of charge.[242] However, it was the missionary hospitals that treated the largest number of patients, until the establishment of the APOC hospitals. The American missionaries, for example, had a total of about 188 beds by 1920 and treated more than 30,000 patients per year. They only charged money for drugs, if the patient was rich; the poor received both treatment and drugs free-of-charge.[243] It was not only Europeans who provided medical assistance. For example, the medical assistance provided to the poor in the various British consulates was in most cases carried out by Indian medical orderlies, assisting British physicians, while the missionaries were assisted by Iranian Christian physicians and nurses, whom they had trained themselves.[244] Although patients were treated free of charge at the mission hospitals and dispensaries, they nevertheless felt that the physicians also gained something, viz., an enhanced spiritual position because of having done a good deed or *ṯavāb*.[245] Rich Persian patients paid, of course, for

---

240 Elgood 1951, p. 441.

241 Elgood 1951, pp. 533–535.

242 Serena 1883, p. 142; Collins 1896, p. 276; Andreeva 2007, p. 193.

243 'Ayn al-Salṭana 1376, vol. 1, pp. 377, 865; Kumīsiyūn 1343, vol. 2, p. 1451; Elgood 1951, pp. 511–512, 534; *One Hundred Seventeenth Annual Report of the Home Missions of the Presbyterian Church of the U.S.A.*, 1919, pp. 270, 280; *The Eighty-third Annual Report of the Board of Foreign Missions of the Presbyterian Church in the U.S.A.*, 1920, pp. 321, 332, 327; *The Eighty-fifth Annual Report of the Board of Foreign Missions of the Presbyterian Church in the U.S.A.*, 1922, pp. 372, 378.

244 Wright 2001, p. 118. Mrs. Rice writes, "During the war, when Europeans had to leave Persia, the Armenian helpers, both nurses and teachers, courageously carried on the work as well as they could." Linton *et al.* 1921, p. 16, note. For similar laudatory observations about the contribution made by the local medical staff see Wood 1922, pp. 60–61; Cash 1930, p. 31. For the training of nurses as of 1936 see Setzler 1941, pp. 520–525.

245 Malcolm 1911, p. 55.

their medical service and medicines: "In fact, what might be called the private practice of the doctors largely pays for the upkeep of the hospitals, with their thousands of patients."[246] Moreover, the rich also contributed in another way—the construction of many of the mission hospitals and schools had been made possible by the largesse of Persian merchants and other wealthy individuals, both Muslim and non-Muslim.[247]

The Indo-European Telegraph Department (IETD), which was established in 1865, employed a number of physicians, who also operated some dispensaries for the poor. Of course, the main task of these physicians was to keep IETD staff healthy. Some telegraph station managers also provided help.[248] The quarantine stations operated by the British government in the Persian Gulf and by the Russian government at the northern border on behalf of the government of Iran also provided medical assistance to the local population, in particular the poor.[249] However, this only happened when there was no room in the consulate or a dedicated dispensary.

In 1920 in Iran, the situation of foreign hospitals and dispensary activities is represented in Table 15. The number of foreign hospitals was reduced after World War I. Due to the Russian Revolution all Russian hospitals were closed, while the French missionary service, run by the *Filles de la charité*, interrupted its medical operations. While German medical staff did not return, this loss was more than offset by the vastly increased number of Russian and Armenian physicians in the North.[250] After the Great War the British CMS continued its operations in four locations where it had one hospital each,[251] while the American Presbyterian Missionary Society operated seven hospitals by 1920. A new operator was the APOC, which opened a number of new hospitals and dispensaries as of 1914.

---

246 Rice 1916, p. 134. This was not always the case, for Dr. Burlie at Bandar 'Abbas said about his well-to-do patients: "The Persian gentleman's or lady's idea seems to be that if you get well it is the hand of God and so *Shukr Allah*!—thanks be to God. If you don't improve it is the fault of the Doctor-then why pay?", Cursetjee 2001, p. 44.

247 Linton 1923, p. 73; Rice 1916, pp. 133–134; Stuart n.d., p. 19.

248 Wright 2001, p. 126; Rubin 1999, pp. 295–299; Collins 1896, p. 109; see also pp. 162, 276.

249 Sadīd al-Salṭana 1342, p. 169.

250 According to Schmidel n.d., pp. 137, 164 there were thousands of Russian physicians in Iran in the early 1920s who, because there were too many of them, eked out a subsistence living.

251 See also Rice 1923, pp. 261–262 as to the equipment of the CMS hospitals. The CMS also operated a dispensary in Shahr-e Kord from 1920–1923; see Amīr Ḥusaynī 1357, p. 47.

Table 15: Foreign Hospitals and Private Modern Physicians in Iran in 1920

| Nationality | Type of organization | Location | Type of service | Staff |
|---|---|---|---|---|
| American | Presbyterian Mission | Urmiyeh, Tabriz, Rasht, Tehran, Mashhad, Hamadan; Kermanshah; Qazvin+ | Hospital (plus apothecary): Mashhad (50 beds); Tehran (45 beds); Rasht (5 beds); Hamadan (25 beds); Kermanshah (25 beds); Tabriz (100 beds); Urmiyeh (40 beds); + = dispensary | 11 physicians of whom two female |
| British | British Government | Tehran+, Mashhad, Torbat-e Heydarieh, Naserabad+, Bushire, Kermanshah, Lengeh+, Mohammerah +, Ahvaz | Small hospitals; + = dispensary | At least 10 of whom two female |
| | Church Missionary Society | Isfahan, Kerman, Yazd, Shiraz | Isfahan 180 beds (120 for men and 60 for women) Kerman 80 beds (60 for men and 20 for women) Yazd 80 beds (60 for men and 20 for women); Shiraz 50 beds (new hospital under construction in 1924) | At least 6, of whom two female |
| | APOC | Abadan, Masjed-i Soleyman, Ahvaz, Mohammerah+ | The most modern hospitals in the Middle East; + = dispensary; >200 beds | >20 |
| Russian (until 1918) | Red Cross; Government | Tehran; Mashhad, Torbat-e Heydarieh; Tabriz; Urmiyeh | Small hospital | At least four |
| German (until 1915) | Government | Tehran, Tabriz, Barfurush, Rasht, Hamadan, Senneh, Kermanshah | Legation physician and one that directed the government hospital in Tehran. In the other towns are German apothecaries | Two |
| French | Filles de la charité | Khosrova | Small 8-bed hospital at Khosrova | A Nestorian doctor trained in France |

Source: Grothe 1911, pp. 131–132; Aubin 1908, p. 71; Gilmour 1924, p. 30.

Table 16: Modern Iranian Hospitals and Their Capacity in 1920

| Town | Beds | Remarks | Nature of ownership |
|---|---|---|---|
| Tehran | 172 (civil) 200 (army) | dispensary + pharmacy | State (3), municipal (1), army (2) |
| Enzeli | 10 male + 5 female | dispensary + pharmacy | Municipal |
| Tabriz | 30 | – | Municipal |
| Hamadan | 12 | Only outpatients | Municipal |
| Mashhad | (i) 70; (ii) 20 | – | Two Foundations (i) + (ii) |
| Qazvin | 25–30 | + dispensary | Amini endowment |
| Mohammerah | 20 | – | Šeyḫ Ḫazʿal |
| Malayer | 10 | – | Foundation |
| Sabzavar | ? | – | Built with locally raised funds |

Source: Gilmour 1924, pp. 29–30; q.v. Qazvin and Sabzavar.

The number of modern Iranian hospitals grew especially after 1905, with the largest concentration in Tehran, both in number and size. At first, doctors of foreign legations were looked on with suspicion. But the hostile attitude changed over time. First and foremost there were many Iranian doctors and many mullahs who opposed foreign medical aid. The first because they feared competition, the second because they saw medical aid (especially missionary medical aid) as an instrument aiming to establish foreign domination over Iran and replace Islam with Christianity, an attitude that is still found in writings of Iranian scholars or authors of to-day. Mullahs, therefore, "expressed surprise that Christians should look after patients who could not pay,"[252] for this was further proof of their suspicions about the ulterior motives of these European physicians. Not only were the competitors for people's body and soul wary of the gifts borne by European physicians, so were many of the poor and terribly sick patients. Despite the long presence of the American mission in Christian Urmiyeh in the town itself the Jewish and Muslim communities in 1892 were still "very conservative and wish no European help."[253] These sentiments were reinforced, in the case of Muslims, by their deep-seated conviction

252 Rice 1916, p. 89.

253 Speer 1911, pp. 166, 270, 328–329. It was difficult for women to come and seek help, for their men said: "she's only a woman," and many had "to steal away from their homes to go to the hospital during the absence of their husbands." *The Eighty-fourth Annual Report of the Board of Foreign Missions of the Presbyterian Church in the U.S.A.*, 1921, p. 338.

that non-Muslims were ritually unclean, and therefore, had to force themselves to be touched and swallow medicines prepared by a Christian physician.[254] The same kind of reaction was present in towns such as Yazd and Kerman.[255]

However, initial stand-offishness if not hostility soon turned into acceptance and appreciation. There were still problems such as in 1908, when rumors were spread that operations were carried out in the hospital in Kerman that should not be done. A high-placed British individual even lent credence to these rumors and sent "a vindictive report" to London and, as a result, the CMS considered closing down the Kerman hospital. When the town's people learnt about the pending closure in the autumn of 1907 a letter was written and signed by all the *mujtahids* or leading mullahs, with 700 seals of merchants and townsfolk affixed. The CMS then decided to continue its Kerman operation.[256] Dr. Emmeline Stuart, who elaborated on the initial difficulties to overcome Muslim prejudice with regards to the Christian doctors, wrote around 1923, "No longer have we the same prejudices to contend with. No longer is the *istikhareh*, or omen, indispensable before patients submit to the treatment. It is now as a rule, only consulted by the more bigoted Moslems, or by those who do not really want to come into hospital, or who are afraid to undergo an operation."[257] When Dr. Dodson died of typhoid fever, while caring for his patients in Kerman in 1937, "The Governor of the town, all the officials, and fifteen thousand people lined the narrow streets and went to the bare graveyard in the desert outside the town to do honour to the man who had served them for thirty-four years."[258]

Other beliefs that interfered with effective treatment were ritualistic in nature. The dispensaries and hospitals were almost empty during Ramadan, because the taking of medicine, or the use of drops into the eye, was tantamount to breaking fast. European doctors, therefore, had to be aware to tell the few patients that showed up to take their medicine twice a night instead of twice a day. Also, after Ramadan the dispensaries were

---

254 Richter 1910, p. 321.

255 Malcolm 1905, pp. 55–59; A Friend of Iran 1940, pp. 20–21; Hume-Griffith 1909, pp. 157–161.

256 A Friend of Iran 1940, pp. 52–55.

257 Stuart n.d., p. 23.

258 A Friend of Iran 1940, p. 73.

full of patients who had overeaten at night after having eaten nothing during the day.[259]

The goodwill that was created by this kind of medical assistance was so impressive that a commercial commission sent by the Government of India to Persia in 1904 remarked: "In my journey through Persia I have noticed the very great influence that a medical man possesses, and the good that he does; the appointment of a medical officer, with Hospital Assistants, at all head-quarters is desirable, and I would further suggest that the Consular Agents at Sirjan, Rafsanjan and Bampore be selected from the subordinate medical staff, and have dispensaries at these stations."[260] Similar sentiments were expressed by British Consuls in Lengeh and Ahvaz, who for that reason, wanted to separate the dispensary from the quarantine stations so that the British government and nobody else would get the patients' gratitude, while it was expected to also stimulate British trade. It therefore comes as no surprise that those Iranians who were already suspicious of foreign assistance found vindication for their strongly held feelings in these and similar observations.

The Mission Hospitals and dispensaries as well as the British government charitable dispensaries and Civil Hospitals treated tens of thousands of patients every year a number that by 1925 had grown to more than 350,000 per year, many of whom were repeat visitors, not new patients.[261] The missionary physicians trained native physicians and nurses and also provided education in hygiene.[262] For both at home, in their towns, and in their villages, people lived in an environment that was a breeding place for all kinds of endemic and contagious diseases, the main cause for the many diseases with which people were afflicted. Therefore, "the utter lack of cleanliness" was the main problem, coupled with the need to overcome "the ignorance and prejudices of the people," according to the medical staff in Mohammerah.[263] It was a refrain repeated by their colleagues in Bandar

259 Malcolm 1911, p. 49.

260 Gleadowe-Newcomen 1904, p. 19. In the mid-1830s the British envoy to Iran, Sir John Campbell had made the same argument, but his advice was not heeded. Elgood 1951, p. 472. The Russians also noted the benefit of good-will due to medical assistance. Andreeva 2007, p. 193. In 1904–05, Sykes reported that "During the Mohurram riots it was understood that the British Consulate-General was held invioble by the people on account of the great boon conferred on the population of Khorasan by the work of this [British] hospital", Sykes 1905, p. 22.

261 In 1907 the American hospitals treated 30,000 patients. Grothe 1911, p. 131, while the CSM in Yazd alone did more than 30,000; otherwise see entries per town above.

262 Wilson 1895, p. 310.

263 *Administration Report* 1912, p. 65; Wilson 1932, p. 98.

'Abbas, where it was observed that the inhabitants practiced no sanitation whatsoever. "Advice given on the dangers of these conditions receive a deaf ear."[264] In Urmiyeh the missionary medical staff also tried to teach patients about the importance of hygiene and sanitation, and made an effort to improve the medical knowledge of Galenic physicians and also consulted them to arrive at better medical treatments.[265] People were more susceptible to notions of prevention when it was too late (when there was already another cholera epidemic) and invariably only for as long as the epidemic lasted. There was little preventive follow-up by either the government or the population at large.[266] The APOC made the most concerted sanitation effort in that area, as good public health was vital for its operations and its ability to attract workers. It had special staff to inspect and enforce public health measures; in fact, it performed many functions (such as inspecting the sale of meat and vegetables) that should have been carried out by the government of Iran.[267] A similar concerted effort was made by the British government, on behalf of the government of Iran from 1849 until 1928, by enforcing quarantine rules in the Persian Gulf through five stations to check the spread of epidemics. The costs were borne by the Iranian government. However, the hospitals and its physicians were mainly treating symptoms rather than the underlying causes of the diseases that gave rise to them.

In Iran in 1924, there existed some 35 hospitals with more than 1,400 beds, 40 or more dispensaries, ten quarantine stations,[268] and 945 officially authorized physicians (both foreign and Iranian, of whom 323 practiced in Tehran). Of course, there was insufficient capacity to address the health needs of the 10 million inhabitants of Iran let alone preventing or reducing the prevalence of endemic and contagious diseases. But it was a beginning. However, as in Europe, the incidence and prevalence of most common diseases in Iran was spectacularly and most significantly reduced not by hospitals, but by the spread of sanitation and personal hygiene through

---

264 *Administration Report* 1922, pp. 19–20; *Administration Report* 1921, p. 20; *Administration Report* 1923, p. 36.

265 Wilson 1896, p. 275.

266 See for the panic reaction to a cholera epidemic by the population and the temporary positive reaction to "what to do" pamphlets, for example, Wishard 1908, pp. 220–221.

267 Williamson 1927, pp. 133–138 and Gilmour 1924, p. 29, both give an overview of the types of measures taken. For the towns that had an Iranian public health physician see Gilmour 1924, pp. 24–25 (map).

268 This number also includes the quarantine stations on the Caspian Sea (Enzeli, Mashhad-e Sar) and on the border with the Ottoman Empire (Kermanshah, Qasr-e Shirin) and Russia (Astara, Jolfa). Gilmour 1924, pp. 21–26. Torbat-e Heydarieh (q.v. above) should also be listed among the quarantine stations.

public (uncontaminated water supply; effective sewage and drainage system, etc.) and personal (clean clothes, bedding and homes, washing hands, etc.) policy, practice, and actions after 1950. Neither the traditional *dār al-šifā*, nor the modern hospitals could really solve that problem.

## Bibliography


### A. *Documents and Reports*

Adamec, Ludwig, ed., 1981, *Historical Gazetteer of Iran*, 4 vols., Graz, Akademie.
*Administration Report* = *Administration Report on the Persian Gulf Political Residency for the year (1898–99 to 1925) in Government of India. The Persian Gulf Administration Reports 1873–1947*, 10 vols., Gerrards Cross, Archives Editions, 1986.
Āṣaf al-Dawla, Mīrzā ʿAbd al-Vahhāb Ḫān, 1377/1998, *Asnād*, 2 vols., ʿAbd al-Ḥusayn Navāʾī – Nīlūfar Kasrī, eds., Tehran, Muʾassisa-yi Muṭālaʿāt-i Tārīḫ-i Muʿāṣir-i Īrān.
*DCR* = *Diplomatic and Consular Reports*, Government of Great Britain, Parliamentary Papers:

(a) Miscellaneous Series *DCR* no. 590, "Report on the Trade and General Condition of the City and Province of Kermanshah by Mr. H. L. Rabino", pp. 1–75.
(b) Annual Series: *DCR* no. 4828, "Report from March 21, 1909 to March 20, 1911 on the Trade of the Persian Caspian Provinces by Mr. H. L. Rabino", pp. 1–34.
DCR 3189, "Trade of Kermanshah and District for the year 1903–04 by Mr. H. L Rabino", pp. 1–46.

Gilmour, John, 1924, *Rapport sur la situation sanitaire de la Perse*. Geneva, League of Nations.
Gleadowe-Newcomen, 1904, *Report of a commercial mission to Persia*. Calcutta.
Government of Iran, 1373/1994, *Rūznāma-yi vaqāʾiʿ-yi ittifāqiya*, 4 vols., Tehran.
Lorimer, J. G., 1970, *Gazetteer of the Persian Gulf*. Westmead, Gregg International (Calcutta 1915).
*One Hundred Seventeenth Annual Report of the Home Missions of the Presbyterian Church of the USA*. New York, Presbyterian Church, 1919.
*Report 1920–21* = *The Persian Gulf Trade Reports 1905–1940. Bushire*, 2 vols., Gerrards Cross, Archive Editions, 1987.
Sykes, Major P. Molesworth, 1905, "Report on the Trade of Khorassan for the Year 1904–05". *Diplomatic and Consular Report no. 3499 Annual Series*. London, HMSO.
*The Eighty-third Annual Report of the Board of Foreign Missions of the Presbyterian Church in the U.S.A.* New York, Presbyterian Church, 1920.
*The Eighty-fourth Annual Report of the Board of Foreign Missions of the Presbyterian Church in the U.S.A.* New York, Presbyterian Church, 1921.
*The Eighty-fifth Annual Report of the Board of Foreign Missions of the Presbyterian Church in the U.S.A.* New York, Presbyterian Church, 1922.

### B. *Persian Sources*

Ādamiyat, Faraydūn, 1348 h. š./1969–70, *Amīr Kabīr va Īrān*. Tehran, Ḫvārazm.
Afšār, Īraj, 1354 h. š./1975–6, *Yādgārhā-yi Yazd*, 2 vols., Tehran, Anjuman-i Āṯār-i Millī.
——, 1371 h. š./1992–3, *Ganjīna-yi ʿakshā-yi Īrān*. Tehran, Farhang.
Afżal al-Mulk, Ġulām Ḥusayn, 1361 h. š./1982–3, *Afżal al-tavārīḫ*, Ittiḥādiya Manṣūra – Sīrūs Saʿdvandiyān, eds., Tehran, Tārīḫ.
Amīr Ḥusaynī, Karīm Nīkzād, 1357 h. š./1378–9, *Šināḫt-i sarzamīn-i čār maḥāll*, Isfahan.

Āṣaf, Muḥammad Hāšim (Rustam al-Ḥukamā), 1348 h. š./1969–70, *Rustam al-tavārīḫ*, Muḥammad Mušīrī, ed., Tehran.

ʿAttārdī, ʿAzīz Allāh, 1371 h. š./1992–3, *Tārīḫ-i Astān-i Quds-i Rażavī*, 2 vols., Tehran, Vizārat-i Farhang.

ʿAyn al-Salṭana, Qahramān Mīrzā Sālūr, 1376 h. š./1997–8, *Rūznāma-yi ḫāṭirāt*, 10 vols., Masʿūd Sālūr – Īraj Afšār, eds., Tehran, Asāṭīr.

Bāfqī, Muḥammad Mufīd Mustawfī, 1340 h. š./1961–2, *Jāmiʿ-i Mufīdī*, 3 vols., Īraj Afšār, ed., Tehran.

Bāmdād, Mahdī, 1347 h. š./1968–9, *Šarḥ-i ḥāl-i rijāl-i Īrān dar qurūn-i davāzdahum va sizdahum va čahārdahum hijrī*, 6 vols., Tehran, Zavvār.

Dihgān, Ibrāhim, 1329 h. š./1950–1, *Tārīḫ-i Arāk*, 2 vols., Arak.

Farīd al-Mulk Hamadānī, Mīrzā Muḥammad ʿAlī Ḫān, 1345 h. š./1966–7, *Ḫāṭirāt-i Farīd*, Masʿūd Farīd Qarāguzlū, ed., Tehran, Zavvār.

Fasāʾī, Ḥājj Mīrzā Ḥasan Ḥusaynī, 1367 h. š./1988–9, *Fārsnāma-yi Nāṣirī*, 2 vols., Manṣūr Rāstigar Fasāʾī, ed., Tehran, Amīr Kabīr.

Furṣat-i Šīrāzī, Muḥammad Nāṣir, 1312 h. q./1894–5, *Āṯhār-i ʿAjam*, Bombay, lithograph.

Ġanī, Qāsim, 1367 h. š./1988–9, *Yāddāšthā-yi duktur Qāsim Ġanī*, 9 vols., Sīrūs Ġanī, ed., Tehran, Zavvār.

Ḥakīm al-Mamālik, ʿAlī Naqī ibn Ismaʿīl, 1356 h. š./1977–8, *Rūznāma-yi safar-i Ḫurāsān*. Tehran, Farhang-i Īrān-Zamīn.

Hamadānī, Āyat Allah Ṣabirī, 1382 h. š./2003–4, *Tārīḫ-i mufaṣṣal-i Hamadān*, 3 vols., Qom, Šākir.

Hidāyat, Rižā Qulī Ḫān, 1339 h. š./1960–1, *Tārīḫ-i rawżat al-ṣafā-yi Nāṣirī*, 10 vols., Tehran, Ḫayyām.

Išrāqī, Fīrūz, 1383 h. š./2004–5, *Golpaygān dar āʾīna-yi tārīḫ*. Isfahan, Čahār Bāġ.

Iʿtimād al-Salṭana (Ṣanīʿ al-Dawla), Muḥammad Ḥasan Ḫān, 1294–97 h. q./1877–80, *Mirʾat al-buldān*, 4 vols., Tehran, lithograph.

——, 1300 h. q./1882–3, *Muntaẓam-i Nāṣirī*, 3 vols., Tehran, lithograph.

——, 1301–03 h. q./1883–86, *Maṭlaʿ al-šams*. Tehran, lithograph.

——, 1306 h. q./1888–9, *Kitāb al-maʾāṯir va al-āṯār*. Tehran, lithograph.

——, 1345 h. š./1967–8, *Rūznāma-yi ḫāṭirāt*, Īraj Afšār, ed., Tehran, Amīr Kabīr.

Jābarī-Anṣārī, Ḥājj Mīrzā Ḥasan Ḫān, 1373 h. š./1994–5, *Tārīḫ-i Iṣfahān*. Isfahan.

Jurjānī, Ismaʿīl ibn Ḥasan, 2535/1976–7, *Ḏaḫīra-yi Ḫvārazmšāhī*, Saʿīdī Sīrjānī, ed., Tehran, Bunyād-i Farhang-i Millī.

Kumīsiyūn = Kumīsiyūn-i Millī-i Yūniskū-yi Īrān, 1343 h. š./1964–5. *Īrānšāhr*, 22, Tehran.

Munšī, Iskandar Beg, 1350 h. š./1971–2, *Tārīḫ-i ʿālamārā-yi ʿAbbāsī*, 2 vols., Īraj Afšār, ed., Tehran; English translation: *History of Shah ʿAbbas the Great*, 2 vols., R. M. Savory, trad., Boulder, 1978.

Musṭafavī, Muḥammad Taqī, 1343 h. š./1964–5, *Iqlīm-i Pārs*. Tehran, Anjuman-i Āṯār-i Millī.

Muʾtaman, ʿAlī, 1348 h. š./1969–70, *Rāhnamā yā tārīḫ va tawṣīf-i darbār-i vilāyatmadār-i rażavī*. Tehran.

Muʿtamid al-Vizāra, Raḥmat Allah Ḫān, 1379 h. š./2000–1, *Ūrūmiya dar muḥāraba-yi ʿālamsūz*, Kāvih Bayāt, ed., Tehran.

Muʿtamadī, Muḥsin, 1381 h. š./2002–3, *Juġrāfiyā-yi tārīḫī-i Tehrān*. Tehran, Dānišgāhī.

Nafīsī, Saʿīd, 1325 h. š./1946–7, "Duktur ʿAlī Akbar Nafīsī Nāẓim al-Aṭibbā". *Yādgār* 3/4, pp. 52–65.

——, 1329–31 h. š./1950–53, "Tāriḫ-i bīmāristānhā-yi Īrān". *Majalla-yi Šīr-u ḫuršīd-i surḫ-i Īrān*, 3/9–10, pp. 12–23.

Naḫjavānī, Muḥammad ibn Hindūšāh, 1964, *Dastūr al-kātib fī taʿyīn al-marātib*, 2 vols. in 3 parts, A. ʿAlī-Zada, ed., Moscow, Nauka.

Nasīrī, Muḥammad Ibrāhīm ibn Zayn al-ʿĀbidīn, 1373 h. š./1994–5, *Dastūr-i šahriyār*, Muḥammad Nādir Nasīrī Muqaddam, ed., Tehran.

Naṣrābādī, Mīrzā Muḥammad Ṭāhir, 1361 h. š./1982–3, *Taḏkira-yi Naṣrābādī*, Vaḥīd Dastgirdī, ed., Tehran.

Rustā'ī, Muḥsin, 1382 h. š./2003–4, *Tārīḫ-i ṭibb va ṭibābat dar Īrān*, 2 vols., Tehran, Sāzmān-i Asnād.
*Rūznāma-yi Īrān*, 1374–78 h. š./1995–99, 5 vols., Tehran, Kitābḫāna-yi Millī.
*Rūznāma-yi sulṭānī va Īrān*, 1380 h. š./2001–2, Tehran, Kitābḫāna-yi Millī.
Sadīd al-Salṭana, Muḥammad 'Alī, 1342 h. š./1963–4, *Bandar 'Abbās va Ḫalīj-i Fārs*, 2 vols. in one, Aḥmad Iqtidārī, ed., Tehran, Amīr Kabīr.
Sa'dvandiyān, Sīrūs – Ittiḥādiya (Niẓām-Māfī), Manṣūra, 1368 h. š./1989–90, *Āmār-i Dār al-ḫilāfa*. Tehran, Našr-i Tārīḫ.
Ṣafarī, Bābā, 1350–62 h. š./1971–83, *Ardabīl dar guḏargāh-i tārīḫ*, 3 vols., Tehran.
Sayyāḥ, Ḥājj, 1347 h. š./1968–9, *Ḫāṭirāt-i Ḥājj Sayyāḥ ya dawra-yi ḫawf-u vaḥšat*, Hamīd Sayyāḥ, ed., Tehran, Ibn Sīnā.
Sipihr, 'Abd al-Ḥusayn, 1368 h. š./1989–90, *Mir'at al-vaqā'i'-yi muẓaffarī va yāddāšthā-yi malik al-muvarriḫīn*, 'Abd al-Ḥusayn Navā'ī, ed., Tehran, Zarrīn.
Sipihr, Muḥammad Taqī Lisān al-Mulk, 1377 h. š./1998–9, *Nāsiḫ al-tavārīḫ*, 3 vols., Jamšīd Kayānfar, ed., Tehran, Asāṭīr.
Šahnī, Dāniš 'Abbāsī, 1374 h. š./1995–6, *Tārīḫ-i Masjid-i Sulaymān*. Tehran, Hīrmand.
Šahrī, Ja'far. 1368 h. š./1989–90, *Tarīḫ-i ijtimā'ī-i Tihrān dar qarn-i sīzdahum*, 6 vols., Tehran, Farhang-Rasā.
Sutūda, Manūčihr, ed., 1366 h. š./1987–9, *Az Astārā ta Astārābād*, 10 vols., Tehran, Anjuman-i Āṯār va Mafāḫir-i Farhang.
Sulṭānī, Muḥammad 'Alī, 1370 h. š./1991–2, *Juġrāfiyā-yi tārīḫī va tārīḫ-i mufaṣṣal-i Kirmānšāhān*, 3 vols., Tehran.
Šūštarī, Mīr 'Abd al-Laṭīf Ḫān, 1363 h. š./1984–5, *Tuḥfat al-'ālam va ḏayl al-tuḥfa*, Ṣamad Muvaḥḥid, ed., Tehran.
Ṭabāṭabā'ī, Mudarrisī Ḥusayn, 2535/1976–7, *Turbat-i pākān*, 2 vols., Qom.
Tabrīzī, Rižā Vakīlī Ṭabāṭabā'ī Ḥājj Mīrzā Rižā Ḫān, 1345–46 h. š./1966–67, "Tārīḫ-i 'Araq (Arāk)", Manūčihr Sutūda, ed., *Īrān Farhang-Zamīn*, 14, pp. 362–460.
Tadjbakhsh, Hasan, 1379 h. š./2000–1, *Tārīḫ-i bīmāristānhā-yi Īrān*. Tehran, Pažūhišgāh-i 'ulūm-i insānī va muṭāla'āt-i farhangī.
Tamaddun, Muḥammad, 1350 h. š./1971–2, *Awzā'-yi Īrān dar jang-i avval ya tārīḫ-i Rižāya*. Tehran.
Ṭavīlī, 'Azīz, 1371 h. š./1992–3, *Tārīḫ-i jāmi'-i Bandar-i Anzalī*, 2 vols., Rasht.
Taymūrī, Ibrāhīm, 1363 h. š./1984–5, *'Aṣr-i bīḫabarī*. Tehran.
Varjāvand, Parvīz, 1377 h. š./1998–9, *Sīmā-yi tārīḫ va farhang-i Qazvīn*, 3 vols., Tehran, Našr-i nay.
Ẓahīr al-Dawla, 1351/1972, *Ḫāṭirāt va Asnād-i Ẓahīr al-Dawla*, Īraj Afšār, ed., Tehran.

### C. *European Language Sources*

Abbott, Keith Edward, 1855, "Geographical Notes taken during a Journey in Persia in 1840 and 1850". *Journal of the Royal Geographical Society*, XXV, pp. 1–78.
A Friend of Iran, 1940, *"Dawdson," The Doctor. G.E. Dodson of Iran*. London, Highway Press.
Andreeva, Elena 2007. *Russia and Iran in the Great Game*. London – New York: Routledge.
Aubin, Eugène, 1908, *La Perse d'aujourd'hui*. Paris, Armand Colin.
Aubin, Jean, 2000, "Ormuz au jour le jour à travers un register de Luís Figueira 1516–1518", in: F. Aubin, ed., *Le latin et l'astrolabe*. Lisbon, Centre culturel Calouste Gulbenkian—Commission nationale pour les commémorations des découvertes portugaises, vol. 2, pp. 393–415.
Barbaro, Joseph – Contarini, Ambrogio, 1873, *Travels to Tana and Persia*, 2 vols., Lord Stanley, trad., London, Hakluyt.
Bricteux, Auguste, 1912, *Voyage en Perse. Au pays du lion et du soleil*. Brussels, Falk Fils.
Burrell, R. M., 1988, "The 1904 epidemic of cholera in Persia: some aspects of Qajar society". *Bulletin of the School of Oriental and African Studies*, 51/2, pp. 258–270.
Cash, W. Wilson, 1930, *Persia Old and New*. London, CMS.

Chardin, Jean, 1811, *Voyages*, 10 vols., L. Langlès, ed., Paris.
Coan, Frederick G., 1939, *Yesterdays in Persia and Kurdistan*. Claremont.
Collins, Edward Treacher, 1896, *In the Kingdom of the Shah*. London, T. F. Unwin.
Collins, Henry W., 1925, *From Pigeon Post to Wireless*. London, Hodden and Stoughton.
"Current Topics". *Moslem World*, 14, 1924, p. 182.
Curzon, George Nathanial, 1892, *Persia and the Persian Question*, 2 vols., London.
Cursetjee, C. M., 2001, *The Land of the Date*. New York.
Daniel, Mooshie G., 1901, *Modern Persia*. Toronto, Carswell Co.
De Warzeé, Dorothy, 1913, *Peeps into Persia*. London.
Donaldson, Bess Allen, 1972, *Prairie Girl in Iran and India*. Galesburg, Il.
Du Mans, Raphael, 1890, *Estat de la Perse en 1660*, Charles Schefer, ed., Paris, E. Leroux.
Eastwick, Edward B. 1976, *Journal of a Diplomat's Three Years' Residence in Persia*, 2 vols. in one, Tehran, Imperial Organization for Social Services.
Ebrahimnejad, Hormoz, 2000, "Theory and Practice in Nineteenth-Century Persian Medicine: Intellectual and Institutional Reforms". *History of Science*, 38, pp. 171–178.
——, 2004, *Medicine, Public Health and the Qājār State: Patterns of Medical Modernization in Nineteenth-Century Iran*. Leiden, E. J. Brill.
Elgood, Cyril, 1951, *A Medical History of Persia and the Eastern Caliphate*. Cambridge, Cambridge University Press.
——, 1970, *Safavid Medical Practice*. London, Luzac & Co.
Floor, Willem, 2000, *The Economy of Safavid Persia*. Wiesbaden, Reichert.
——, 2003, *Agriculture in Qajar Iran*. Washington DC, MAGE.
——, 2004, *Public Health in Qajar Iran*. Washington DC, MAGE. Persian translation: *Salāmat-i mardum dar Īrān-i Qājār*, Iraj Nabipur, trad., Bushire, Dānišgāh-i ʿUlūm-i Piziškī-i Bušihr, 1386/2007.
——, 2006, *The Persian Gulf. A Political and Economic History*. Washington DC, MAGE.
Fryer, John, 1909–15, *A New Account of East India and Persia Being Nine Years' Travels, 1672–1681*, 3 vols., London, Hakluyt.
Funk, J. Arthur, 1920, "The Missionary Problem in Persia". *Muslim World*, X, pp. 138–143.
Gaube, H. – Wirth, E., 1978, *Der Bazar von Isfahan*. Wiesbaden, Reichert.
Gilbar, Gad G., 1976, "Demographic Development in late Qajar Persia, 1870–1906". *Asian and African Studies* 11, pp. 125–156.
Griscom, Mary W., 1921, "A medical motor trip through Persia". *Asia. The American Magazine on the Orient*, March, pp. 233–240.
Grothe, Hugo, 1911, *Zur Natur und Wirtschaft von Vorderasien. I. Persien*. Halle, Gebauer-Schwetschke.
Hamilton, Alexander, 1930, *A New Account of the East Indies*, 2 vols., London.
Häntzsche, J. C., 1869, "Specialstatistik von Persien". *Zeitschrift der Gesellschaft für Erdkunde zu Berlin*, 4, pp. 429–449.
Hassendorfer, Colonel, 1954, "Les médecins militaries français fondateurs et organisateurs de l'Enseignement Médical et de la Santé Publique en Iran". *Histoire de la médicine*, 4/7, pp. 57–63.
Hellot, Florence, 1996, "L'ambulance française d'Urmia (1917–1918) ou le ressac de la grande guerre en Perse". *Studia Iranica*, 25, pp. 45–82.
——, 2002, "La première guerre mondiale à l'ouest de lac d'Urumiye" in: Olivier Bast, ed., *La Perse et la Grande Guerre*. Tehran, Institut Français de Recherche en Iran.
Hemmati, Abouzardjomehr, n. d., *Die abenländische Medizin in Persien*, unpublished dissertation, University of Bonn.
Holmes, W. R., 1845, *Sketches on the Shores of the Caspian, Descriptive and Pictorial*. London, Richard Bentley.
Hume-Griffith, M. E., 1909, *Behind the Veil in Persia and Turkish Arabia*. Philadelphia, J. B. Lippincott.
Jackson, A. V. Williams, 1909, *Persia Past and Present*. New York.
Kaempfer, Engelbert, 1968, *Die Reisetagebücher*, K. Meier-Lemgo, ed., Wiesbaden.

Kazembeyki, Mohammad Ali, 2003, *Society, Politics and Economics in Mazandaran, Iran, 1848–1914*. London, Routledge – Curzon.
Linton, J. H. *et al.*, 1921, *Persian Pie. Stories and articles by people who have lived in Persia*. London, CMS.
Linton, J. H., 1923, *Persian Sketches*. London, CMS.
Litten, Wilhelm, 1925, *Persische Flitterwochen*. Berlin, Georg Stilke.
Malcolm, Napier, 1905, *Five Years in a Persian Town*. London, John Murray.
Malcolm, Mrs. Napier, 1911, *Children of Persia*. Edinburgh, Oliphant Anderson & Ferrier.
Martin, François, 1990, *Mémoires de François Martin, fondateur de Pondicherry*, 3 vols. A. Martineau, ed., (Paris 1931–1934); English translation of vol. 1 and part of vol. 2 as *François Martin Mémoires Travels to Africa, Persia & India*, Aniruddha Ray, trad., Calcutta.
Melgunof, Greogorii Valerianiovich, 1868, *Das südliche Ufer des Kaspischen Meeres*. Leipzig, Leopold Voss.
Miller, William McElwee, 1989, *My Persian Pilgrimage*. Pasadena, William Carey.
Moghtader, Réza, 1992, "Teheran dans ses murailles (1553–1930)", in: Adle, Charyar – Hourcade, Bernard, eds., *Téhéran capitale bicentenaire*, Tehran – Paris, Institut Français de Recherche en Iran (Bibliotheque iranienne 37), pp. 39–49.
Momeni, Mostafa, 1976, *Malayer und sein Umland*. Marburg – Lain.
Morton, Rosalie Slaughter, 1940, *A Doctor's Holiday in Iran*. New York, Funk & Wagnalls.
Muirhead. A. L., 1913, *Western Medical Review*, XVIII, Omaha (Nebraska).
Polak, J. E., 1865, *Persien, das Land und seine Bewohner*. Leipzig.
——, 1859, "Medicinische Briefe aus Persien". *Zeitschrift der k.k. Gesellschaft der Aerzte zu Wien*, 9, pp. 138–140.
Rabino, H. L., 1928, *Mazandaran and Astarabad*. London, Luzac.
Rice, Clara, 1916, *Mary Bird in Persia*. London, CMS.
——, 1923, *Persian Women and Their Ways*. London.
Richard, Francis, ed., 1995, *Raphael du Mans, missionnaire en Perse au XVII*e s., 2 vols., Paris, Société d'Histoire de l'Orient—L'Harmattan.
Richter, Julius, 1910, *A History of Protestant Missions in the Near East*. Edinburgh – London, Oliphant Anderson & Ferrier.
"Royal philanthropy in Persia: a prince and his hospital", 1905, *The Graphic*, 7 October, p. 458.
Rubin, Michael Allen, 1999, *The Formation of Modern Iran, 1858–1909: Communication, Telegraph and Society*, unpublished thesis, Yale University.
Rühling, R., 1934, *Quer durch Persien*. Hamburg, Advent Verlag.
Sajjādī, Ṣādeq, 1990, "Bīmārestān". *Encyclopaedia Iranica*, vol. 4, pp. 257–259. (on line version: www.iranica.com)
Salsali, M., 1991, "Nursing and nursing education in Iran". *Image: The Journal of Nursing Scholarship*, 31, pp. 190–193.
Schmidel, Justus, n. d. [1926], *Durch Russland und Persien*. Berlin, Deutscher Wille.
Serena, C., 1883, *Hommes et choses en Perse*. Paris, G. Charpentier.
Setzler, Lorraine, 1941, "In Iran: The development of a nursing school in Shiraz". *The American Journal of Nursing*, 41/5, pp. 520–525.
Shepherd, William Ashton, 1857, *From Bombay to Bushire and Bussora: Including an Account of the Present State of Persia and Notes on the Persian War*. London, Bentley.
Shedd, Mary Lewis, 1922, *The Measure of a Man*. New York, George H. Doran.
Speer, Robert E., 1911, *Hakim Sahib, the foreign doctor; a biography of Joseph Plumb Cochran*. New York, Revell.
——, 1920, "Persia" in: *Foreign Missions Yearbook of North America 1920*, Roderick Beach, ed., New York, Foreign Missions Conference.
Speer, Robert E. – Russell, Carter, 1922, *Report on India and Persia*. New York, Board of Foreign Missions.
Stileman, Rev. Charles Harvey, 1902, *The Subjects of the Shah*. London, CMS.
St. Joseph, Ange de, 1985, *Souvenir de la Perse safavide et autres lieux de l'Orient* (1664–1678), Michel Bastiaensen, translated and annotated, Brussels.

Stuart, Emmeline M., n.d., *Doctors in Persia*. London, CMS.
Tchalenko, John, 2006, *Images from the Endgame. Persia through a Russian Lens 1901–1914*. London.
Tavassoli, Mahmoud – Naser, Bonyadi, 1371/1992, *Urban Space Design*. Tehran.
Tavernier, Jean-Baptiste, 1930, *Voyages en Perse et description de ce Royaume*. Paris, Éditions du Carrefour.
Werner, Christoph, 2000, *An Iranian Town in Transition*. Wiesbaden, Harrassowitz.
Williamson, J. W., 1927, *In A Persian Oil Field. A Study in Scientific and Industrial Development*. London, Ernest Benn.
Wills, C. J., 1893, *In the Land of the Lion and the Sun*. London, Ward, Lock & Bowden.
Wilson, Arnord T., 1928, *Persian Gulf*. London.
——, 1932, *Persia*, London, Ernest Benn.
Wilson, S. G., 1895, *Persian Life and Customs*. New York, Revell.
——, 1896, *Persia: Western Mission*. Philadelphia, Presbyterian Board.
Wishard, John G., 1908, *Twenty Years in Persia. A Narrative of Life under the Last Three Shahs*. New York, Fleming H. Revell.
Wood, M. M., 1922, *Glimpses of Persia*. London, CMS.
Wright, Denis, 2001, *The English Amongst the Persians*. London, I. B. Tauris.
Williams, Maud Hannah (Molly), 1994, *The Rich Tapestry of my Persian Years*. Bendigo (Victoria).
Yate, C. E., 1900, *Khurasan and Seistan*. London, Blackwood & Sons.
Zahereddini, Badri, 1966, *Medizinische Topographie der iranischen Stadt Malayer*. Erlangen.
Zavie, Emile 1927, *D'Archangel au Golfe persique*. Paris.

# DES PARTICULIERS AU SERVICE DU PEUPLE. LE RÔLE DES *VAQF* DANS LA FONDATION D'HÔPITAUX EN IRAN AU DÉBUT DU XXe SIÈCLE[1]

Omid Rezai

Le but de cet article est d'analyser le rôle du *vaqf* (pl. *awqāf*, fondation de mainmorte[2]) établi par des particuliers dans la création d'hôpitaux en Iran à la fin de l'époque qajare. L'institution des *vaqf* a joué un rôle important dans l'établissement d'hôpitaux au sein du monde musulman, à diverses époques et dans diverses régions, mais sur ce sujet de nombreuses sources restent encore peu connues et peu étudiées. En ce qui concerne l'Iran de l'époque qajare (1794–1925), les sources présentées dans cet article révèlent que, vers la fin de cette période, plusieurs hôpitaux sont établis grâce à des donations en *vaqf*, or la plupart de ces *vaqf*, n'ont à ce jour fait l'objet d'aucune étude.

Nous examinerons seulement des *vaqf* d'intérêt public (*vaqf-i ʿāmm*, *vaqf-i ḫayriya*) constitués par des particuliers, en montrant le rôle que ces derniers jouèrent pour l'établissement d'hôpitaux à cette époque, et notamment dans les villes de province. Ces donateurs (sing. *vāqif*) étaient des notables, des hommes politiques, des propriétaires fonciers et des membres de l'élite religieuse. Pour certains de ces hôpitaux furent édifiés des bâtiments nouveaux, conçus pour cette fonction, tandis que dans d'autres circonstances un jardin ou un caravansérail furent détournés de leur fonction originelle pour être transformés en centres de soins. Toutes les institutions et les actes (*vaqf-nāma*[3]) de ce type dont on a retrouvé les données, proviennent d'une période plutôt brève, de vingt ans environ, commençant au début du XXème siècle. L'on présentera également des traductions de ces actes de donation en *vaqf* effectuée par des particuliers.

---

[1] Traduction du persan de Yolande Momtaz et Fabrizio Speziale.

[2] Le *vaqf* est une donation de l'usufruit d'un bien ou d'une propriété au profit de fondations créées dans un but pieux ou d'utilité publique.

[3] Document légal de donation en *vaqf*.

À cette époque, les missions chrétiennes britanniques et américaines et le South Persian Rifles (S.P.R.)[4] géraient en Iran des centres médicaux qui étaient surtout concentrés dans les villes de province[5]. Leur affiliation au prosélitisme religieux et au colonialisme suscita chez les oulémas iraniens une vive opposition[6]. Malgré cela, les malades continuèrent à affluer vers les centres de soins de ces associations, en raison de la pénurie d'hôpitaux publics. Afin d'endiguer l'influence des services médicaux des missionnaires, certains oulémas encouragèrent alors les élites qajares à créer des hôpitaux de bienfaisance (*ḫayriya*). En 1910, fut publié le *Mukālamāt-i muqīm va musāfir* de Ḥājjī Aqā Nūr Allāh (m. 1306 h. š./1927–8), un important *mujtahid*[7] d'Ispahan. Dans ce livre Aqā Nūr Allāh souligne la nécessité de créer des hôpitaux afin que les musulmans, et particulièrement les femmes, n'aient plus à recourir aux services des centres de soins des missionnaires chrétiens[8]. Les trois *vaqf-nāma* qui sont traduits plus bas, relatifs aux hôpitaux de Téhéran, Qazvin et Sari, précisent que ces hôpitaux étaient fondés pour les malades musulmans.

## Les premiers hôpitaux de bienfaisance de la capitale

C'est dans ces circonstances que des notables de l'époque qajare décidèrent de fonder des hôpitaux à Téhéran. Mīrzā ʿĪsā Tafrašī (m. 1310 h. q./1892), qui fut par deux fois *vazīr* de la ville de Téhéran sous le règne de Nāṣir al-Dīn Šāh (r. 1848–1896), légua avant sa mort une partie de ses richesses pour financer l'établissement d'un hôpital[9]. L'éminent *mujtahid* Šayḫ Hādī Najmābādī (1834–1902) fut chargé de l'administration de cette donation et de la construction de l'hôpital (*marīż-ḫāna*, lit. maison du malade). Le Marīż-ḫāna-yi Vazīrī, connu également sous le nom de Marīż-ḫāna-yi

[4] Corps expéditionnaire commandé par des Britanniques au Sud de l'Iran, de 1916 à 1920. Cf. Tadjbakhsh 1379, pp. 203–212, cf. également les photographies sur l'activité médicale du S.P.R. à Chiraz en 1917, dans Ṣaniʿ 1380, pp. 56–57.

[5] Cf. l'article de Willem Floor dans ce volume ; cf. aussi Sajjādī 1990 ; Ebrahimnejad 2004, p. 79 ; Borumand 1381 ; Wright 1998 ; Wright 1999.

[6] Cf. Elgood 1951, p. 535 ; Borumand 1381, pp. 187–188.

[7] Un clerc apte à exercer l'*ijtihād*, l'effort d'interprétation en matière de droit religieux (*fiqh*).

[8] Cf. Borumand 1381, p. 188.

[9] Sur Mīrzā ʿĪsā Tafrašī, désigné par Mīrzā ʿĪsā Vazīr, cf. Bāmdād 1378, vol. 2, pp. 514–515 ; Dihḫudā 1373, pp. 20612–20613. Comme Vajīh Allāh Mīrzā Sipahsālār, lui aussi décéda à cause du choléra.

Šayḫ Hādī, fut terminé en 1318 h. q./1900 et comptait 30 lits[10]. Pour ce qui concerne l'histoire du *vaqf* de cet hôpital, il faut ajouter que Šayḫ Hādī Najmābādī n'avait pas officiellement fait consigner dans un document la nature de *vaqf* de ce *marīż-ḫāna* avant sa mort, ainsi ce furent ses héritiers qui le 19 *jumādā al-ṯānī* 1320/23 septembre 1902 firent rédiger le *vaqf-nāma* de l'hôpital[11].

Un autre hôpital fut établi par Vajīh Allāh Mīrzā Sipahsālār (1271 h. q./1854–5–1322/1904–5), également dénommé Amīr Ḫān Sardār, alors ministre de la guerre[12]. Vajīh Allāh Mīrzā Sipahsālār constitua le *vaqf* de son hôpital en présence des oulémas de la capitale. L'hôpital fut bâti sur un grand terrain de 15 000 *ḏar'* carrés (soit un peu plus de 15 000 mé) situé à Yūsufābād et fut ouvert durant le mois de *ša'bān* 1321/octobre-novembre 1903. Voici la partie principale du texte du *vaqf-nāma* :

> [Formules eulogiques]
>
> Amīr Ḫān Sardār, ministre de la guerre et commandant en chef très respecté, Vajīh Allāh Mīrzā Sipahsālār [...] déclare constituer en *vaqf* perpétuel (*mu'abbad*) et conforme à la loi islamique l'intégralité d'un terrain clôturé situé sur les terres de Yūsufābād au nord-ouest de la porte de Téhéran *Dār al-ḫilāfa*, d'une surface de 15 000 *ḏar'* carrés, sur lequel a été édifié un hôpital (*marīż-ḫāna*), et incluant les constructions s'y trouvant, ainsi que tous les droits conférés par la loi religieuse et la coutume (*šarī'a va 'urfiya*) au terrain susmentionné. Que cet hôpital soit ouvert à tous les malades et blessés musulmans, conformément à un document distinct, et s'engage à leur assurer soins, médicaments (*davā*) et nourriture. De même, sont constitués en *vaqf* perpétuel et conforme à la loi religieuse les droits en vigueur de trois *dāng*[13] des quatre *qanāt*[14] de Yūsufābād, y compris leurs cinq moulins, dont un ancien et quatre nouveaux édifiés par Ḥażrat-i Vālā [Amīr Ḫān Sardār], chacun situé dans un périmètre de 10 *ḏar'* carrés et à l'un des quatre points cardinaux, avec l'ensemble des dépendances et annexes des biens susdits, entièrement définis en leurs lieux et périmètres et destinés aux malades et blessés de l'hôpital. Le produit de leur revenu annuel, après acquittement des frais engendrés par leur réparation ou réfection et par le nettoyage des *qanāt*, et après acquittement des salaires (*ḥaqq*) du gestionnaire (*tawliat*) et du contrôleur (*naẓāra*), selon un document distinct, devra être consacré

---

10 Sur l'hôpital Vazīrī, où il y avait aussi une mosquée et la tombe de Mīrzā 'Īsā Vazīr, cf. aussi l'article de Willem Floor dans ce volume.

11 Cf. le *vaqf-nāma* contenu dans le dossier Téhéran nº 17, Daftar-i asnād va šināsā'ī-i mawqūfāt, Téhéran.

12 L'hôpital établi par Vajīh Allāh Mīrzā Sipahsālār n'est généralement pas mentionné par les études sur l'histoire de la médecine en Iran. Sur Vajīh Allāh Mīrzā Sipahsālār cf. Bāmdād 1378, vol. 4, pp. 391–405 ; Sulaymānī 1379, vol. 1, p. 85.

13 Le *dāng* représente un sixième d'un bien immobilier.

14 Canal d'irrigation souterrain.

aux dépenses de nourriture, médicaments, rétribution du médecin (*ṭabīb*) et autres fournitures nécessaires à l'hôpital ainsi qu'aux malades et blessés.

*Šaʿbān* 1320 h. q./novembre-décembre 1902

[Sceau :] Amīr Ḫān Sardār[15]

Le coût pour l'édification de l'hôpital fut d'environ 15 000 tomans, les revenus annuels des quatre *qanāt* constitués en *vaqf* s'élevaient à 3 750 tomans et ceux des cinq moulins à 1 600 tomans, soit au total 5 350 tomans, ce qui représentait alors des sommes non négligeables. Nous n'avons trouvé aucun détail relatif au montant exact de chacun des postes de dépenses mentionnés dans l'acte de *vaqf*, comme les frais de nourriture, remèdes et honoraires du médecin. Vajīh Allāh Mīrzā Sipahsālār mourut du choléra peu après l'ouverture de l'hôpital. Le document indique qu'il avait désigné, après sa mort, ses enfants comme administrateurs, ainsi que trois personnes, dont le ministre des affaires étrangères et le ministre des sciences, en tant que contrôleurs[16].

## L'hôpital Ṣamṣāmiya-yi Bayāt à Ḥiṣār

Quelques années après la fondation de ces établissements à Téhéran, un hôpital de bienfaisance fut édifié dans le village d'Ḥiṣār, situé à 35 km de la ville d'Arāk[17], par un notable de la région. Ce *marīż-ḫāna* fut fondé par Ḥājj Ḏū al-Faqār Ḫān Bayāt, surnommé Ṣamṣām al-Mulk Amīr Tūmān et mis au service d'Ḥiṣār et des villages environnants. Dans ce cas aussi, un bâtiment neuf fut édifié dans le but d'accueillir l'hôpital[18]. Le *vaqf-nāma* rédigé par Ṣamṣām al-Mulk nous apprend qu'il prit la décision d'établir ce hôpital au terme de soixante années consacrées au service de l'Etat[19]. L'hôpital fut nommé Marīż-ḫāna-yi Ṣamṣāmiya-yi Bayāt, du nom de son fondateur.

Le *vaqf-nāma* de l'hôpital Ṣamṣāmiya fut rédigé au mois de *muḥarram* 1323/mars-avril 1905. Cet acte de donation, parmi tous ceux évoqués dans cet article, est l'un des rares documents de ce type à nous livrer des infor-

---

15 Cf. le *vaqf-nāma* dans le dossier Téhéran nº 663, Daftar-i asnād va šināsā'ī-i mawqūfāt, Téhéran.

16 Cf. le *vaqf-nāma* dans le dossier Téhéran nº 663, Daftar-i asnād va šināsā'ī-i mawqūfāt.

17 Ḥiṣār est localisé dans l'arrondissement de Šāzand, la région d'Arak borde la région de Téhéran.

18 Le bâtiment de cet hôpital existe encore et est aujourd'hui abandonné, sur la porte d'entrée figure encore une petite inscription portant le nom de l'hôpital.

19 Le *vaqf-nāma* du Marīż-ḫāna-yi Ṣamṣāmiya est conservé au Daftar-i asnād va šināsā'ī-i mawqūfāt, Téhéran, dossier Markazī nº 526.

Tableau 1. Dépenses consignées dans le *vaqf-nāma* de l'hôpital Ṣamṣāmiya

<table>
<tr><th>Titre général</th><th>Détail des dépenses</th><th colspan="2">Total annuel en tomans</th></tr>
<tr><td>Droits d'administration</td><td></td><td colspan="2">1 *ʿušr* (346,25 *tūmān*)</td></tr>
<tr><td rowspan="5">Dépenses de l'hôpital</td><td>Honoraires du médecin</td><td>600 *tūmān*</td><td rowspan="5">4 *ʿušr* (1 385 *tūmān*)</td></tr>
<tr><td>Salaires du personnel et frais de blanchisserie</td><td>50 *tūmān*</td></tr>
<tr><td>Salaire du cuisinier</td><td>15 *tūmān*</td></tr>
<tr><td>Médicaments, alimentation et effets du médecin</td><td>700 *tūmān*</td></tr>
<tr><td>Gardien</td><td>20 *tūmān*</td></tr>
<tr><td>Total</td><td colspan="3">1.731,25 *tūmān*</td></tr>
</table>

mations un peu plus détaillées sur les diverses dépenses concernant la gestion. L'hôpital Ṣamṣāmiya bénéficiait également des revenus d'autres fondations de mainmorte, dont plusieurs villages et terres cultivées situés à proximité, qui couvraient les frais de fonctionnement. Le détail des dépenses annuelles de l'hôpital donné par le texte du *vaqf-nāma* est reproduit dans le tableau 1[20].

Le personnel de l'hôpital Ṣamṣāmiya était composé d'un administrateur (*mutavallī*), un médecin (*ṭabīb*), un cuisinier (*ṭabbāḫ*), un blanchisseur, un serviteur (*ḫādim*) et un gardien. La charge de *mutavallī* de l'hôpital fut prise par Ṣamṣām al-Mulk lui-même. Par ailleurs, il semble qu'à l'hôpital Ṣamṣāmiya il n'existait pas de poste de directeur. Il est alors possible que Ṣamṣām al-Mulk lui-même en occupât également la fonction. En l'occurrence, l'administrateur, outre la responsabilité de louer et de recouvrer les loyers, pouvait surveiller parallèlement la gestion de l'hôpital en tant que partie intégrante des biens constitués en *vaqf*.

## L'hôpital de Ḥājjī ʿIzz al-Mulk à Chiraz

Il n'existait à Chiraz aucun hôpital avant qu'un particulier, Ḥaydar ʿAlī Ḫān Šīrāzī, plus connu sous le nom de Ḥājjī ʿIzz al-Mulk n'entreprît de constituer un *vaqf* entre 1910 et 1912. Les circonstances entourant l'institution de cet hôpital à Chiraz nous fournissent un autre témoignage important

[20] Cf. le *vaqf-nāma* dans le dossier Markazī nº 526, Daftar-i asnād va šināsā'ī-i mawqūfāt.

de l'action convergente des bienfaiteurs privés en ce qui concerne les donations et les oulémas qui les y exhortaient. 'Izz al-Mulk était originaire de Chiraz mais s'établit pour un temps à Ispahan, avant de regagner sa ville d'origine. À Ispahan, il fit rédiger par le *mujtahid* Aqā Najafī Iṣfahānī (m. 1332 h. q./1913–4), l'un des célèbres oulémas de son temps, le *vaqf-nama* en vue de la construction d'un hôpital à Chiraz. Ce *vaqf-nāma* a été rédigé le 10 du mois de *šavāl* 1328 h. q./15 octobre 1910. Nous savons qu'Aqā Najafī avait fait connaître, dans une lettre adressée à Ẓill al-Sulṭān, gouverneur d'Ispahan, son opposition aux démarches des missionnaires visant à créer une imprimerie ainsi qu'aux activités médicales de leurs agents, hommes et femmes[21].

'Izz al-Mulk donna en *vaqf* la moitié (5,5 *'ušr* – c'est-à-dire dixièmes) des revenus de deux villages en vue de l'acquisition d'une maison valant la peine et la dépense d'être aménagée en hôpital[22]. Or cette initiative s'est trouvée ajournée jusqu'à l'année 1330 h. q./1912, date à laquelle le donateur fit l'acquisition d'un jardin[23] situé à l'extérieur de la porte Bāġšāh, connu sous le nom de Bāġča-yi Mīrzā Muḥammad Rižā Mustawfī, où l'hôpital fut installé[24]. 'Izz al-Mulk n'eut donc pas à construire un nouveau bâtiment, il modifia simplement l'usage d'un jardin d'agrément et du bâtiment qui s'y trouvait. Tout comme Ṣamṣām al-Mulk, il aura consacré près de la moitié des revenus de ses biens constitués en *vaqf* aux dépenses de son hôpital. Le tableau des dépenses annuelles de cet hôpital dans la période 1910–1912, figurant dans le tableau 2, met en évidence leur similitude avec celles de l'hôpital Ṣamṣāmiya.

Comme nous l'avons remarqué, il est vraisemblable que 'Izz al-Mulk a établi son hôpital sous l'influence des exhortations des oulémas. On peut noter que le *vaqf-nāma* de cet hôpital a été rédigé quelques mois seulement après la parution de l'ouvrage de Ḥājjī Aqā Nūr Allāh, *Mukālamāt-i muqīm va musāfir*. Le fait que 'Izz al-Mulk ait figuré au nombre des disciples du *mujtahid* Aqā Najafī éclaire bien des points : d'abord, son choix de résider à Ispahan, puis son *vaqf-nāma* pour l'hôpital déposé à l'étude de ce dernier. C'est probablement à cause de l'influence de ce *mujtahid*

---

21 Cf. Borumand 1381, p. 187.

22 Cf. le *vaqf-nāma* dans le dossier Fars nº 83, Daftar-i asnād va šināsā'ī-i mawqūfāt; sur cet hôpital cf. aussi Rezai 1382a, pp. 17–20.

23 Sur la situation de ce jardin cf. Āryānpūr 1365, vol. 1.

24 L'*iqrār-nāma* (contrat) rédigé par 'Izz al-Mulk, en date du mois de *rajab* 1330 h. q./ juin-juillet 1912, est conservé au Daftar-i asnād va šināsā'ī-i mawqūfāt, dossier Fars nº 83.

25 Cf. l'*iqrār-nāma* dans le dossier Fars nº 83, Daftar-i asnād va šināsā'ī-i mawqūfāt.

Tableau 2. Dépenses annuelles de l'hôpital de Ḥājjī ʿIzz al-Mulk à Chiraz pour la période 1910–1912[25]

| Rubriques générales | Détail des dépenses | Sommes annuelles |
|---|---|---|
| Administration et surveillance | Comptable et intendant de l'hôpital | 1 *ʿušr* |
| Travaux de réparation | Réfection, nettoyage | Un demi *ʿušr* |
| Dépenses de l'hôpital | Honoraires du médecin<br>Dépenses en personnel<br>Médicaments, nourriture<br>Equipement et ustensiles | 4 *ʿušr* |
| Total | | 1 980 *tūmān* |

également que ʿIzz al-Mulk accordait la priorité aux dépenses générées par l'hôpital, y compris sur celles destinées aux cérémonies de deuil de l'Imam Ḥusayn.

## Le Marīż-ḫāna-yi Amīnī à Qazvin

Dans la ville de Qazvin, un hôpital *vaqfī* doté de 30 lits fut fondé en 1335 h. q./1917 par un propriétaire foncier du nom de Ḥājj Muḥammad ʿAlī Aqā Amīnī Qazvīnī. Un bâtiment nouveau fut édifié pour héberger cet hôpital. Il est intéressant de remarquer que le texte de ce *vaqf-nāma* nous indique que Muḥammad Amīnī ne voulait pas créer un lieu exclusivement aménagé pour dispenser des soins aux malades. Il était convaincu de la nécessité pour eux d'avoir un environnement gai et agréable, et pour ce faire il avait voulu agrémenter d'arbres et de massifs de fleurs les lieux fréquentés par les malades. Nous donnons ici la partie principale du texte du *vaqf-nāma* que Ḥājj Muḥammad Amīnī fit rédiger le 20 *šaʿbān* 1337 h. q./21 mai 1919, deux ans environ après l'ouverture de l'hôpital :

> [Formules eulogiques]
> Ḥājj Muḥammad ʿAlī Aqā Amīnī Qazvīnī [...] constitue en *vaqf* la totalité d'un terrain enclos m'appartenant, situé dans le secteur de Bāġ-i šāh du quartier Dār al-sulṭān de Qazvin [...] au bénéfice d'un hôpital (*marīż-ḫāna*) composé de plusieurs bâtiments, d'une cuisine, d'un réservoir d'eau (*ambār-i āb*) et de chambres exposées au nord, et au sud pour les femmes ; d'une galerie surplombée par des chambres au nord et au sud et de petits espaces, dont l'un, situé à l'est des chambres et de l'édifice, sert d'entrée vers

> les bâtiments et de sortie vers la vaste cour (*ḥayāṭ*) qui les précède ainsi que la grande cour du jardin (*bāġ*), située au nord de l'édifice ; un autre espace, à l'ouest de l'édifice et des chambres, reconnu pour être celui de la cuisine. Concernant les deux grandes cours susmentionnées, l'une est réservée aux malades et autres, et l'autre, à savoir celle qui est située au nord des chambres, où sont plantés des arbres et aménagés des massifs (*bāġča-bandī*) de fleurs, de plantes aromatiques, de céréales, etc. est destinée à la promenade des malades. Tout ce qui se trouve sur cette parcelle de terre est mis au nom de l'hôpital qui y a été édifié afin que, avec l'autorisation de l'administrateur du moment, y soient toujours amenés les malades musulmans pour, autant que faire se peut, y être soignés et que, une fois guéris, sur l'autorisation du médecin (*ṭabīb*) de l'hôpital et après en avoir informé le directeur (*mudīr*) nommé par l'administrateur (*mutavallī*), ils puissent en sortir et laisser leur place à d'autres malades qui y seront admis de la façon décrite. C'est ainsi qu'il sera procédé dans cet hôpital [...] et que l'existence du très respecté donateur (*vāqif*) et de ses parents en soit récompensée. Le détail des bâtiments, des chambres, des caves, etc. et des cours composant ce *marīż-ḫāna* est consigné ci-après et enregistré, a force de loi et qu'il soit bien clair que cette parcelle de terre clôturée et le bâtiment qui s'y trouve, le jardin, la cour et autres, et même la grande porte d'entrée du jardin et le local la surplombant ainsi que les boutiques y attenantes, la petite porte, etc. sont dans leur intégrité au nom de l'hôpital.
>
> 20 *Šaʿbān* 1337 h. q./21 mai 1919
>
> [Sceau :] Ḥājj Muḥammad ʿAlī Aqā Amīnī[26]

Pour la réalisation de cet établissement hospitalier Muḥammad Amīnī céda une parcelle de terre enclose comprenant plusieurs bâtiments et deux cours, d'une surface approximative de 4 500 m$^2$. Il constitua donc en *vaqf* cette propriété située dans le quartier de Bāġ-i šāh avec, en sus, un certain volume d'eau du grand *qanāt*. En outre, il donna deux des quatre parts des revenus de trois villages situés dans le district de Qāqazān, dépendant de Qazvin, pour couvrir les rémunérations de l'administrateur, des médecins, du personnel, les frais de médicaments, de nourriture, des meubles et ustensiles de l'hôpital. Ces revenus, étant donné les exigences particulières inhérentes aux malades et à l'hôpital, allaient devoir être versés chaque mois. Le document fait évidemment mention du poste de directeur (*mudīr*) de l'hôpital qui est choisi sur avis de l'administrateur (*mutavallī*)[27].

---

26 Cf le *vaqf-nāma* dans le dossier Qazvin nº 9, Daftar-i asnād va šināsā'ī-i mawqūfāt.

27 Cf. le *vaqf-nāma* dans le dossier Qazvin nº 9, Daftar-i asnād va šināsā'ī-i mawqūfāt; bien qu'il soit stipulé dans le *vaqf-nāma* que le détail des dépenses de l'hôpital figure dans le testament (*vaṣiyat-nāma*), rédigé au mois de *šaʿbān* 1337 h. q./1919, il n'y paraît pas ; cf. également Varjāvand 1377, pp. 1819–1820.

## L'hôpital Mahdavī de Sari

Le premier hôpital civil de Sari fut établi grâce à un *vaqf* constitué par Ḥasan Ẓahīr al-Mulk, qui était gouverneur du Mazandaran[28]. Il se mit à la recherche, avec l'aide d'experts, d'un lieu adéquat pour la fondation d'un hôpital et finalement, le 28 *rabīʿ al-ṯānī* 1338/20 janvier 1920, il acheta pour le prix de 1 700 *tūmān* aux neuf bénéficiaires de la succession de Ḥājj Ḥusayn, commerçant de Sari, un caravansérail situé à l'extérieur de la ville. Quelques jours plus tard, il constitua cette propriété en *vaqf* au profit d'un hôpital public pour les musulmans. Ce caravansérail, situé au-delà de la porte de Bārfurūš, face à la colline de Jaʿfarābād, était appelé le caravansérail de Mīrzā ʿAbd Allāh Ḫān Nūrī. À la fin du *vaqf-nāma*, Ḥasan Ẓahīr al-Mulk le renomma : « Marīż-ḫāna-yi Mahdavī ». Ce *vaqf-nāma* est reproduit dans la figure 1, et nous donnons ici la traduction partielle du texte de ce acte de donation :

> [Formules eulogiques]
> Ẓahīr al-Mulk, gouverneur du Mazandaran, a toujours été habité par une profonde affection à l'égard de toute la population de cette province, et donc par le désir de lui apporter des bienfaits, d'améliorer sa condition et d'offrir le bien-être [...] à tous les musulmans, en particulier aux habitants de Sari. L'absence d'un hôpital pour tous, institution pourtant nécessaire à la vie en société, était de ces carences dont le comblement était pour lui prioritaire et auquel aspiraient son instruction et sa générosité. Par conséquent, sa juste décision, brillante idée approuvée par un grand nombre de croyants, dépendait pour sa réalisation de l'acquisition d'un emplacement convenant parfaitement, tant du point de vue de la sauvegarde de la santé et de la guérison des malades que de tout autre point de vue s'y rapportant. Il a ainsi choisi ce caravansérail (*ḫān*) et ce jardin (*bāġ*) attenant et [...] les a constitués en *vaqf* légal et perpétuel pour en faire un hôpital (*marīż-ḫāna*) pour tous les pauvres parmi les malades iraniens, les musulmans, et, bien légitimement, les habitants de la province et tous autres nécessiteux. Tant qu'ils sont malades et quelle que soit leur maladie, qu'ils demeurent dans cet hôpital et ne le quittent qu'après leur rétablissement et leur temps de convalescence.
> 3 *jumāda al-avval* 1338/24 janvier 1920
> [Sceau :] Ḥasan Ẓahīr al-Mulk[29]

---

[28] L'armée des Européens chercha à se doter d'un hôpital militaire avant son entrée au Mazandaran. Dans l'accord politico-militaire conclu le 19 juin 1918 entre l'empire austro-hongrois et Muḥammad Ismāʿīl Ḫān Amīr Mu'ayyid, il était prévu que des hommes du détachement austro-hongrois s'occuperaient du dispensaire et que l'un des officiers ferait office de directeur, cf. Turkamān 1378, pp. 204–211.

[29] Cf. le *muṣālaḥa-nāma* (compromis) avec le *vaqf-nāma* en marge dans le dossier Mazandaran nº 259, Daftar-i asnād va šināsā'ī-i mawqūfāt.

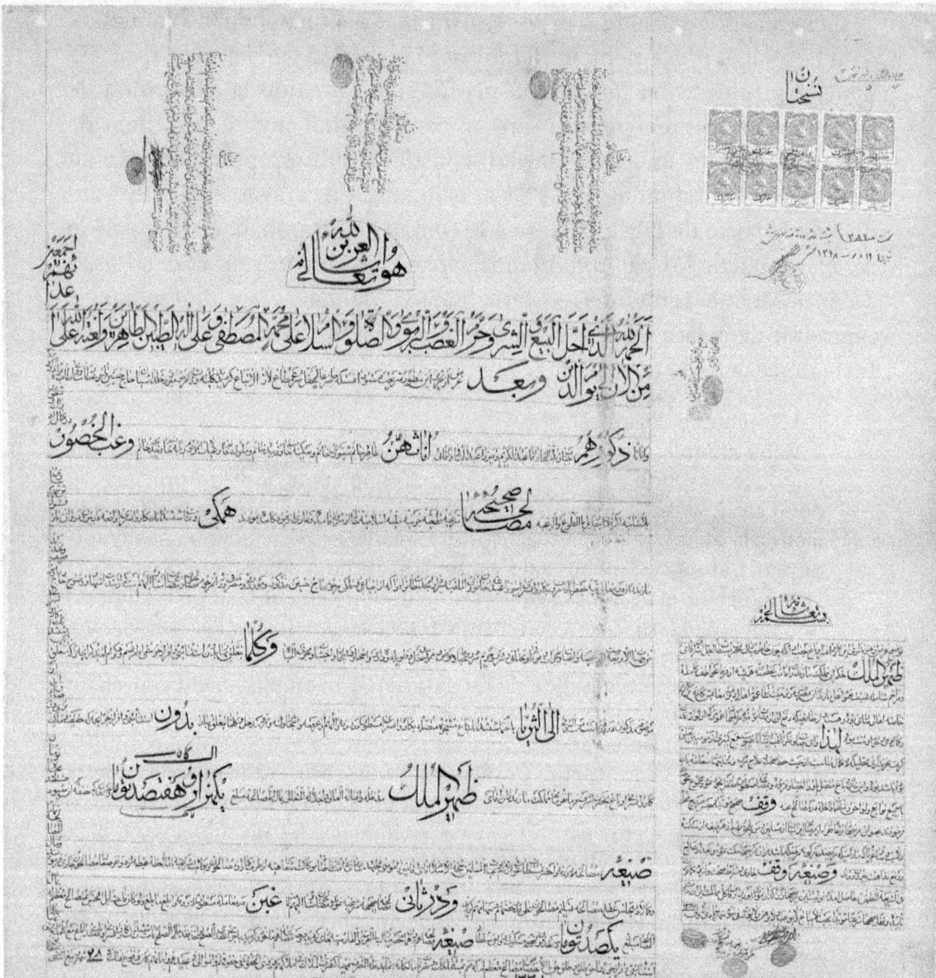

Figure 1. Le *vaqf-nāma* de l'hôpital Mahdavī de Sari, rédigé à la demande du gouverneur du Mazandaran Ḥasan Ẓahīr al-Mulk et daté du 24 janvier 1920.

Des enquêtes menées sur place ont mis en évidence que la surface approximative de cet établissement était de deux hectares, à savoir celle de l'actuel hôpital Imam Khomeyni, anciennement appelé Pahlavī, qui a été édifié sur les fondations de l'hôpital Mahdavī[30]. Parmi les hôpitaux fondés grâce à un *vaqf* que nous avons passés en revue, l'hôpital Mahdavī était le seul pour lequel le donateur n'avait prévu aucune source de revenus, ce qui générait inéluctablement des perturbations dans la bonne marche de ses services et affaires courantes. Ainsi, au début de l'époque pahlavi, entre 1308 h. š./1929 et 1312 h. š./1933, on trouve divers biens qui furent constitués en *vaqf* au bénéfice de cet hôpital[31]. Dans ces différents *vaqf-nāma*, il est appelé Marīż-ḫāna-yi Pahlavī de Sari, nouvelle dénomination conséquente à la politique d'annulation des anciens titres et de modification des noms de lieux de l'époque.

## L'hôpital Nūriya à Kerman

L'hôpital Nūriya de Kerman nous offre un autre témoignage du rapport de ces donateurs avec le milieu religieux de l'époque qajare. Ce fut en 1338 h. q./1920 qu'un propriétaire foncier de Kerman décida d'établir un *vaqf* pour la création d'un hôpital, le Marīż-ḫāna-yi Nūriya[32]. Le donateur en était Nūr Allāh Ḫān Qājār, surnommé Ẓahīr al-Mulk, petit-fils du gouverneur de Kerman Ẓāhir al-Dawla[33] et membre de l'école *šayḫī*. L'école théologico-mystique *šayḫī* était particulièrement présente à Kerman où résidait alors son maître, Zayn al-ʿĀbidīn Ḫān Ibrāhīmī Kirmānī (m. 1360 h. q./1942). Il faut signaler que Muḥammad Karīm Ḫān (m. 1288 h. q./1871), le troisième maître de l'école *šayḫī*, avait été l'auteur de plusieurs traités sur la médecine traditionnelle avicennienne[34]. En outre, Muḥammad Karīm Ḫān critiqua explicitement le Dār al-funūn et l'influence grandissante de la science

---

30 Cf. la lettre n° 15722, datée du 19/7/1385 h. š., de l'Idāra-yi kull-i awqāf va umūr-i ḫayriya (Direction générale des *vaqf* et affaires de bienfaisance) de la province du Mazandaran, envoyée au Daftar-i asnād va šināsā'ī-i mawqūfāt (Bureau des documents et identifications des biens en *vaqf*), la lettre est conservée au Daftar-i asnād va šināsā'ī-i mawqūfāt de Téhéran.

31 Ṣaḥrā'ī Ardakānī 1380, pp. 16–32.

32 Sur le rôle du *vaqf* dans la formation de la communauté *šayḫī* de Kerman à l'époque qajare cf. Hermann-Rezai 2007.

33 Ebrahimnejad 2004, p. 74.

34 Muḥammad Karīm Ḫān fut l'auteur de *Javāmiʿ al-ʿilāj*, rédigé en 1269 h. q./1852, *Ḥaqā'iq al-ṭibb*, complété en 1264 h. q./1848, *Daqā'iq al-ʿilāj*, du 1267 h. q./1850, et d'un traité concis sur l'analyse du pouls intitulé *Risāla fī javāb su'āl fī al-nabḍ fī javāb al-Mīrzā Zayn al-ʿĀbidīn al-Ṭabīb*, complété en 1265 h. q./1849.

moderne des Occidentaux en Iran[35]. On ne peut pas exclure qu'à l'hôpital Nūriya des remèdes tirés de la pharmacopée traditionnelle eussent parfois encore été utilisés.

Nūr Allāh Ḫān constitua en *vaqf* de nombreux domaines qu'il possédait à Kerman et dans le village de Rafsanjān, afin que soient bâtis un hôpital pour les malades et les blessés chiites duodécimains et une école de médecine. Pour ce faire, il avait retenu les terres dites de Šāh Murād Ḫānī[36]. Ġaffārīnižad et Nīkpūr rapportent dans leur ouvrage que le *vafq-nāma* de cet hôpital fut rédigé en 1335 h. q./1917 et que l'hôpital fut inauguré en 1338 h. q./1920, or ces dates nous paraissent incorrectes d'après la lecture de ce *vafq-nāma*, daté de 1920, qui nous informe que cette année là, un terrain fut seulement désigné pour la construction d'un hôpital.[37]

Il faut remarquer deux points importants concernant le *vaqf-nāma* de l'hôpital établi par Nūr Allāh Ḫān, si on le compare aux autres actes des hôpitaux précités. D'abord, Nūr Allāh Ḫān y a dès le départ stipulé que femmes et hommes devaient disposer de sections séparées. Deuxièmement, et cela était nouveau par rapport aux autres hôpitaux fondés à cette époque par des particuliers, il avait été prévu un centre d'enseignement annexe pour former médecins et infirmiers. Le but en était probablement d'assurer ainsi le personnel pour l'hôpital et en même temps de favoriser l'enseignement pour les étudiants à travers la pratique au sein de l'hôpital. Le bâtiment du Marīż-ḫāna-yi Nūriya existe toujours et est encore utilisé aujourd'hui comme hôpital et comme centre pour l'enseignement médical.[38]

## Conclusion

Suite à l'avènement de Rižā Šāh Pahlavī en 1925, la situation de certains de ces hôpitaux allait connaître des bouleversements importants. L'armée s'empara du contrôle et de l'administration de l'hôpital de Vajīh Allāh Mīrzā Sipahsālār à Téhéran ainsi que de l'hôpital Amīnī de Qazvin. Ainsi, peu de temps après la fondation de ces établissements, se réalisa une muta-

---

[35] Cf. à ce sujet Hermann 2007, pp. 195–198, 209, 216–218.

[36] Cf. le *vaqf-nāma* dans le dossier Kerman nº 49, Daftar-i asnād va šināsā'ī-i mawqūfāt.

[37] Cf. Ġaffārīnižād–Nīkpūr 1377 p. 88, cf. également Bāstānī-Pārīzī 1362 p. 372 ; Rezai 1382b, pp. 99–100.

[38] Il est connu jusqu'à aujourd'hui sous le nom de Marīż-ḫāna-yi Nūriya et est localisé sur la ḫyābān-i Zarīsf, čahārrāh-i Mudīriyat.

tion importante de leur nature juridique, lorsqu'ils devinrent des biens de l'Etat. Cela contribua à faire oublier le fait que ces institutions étaient à l'origine des fondations de mainmorte établies par des particuliers et non par l'Etat. La politique pahlavi de changement des noms anciens contribua également à cet oubli, ainsi l'hôpital de Mīrzā Sipahsālār fut rebaptisé Marīż-ḫāna-yi Artiš (hôpital de l'armée) tandis que l'hôpital Mahdavī de Sari prit le nom d'hôpital Pahlavī.

Dans cette étude, nous avons mis en évidence le rôle qu'a tenu la constitution de *vaqf* par des particuliers dans la fondation de hôpitaux de bienfaisance dans plusieurs villes d'Iran à la fin de l'époque qajare. Nous nous sommes concentré sur une période d'une vingtaine d'années, allant de la fondation de l'hôpital établi à Téhéran en 1900 par Mīrzā ʿĪsā Vazīr et le *mujtahid* Šayḫ Hādī Najmābādī, et ce jusqu'à 1920, année de l'acte de donation de Nūr Allāh Ḫān Qājār de Kerman. Les sources présentées ici nous indiquent que cette période, assez brève, est caractérisée par un véritable mouvement de fondation d'hôpitaux, grâce à des donations pieuses issues des particuliers. La distribution de ces institutions nous montre que cette activité ne fut pas limitée à la capitale, mais concerna également diverses villes provinciales du pays. Quant au type de médecine employée dans ces hôpitaux, les documents examinés ici ne nous apprennent rien à ce sujet. Cependant, considérant que le Dār al-funūn de Téhéran avait été ouvert un demi-siècle auparavant, il est vraisemblable de penser que la médecine pratiquée dans ces établissements était de type moderne et occidental. Seules des recherches futures pourront nous donner une connaissance plus approfondie et complète de ces activités de bienfaisance, et nous apprendront si des institutions similaires furent également établies dans d'autres centres provinciaux.

Les hôpitaux que nous avons évoqués dans cet article furent surtout institués par des notables et des propriétaires fonciers de l'époque. Comme nous l'avons souligné, parmi les facteurs qui contribuèrent à inspirer les activités de bienfaisance de ces notables figuraient les exhortations de certains oulémas pour s'opposer à l'hégémonie des Occidentaux dans l'établissement de centres de soins. Ce fut par le biais des *vaqf* qu'à cette époque sensible, contemporaine de l'expansion des activités missionnaires en Iran, des membres de l'élite économique et religieuse s'efforcèrent de s'opposer aux missionnaires qui utilisaient les hôpitaux comme moyen de prosélytisme. Dans ces conditions, il serait réducteur d'interpréter de telles activités comme procédant en premier lieu d'une inspiration moderne et occidentalisée de la part des élites locales. Certains de ces hôpitaux en particulier ne paraissent pas résulter d'un mouvement culturel ou scientifique ayant pour but principal d'augmenter la pénétration du savoir scientifique moderne occidental dans la société iranienne. Du point de vue des dynamiques culturelles de l'époque, ils semblent plutôt procéder de la part des notables locaux d'une forme d'évergétisme qui fut stimulée par les injonctions des religieux pour limiter les effets du prosélytisme des missionnaires : l'établissement de centres de soins comptant parmi les instruments les plus efficaces de ce prosélytisme.

## Bibliographie

### I. *Sources d'archives*

Dossier Fars nº 83. Téhéran, Daftar-i asnād va šināsā'ī-i mawqūfāt, Sāzmān-i awqāf va umūr-i ḫayriya.

Dossier Kerman nº 49. Téhéran, Daftar-i asnād va šināsā'ī-i mawqūfāt, Sāzmān-i awqāf va umūr-i ḫayriya.

Dossier Markazī nº 526. Téhéran, Daftar-i asnād va šināsā'ī-i mawqūfāt, Sāzmān-i awqāf va umūr-i ḫayriya.

Dossier Mazandaran nº 259. Téhéran, Daftar-i asnād va šināsā'ī-i mawqūfāt, Sāzmān-i awqāf va umūr-i ḫayriya.

Dossier Qazvin nº 9. Téhéran, Daftar-i asnād va šināsā'ī-i mawqūfāt, Sāzmān-i awqāf va umūr-i ḫayriya.

Dossier Téhéran nº 17. Téhéran, Daftar-i asnād va šināsā'ī-i mawqūfāt, Sāzmān-i awqāf va umūr-i ḫayriya.

Dossier Téhéran nº 663. Téhéran, Daftar-i asnād va šināsā'ī-i mawqūfāt, Sāzmān-i awqāf va umūr-i ḫayriya.

Lettre nº 15722, dossier Mazandaran. Téhéran, Daftar-i asnād va šināsā'ī-i mawqūfāt, Sāzmān-i awqāf va umūr-i ḫayriya.

### II. *Sources éditées*

'Abd al-Ġaffār, 1363 h. š./1984–5, *Naqša-yi šahr-i Dār al-ḫilāfa-yi nāṣirī.* Téhéran Intišārāt-i saḥāb.

Āryānpūr, 'Alī-Riżā, 1365 h. š./1986–7, *Pažūhišī dar bāġhā-yi Īrān va bāġhā-yi Šīrāz.* Téhéran, Farhangsarā.

Bāmdād, Mahdī, 1378 h. š./1999–2000, *Šarḥ-i ḥāl-i rijāl-i Irān dar qurūn-i davāzdahum va sizdahum va čahārdahum hijrī,* 6 vols., Tehran, Zavvār.

Bāstānī-Pārīzī, Ibrāhīm, 1362 h. š./1983–4, *Āsiā-yi haft rang.* Téhéran, Instišārāt-i dāniš.

Borumand, Ṣafūrā, 1381 h. š./2002–3, *Pažūhišī bar fa'āliyat-i anjuman-i tablīġī-i kalīsā C.M.S. dar dawra-yi qājār.* Téhéran, Mu'assisa-yi muṭāla'āt-i tārīḫ-i mu'āṣir-i Īrān.

Dihḫudā, 'Alī Akbar, 1373 h. š./1994–5, *Luġat-nāma.* Téhéran, Intišārāt-i dānišgāh-i Tihrān.

Ebrahimnejad, Hormoz, 2004, *Medicine, Public Health and the Qājār State: Patterns of Medical Modernization in Nineteenth-Century Iran.* Leiden, E. J. Brill.

Elgood, Cyril, 1951, *A Medical History of Persia and the Eastern Caliphate.* Cambridge, Cambridge University Press.

Ġaffārīnižād, 'Alī Riżā - Nīkpūr, Majīd, 1377 h. š./1998–9, *Pīšīna-yi piziškī-i Kirmān dar sada-yi aḫīr 1280–1377.* Kerman, Sāzmān-i asnād-i millī.

Hermann, Denis, 2007, *Aspects de l'histoire sociale et doctrinale de l'école šayḫi au cours de la période qājār (1843–1911).* EPHE, Paris, thèse non publiée.

Hermann, Denis - Rezai, Omid, 2007, « Le rôle du *vaqf* dans la formation de la communauté *shaykhī kermānī* à l'époque qājār (1259–1324/1843–1906) ». *Studia Iranica* 36/1, pp. 87–131.

Rezai, Omid, 1381 h. š./2002–3, « Āšnā'ī bā daftar-i asnād va šināsā'ī-i mawqūfāt ». *Vaqf mīrāṯ-i jāvīdān*, 37, pp. 41–46.

——, 1382a h. š./2003–4, « Pīšgāmān-i rāhandāzī-i si marīż-ḫāna-yi mujahhaz dar Šīrāz » *Vaqf mīrāṯ-i jāvīdān*, 41–42, pp. 17–20.

——, 1382b h. š./2003–4, *Fihrist-i asnād-i mawqūfāt-i Īrān, vol. II. Ustān-i Kirmān*. Téhéran, Mu'āvanat-i farhangī-i sāzmān-i awqāf va umūr-i ḫayriya.

Ṣaḥrā'ī Ardakānī, 'Abbās, 1380 h. š./2001–2, *Mīrāṯ-i māndgār*. Téhéran, Našr-i tandīs.

Sajjādī, Ṣādeq, 1990, « Bīmārestān ». *Encyclopaedia Iranica*, vol. 4, pp. 257–259. (version en ligne : www.iranica.com)

Ṣāni', Manṣūr, 1380 h. š./2001–2, *Ba-yād-i Šīrāz. 'Akshā-yi Šīrāz-i qadīm*. Téhéran.

Sulaymānī, Karīm, 1379 h. š./2000–1, *Alqāb-i rijāl-i dawra-yi qājāriya*. Téhéran, Našr-i nay, vol. 1.

Tadjbakhsh, Hasan, 1379 h. š./2000–1, *Tārīḫ-i bīmāristānhā-yi Īrān*. Téhéran, Pažūhišgāh-i 'ulūm-i insānī va muṭāla'āt-i farhangī.

Turkamān, Muḥammad, 1378 h. š./1999–2000, *Asnād-i Amīr Mu'ayyid Savādkūhī*. Téhéran, Našr-i nay.

Varjāvand, Parvīz, 1377 h. š./1998–9, *Sīmā-yi tārīḫ va farhang-i Qazvīn*. Téhéran, Našr-i nay.

Wright, Denis, 1998, « Burials and Memorials of the British in Persia ». *Iran*, 36, pp. 165–173.

——, 1999, « Burials and Memorials of the British in Persia: Further Notes and Photographs ». *Iran*, 37, pp. 173–174.

# TOGETHER AND APART: CATHOLIC HOSPITALS IN PLURAL GOA[1]

Cristiana Bastos

## The Royal Hospital of Goa and Its Wonders

Among the wonders and evils of the exotic places depicted in the *Voyage of Pyrard de Laval to the East Indies* (*1601–1611*), the Royal Hospital of Goa stands in magnificence and grandeur. After a long journey through the world, the French traveller François Pyrard arrived in Goa in 1608 feeling ill. Together with some of his shipmates, he was taken to the Royal Hospital. Its grandeur mesmerized them: "We could hardly believe that this was a hospital, when seeing it from the outside, as it looked like a grand palace, except for the inscription *Hospital do Rey Nosso Senhor.*"[2] The high quantity and "quality" of the people (*gens de qualité*) who looked for the hospital services impressed Pyrard, for many of them had arrived in palanquins, a means of transportation typically used by the rich and influential.

Pyrard's travel memories contain many laudatory remarks about the layout and functions of the hospital. The stone stairwell was high and quite magnificent (*fort magnifique*), leading to an upper floor where, in normal times, the patients were lodged. There were also times when demand was exceptional, such as when the caravels arrived filled with hundreds of people suffering from all kinds of ailments picked up at sea and on land, from scurvy to assorted fevers and stomach disorders. On

[1] This article results from the research project *Empire, centers and provinces: the circulation of medical knowledge* (FCT PTDC/HCT/72143/2006) and benefits from earlier research conducted within the scope of the project *Medicina Colonial, Estruturas do Império e Vidas Pós-coloniais em Português* (POCTI/41075/ANT/2001), both funded by Fundação para a Ciência e Tecnologia and hosted by the Institute of Social Sciences, University of Lisbon. I would like to mention a special acknowledgement to the warm support provided by the librarians of Arquivo Histórico Ultramarino, in Lisbon, Sociedade de Geografia de Lisboa, Biblioteca Nacional de Portugal, particularly to João Zink, and the Public Library in Pangim, Goa, specially to Lourdes Bravo da Costa. Warm thanks to the careful and patient editorial comments of Fabrizio Speziale, editor of this volume.

[2] Pyrard 1998, Vol. 2, p. 524.

those occasions, the hospital reportedly lodged up to 3,000 at once.[3] When François Pyrard was there, he estimated that the occupation was of 1,500 patients.[4]

Those numbers are extraordinary when compared to today's hospitals occupancy, rarely over a thousand beds, and to the main hospital of Lisbon at that time (Todos os Santos), which had capacity for a few hundred—or, in the most generous speculations, up to a thousand.[5] We should also note that only about 1,500 Portuguese and their descendants lived then in the city of Goa, out of a total of 75,000 people (about 20,000 Hindus and 50,000 local Christians).[6] Clearly, the hospital served more than the local population, and as we shall see, not the local population.

The hospital furniture and decorations were described in detail by Pyrard. The *esquifes* (or *catres*, hospital beds/stretchers) were finished in red lacquer or in golden or multi-colour polish. Beds were made with fresh mats and linen on the arrival of new patients. The bedding, which was changed every three days, consisted of cotton sheets, cotton-filled pillows, mats and covers in cotton and in silk that were decorated with assorted figures and colors. Everything was a true wonder.

The services provided there were also depicted as remarkable: on arrival a barber shaved the patients thoroughly; a servant washed them with warm water, and gave them appropriate clothing and room equipment, including a clay jar, a chamber pot, and a handkerchief. When leaving, they would get a change of clothes suitable for life outside. The patients' needs were thoroughly accommodated by the staff, among whom the upper echelons were Portuguese and the subordinates were "Brahmins or Christian Goa Canarins."[7]

---

[3] Pyrard 1998, Vol. 2, p. 534.

[4] Pyrard 1998, Vol. 2, p. 527.

[5] Although it is hard to estimate the number of beds, we know that in 1672 there were fourteen wards in the All Saints Hospital of Lisbon. Four of them were for people with fevers (three for men and one for women) and then a pair of each (male/female) for the wounded, for the bed-ridden, the ill, the alienated, the convalescent, Santos 1925, p. 54.

[6] Pearson 2001, p. 404.

[7] Pyrard 1998, Vol. 2, pp. 524–525. The term "Canarins" was frequently used by Europeans to refer to the locals in a derogatory manner. Sometimes it was used specifically for local Christians, other times for the Hindus, also referred as "Gentios", which corresponds to "Heathen" or, to keep the tone, "Gentile". Goa scholars have argued that the term "Canarim" should not be taken as derogatory, as it meant, literally, "inhabitant of Kanara" (Kanada, or Karnata), the region south of the Konkan (Goa) and north of the Malabar; it had been mistakenly used by the Europeans to refer also to the peoples of Goa—who, in turn, would better see themselves as "Konkan", a regional and linguistic distinction that is used today as an identity reference for Goa, see Dalgado 1919, vol. I, pp. 197–198.

Pyrard referred to the hospital as "the most beautiful in the world", not only for the quality of the building and annexes, for its orderly cleanliness, the very good care provided to the patients' needs and demands, but also "for the doctors, drugs and remedies used for the recovery of health [...] as well as for the spiritual support provided at any time and moment."[8]

Even more interesting for our purposes are his descriptions of the internal organization of the hospital. The head was a Jesuit priest, who supervised a number of Portuguese officers. Servers and slaves were Christian Indians. The officers had different tasks, as in a big monastery; they readily reprehended the patients who did not abide by the rules. The servers, however, would not dare to do so. The slaves did the menial jobs of laundering and washing, scrubbing the floors, emptying the chamber pots and cleaning the latrines, for which Pyrard used the term "secret places."[9]

Twice a day there were visits from the physicians, surgeons, pharmacists, barbers, and phlebotomists. The pharmacist and some domestics resided in the hospital, while the physicians and surgeons lived outside.[10] The patients were almost exclusively soldiers from Portugal or from other Christian nations. This is a point that should be emphasized—at that time, these were services for Europeans only, and only for certain Europeans. Women and non-Christian men were not allowed in the Royal Hospital. Native Christian men could enter the premises as secondary staff: they could serve there, but not be served. For treatment, noted Pyrard, they had to seek support in the other hospital that existed in the city, one that had a separate building for women.[11]

In sum, to be taken in as a patient of the Royal Hospital one had to be a high status male and a Christian of old stock. Jews and recent converts (*Cristãos novos*) had to pass for old-Christian Portuguese in order to be attended there. On Pyrard's account, "it was for gentlemen and endowed soldiers that those hospitals were established in India."[12]

Non-medical amenities were abundant for the few who could use the place. Water was brought from Banguenim and given to the patients with no restrictions. Incense and other aromatic scents were brought by the

[8] Pyrard 1998, Vol. 2, pp. 525–526.
[9] Pyrard 1998, Vol. 2, p. 526.
[10] Pyrard 1998, Vol. 2, pp. 526–527.
[11] Pyrard 1998, Vol. 2, p. 527. We shall see further on that there were several other hospitals, and their names and number varied along the years.
[12] Pyrard 1998, Vol. 2, p. 535.

servers who followed the physicians in their visits.[13] Food was rich and plenty: regular meals consisted of a whole roasted or boiled chicken—or half a hen—and rice from Surat or Cambay boiled in milk, with jams for dessert; supper included a mutton or chicken soup. Outside visitors could bring food to the patients, if compatible with their prescribed diets, and could share their meals in the hospital. Small bread rolls were one of the most popular items they brought in.[14] Wine—contrary to what happened in Iberia at the time—was rare and by prescription only. Meals were served in Chinese porcelain.[15]

Different diseases were lodged in different rooms.[16] The most recurrent illnesses were the fevers, the dysenteries and the venereal diseases that, according to Pyrard, were rampant in Portuguese India while non-existent elsewhere in the subcontinent.[17] In his estimation, about 1,500 dead bodies left the hospital per year, and "an infinite number" entered. Occupation varied from a minimum of 300–400 to a maximum of over 3,000.[18]

Pyrard was hosted in a brand new hospital. It had not always looked like that—if it ever did—nor would it remain as he described—if it ever was. Linschoten, who stayed in town from 1583 to 1588, refers to a Sprital d'el-rey (Royal Hospital), on the grounds of Santa Catarina[19]—marked as nº 15 in the map reproduced in Figure 1—but there is no mention of the magnificence with which Pyrard depicts it. In a recent academic work about the old hospital, Victor F. Silva estimates its capacity in a few hundred beds, based on the recorded expenses.[20]

The hospital had evolved from a mere row of houses build right after the conquest of Goa by the troops of Albuquerque in 1510. The original setting was meant to be a place where soldiers could restore their health at the expenses of the state and with the assistance of "a nurse, drugs, potions and other needed supplies."[21] As an accommodation for soldiers, the hospital kept some of the elements of the campaign barracks: flexibility, expansion, and contraction. The piled stretchers could easily be turned into beds in order to receive, literally, shiploads of sick soldiers;

---

13 Pyrard 1998, Vol. 2, p. 527.
14 Pyrard 1998, Vol. 2, p. 531.
15 Pyrard 1998, Vol. 2, p. 532.
16 Pyrard 1998, Vol. 2, p. 531.
17 Pyrard 1998, Vol. 2, p. 534.
18 Pyrard 1998, Vol. 2, p. 534.
19 Linschoten 1596, p. 183.
20 Silva 1998.
21 Saldanha 1926, p. 183.

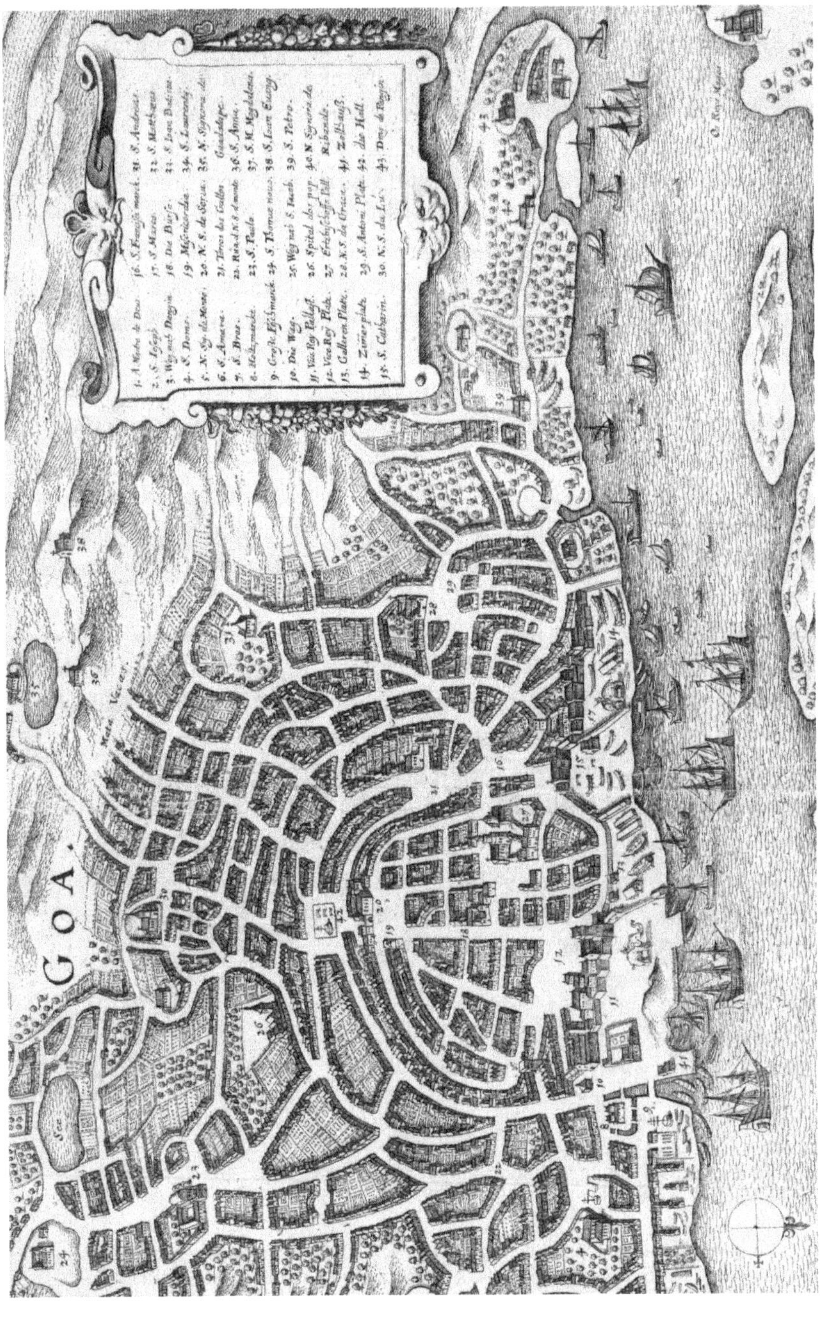


Figure 1. Map of Goa, unknown author, probably a 17th century engraving, Biblioteca Nacional de Portugal. The Royal Hospital was located in Santa Catarina (nº 15). The legend also refers to an hospital for the poor (*Spital dos pop*, nº 26), on which see below. (Reproduced with the kind permission of Biblioteca Nacional de Portugal).

the headquarters could be expanded with the construction of annexes. Apparently, it was reformed already in 1520.[22] In 1524 people would use any lousy excuse, like wounds achieved in street quarrels, or nothing at all, just to get the free amenities given within the hospital.[23]

The construction or renovation that Pyrard came across had reportedly been funded by the revenues of a commercial journey from China in the early 17th century. At the time, the hospital was directly sponsored by the King of Portugal and had the support of the viceroy, of other powerful lords and the archbishop. All of them gave money to the endowment of the hospital.[24] Even if for only a brief period, the hospital was a locus of pomp and grandeur, a good match for the city of Goa, remembered as "the Rome of the Orient."

Yet, while the churches of old city of Goa—now known as Old Goa, as opposed to Goa, the state and former colony, and Nova Goa, another name for Pangim when it became the capital in 1841—are in very good condition today and receive many thousands of Christian pilgrims and tourists every year, there is little left of the grand building of the hospital visited by Pyrard. There is an image (see figure 2) that is sometimes mistakenly used to refer to old Goa Royal Hospital, but in fact it refers to a palace (Casa da Pólvora) where the Royal Hospital was temporarily relocated towards the end of the eighteenth century, in Panelim, a few miles west of the city of Goa. It is a magnificent, whitewashed palace against backdrop of lush green, with the legend "Hospital Real Militar."[25]

We do not know for sure what the grand hospital looked like: all we can find now in the St. Catherine shore in Old Goa are the remains of some of its walls, covered with ivy and overgrown with grass and coconut trees, surrounded by barking dogs, buzzing insects and silent reptiles.[26] We can wonder where did all its riches (and walls) go, and we will attempt to answer the question further on in the text.

---

22 Saldanha 1926, p. 183.

23 Saldanha 1926, p. 184.

24 Pyrard 1998, Vol. 2, p. 535.

25 Reprinted in Carita 1995, p. 29, who correctly refers to the building as Casa da Pólvora. The building is also represented in a lithograph in the volume by Mendes 1886.

26 Many thanks to Lourdes Bravo da Costa Rodrigues for the visit to Old Goa in January 2009.

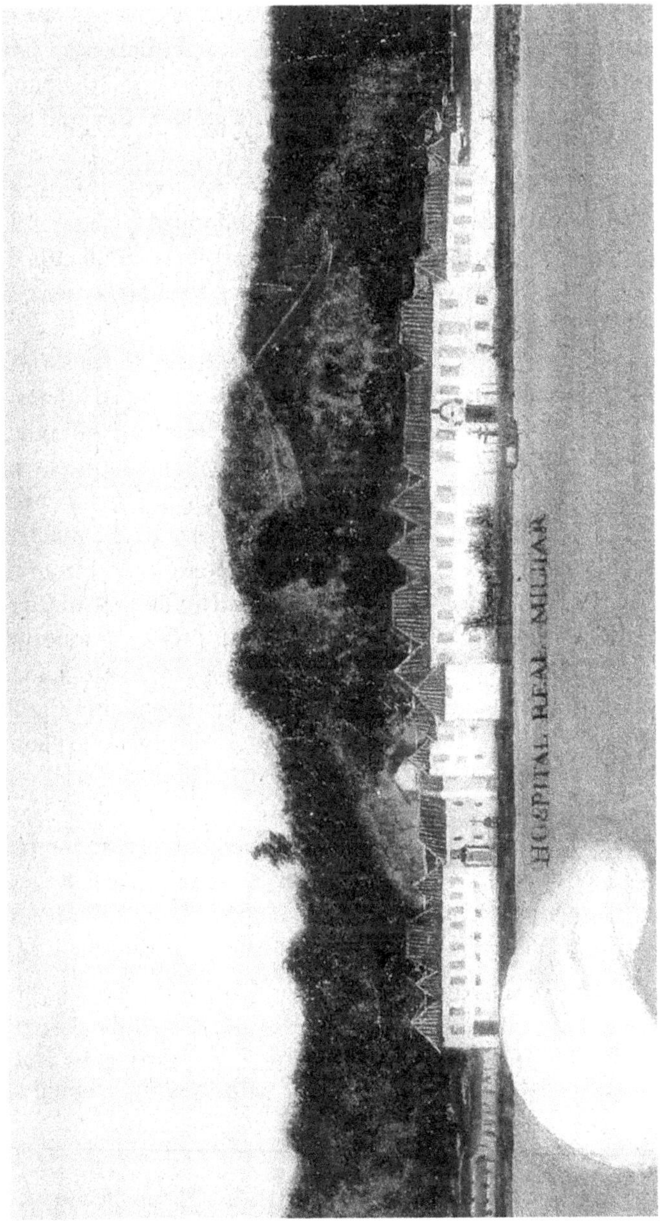


Figure 2. A painting with an image of Casa da Pólvora, with the legend "Hospital Real Militar" (Royal Military Hospital), from Carita 1995, p. 29.

## Beyond the Royal Hospital

The Royal Hospital was not the only one in town. There were a few charity-based hospitals that competed with the local practitioners in providing health care. They also worked towards the conversion of the patients, and catered to a wide number of people. While the Royal Hospital hosted only the military and the gentry of the male European kind, who often were not at all sick, the other hospitals cared for women, non-Europeans, the poor, lepers, the pariahs and the lower status groups in general. Their number is uncertain today; they are depicted either for their function (e.g., leprosy) or for the pious names of Todos os Santos, Piedade, Misericórdia, or merely City hospital.[27]

Father Saldanha's *História de Goa* (1898) and Ferreira Martins' *História da Misericórdia de Goa* (1912) help us in sorting some facts and dates. Saldanha refers to the hospital of Saint Lazarus as a beautiful building that was founded in 1530–31 to treat leprosy but accommodated many other poor people as well—including S. Francis Xavier.[28] In 1551 another hospital for the poor was founded by priest Paulo Camerte in the annexes of the S. Paul's church, and was later transferred to Margão and from there to Rachol.[29] The most famous non-military hospital at the time in Goa was that of Todos os Santos (All Saints), founded in 1547; in 1681 it annexed yet another hospital, the one of Piedade (Piety). Still according to Saldanha, those two merged into what became known as the Hospital of the Poor, run by the Misericórdia, or the order of Mercy. This helps to explain the confusing indistinct references to hospital of Misericórdia, of the Poor, of All Saints, or City hospital.[30]

According to Martins, the Hospital of *Piedade* had been supported by the city, thus the frequent reference to as City hospital (*da cidade*), while the hospital of Todos os Santos had been supported by the Misericórdia, thus the unofficial name of Hospital da Misericórdia. This was also known as hospital "*dos pobres*" (of the poor), or "*gente da terra*" (natives), for it treated the poor and the local people. The official name of Todos os Santos came in 1590 with Fr. Aleixo Meneses. Still according to Martins, there were attempts to merge this hospital with the city hospital since

[27] See Gracias 1994, pp. 118–136, and Pearson 2001, pp. 405–408. The latter suggests that the complete list is still to be established.

[28] Saldanha 1926, p. 191.

[29] Saldanha 1926, p. 193.

[30] Saldanha 1926, p. 192.

1680. The actual merging only took place in 1706, when the official name became Hospital de Todos os Santos e de Nossa Senhora da Piedade (Hospital of All Saints and of Our Lady of Piety).[31]

The proliferation of hospitals for local Christians shows the importance of medical assistance in the process of bringing the local population into the Catholic Church. In her analysis of 16th century Goa triad hospitals-charities-Catholicism, Ângela Barreto Xavier notes that this happened not only in the city, where several Catholic hospitals catered for the poor as a means to expand conversion and guarantee the assistance to the converted, but also in the less studied hinterland of Salcete and Bardez, where medical and spiritual assistance went hand-in-hand in the conquest of native bodies and souls.[32] The role of the Jesuits—who also run hospitals in Cochin, Punnaikayal and Hormuz—in the process of assisting ailing bodies and rescuing the natives' souls in Asia at the time is analyzed by Ines Županov's works.[33]

Hospitals provided care for the ailments and wounds of the bodies, captured the souls, and supported those in need. Ferreira Martins writes that people who were not sick tried to get into the Misericórdia just for the free room and board.[34] The Royal Hospital provided more than mere food and shelter: it gave luxury and grandeur to those who saw themselves dispossessed from the goods and positions they might have previously held.[35] They could find a place to live without losing face in a society like Goa, known for vanity and opulence, even if fake—where, for instance, low-rank soldiers would make a five or six person group subscription of status symbols such as an umbrella, a servant or a velvet outfit, that they used in turns, one at the time, to exhibit a wealth and status they did not own.[36] The splendor and immensity of the Royal Hospital should thus be seen less a sign of its importance as a healing institution, but a direct effect of the other social purposes it also served: on the one hand, stating the grandeur of those who ordered it—the king, the crown, the state—and, on the other hand, providing high-quality room and board, at the expense of the state and donors, to the Portuguese officers and soldiers who could

---

31 Martins 1912, pp. 336–337.

32 Xavier 2007, pp. 258–264. An emphasis on the rural settings of Goa, as opposed to the usual exclusive attention to the maritime commerce, is also given by Souza 1979.

33 Županov 1999, 2008.

34 Martins 1912, p. 340.

35 Martins 1912, pp. 290, 293.

36 Martins 1912; see also Sá 1997, and Abreu 2001.

no longer support themselves in the colony. Along those lines, we could suggest that the hospital was a device to prevent downward mobility and social disgrace among the Portuguese passing by, or stationed for a while. That—more than the development of medicine in Goa—should explain the size, luxury and splendor of the Royal Hospital of Goa.[37]

## Splendor and Fall Revised

With room for 3,000 patients, lacquered beds with fine linen and soft pillows, great food in awesome china, unlimited drinking water and aromatic incenses, the hospital thus portrayed seems more of a legend than a reality. Was Pyrard's description affected by the vapors of the French tavern where, by the fireplace, he told his stories to the scribes who wrote down his travel memoirs? Or, to adopt contemporary canons of interpretation, was the story framed along the lines of the "Golden Goa" mythology, the proto-orientalist tale of a city of unbeatable splendor that once fell from grace?

One thing we know: if the Royal Hospital ever was the wonder depicted by François Pyrard, it was so only for a relatively short period of time; its decline came rapidly, as the depictions provided by international visitors a few decades later report a different reality. In his analysis of state medicine in Goa, Pearson quotes the description of the hospital expressed by Jean-Baptiste Tavernier and Francesco Gemelli Careri, both from the second half of the seventeenth century. Tavernier claimed that since his first visit the quality of services had declined dramatically, and that "many Europeans who enter it do not leave it save to be carried to the tomb"; some patients suffered terribly from thirst, cried out for help, and begged for a little water to drink, only to find avaricious servers—here Tavernier shows his prejudice against the staff of "blacks and Mestifs"—who would "not give a drop without receiving something, that is to say, unless some money is placed in their hands, and to give color to this wickedness they give it only in secret, saying that the physician forbids it."[38]

Nicolò Manucci, who was in Goa just a few years after Tavernier, made very critical remarks about almost anything he came across. The Portuguese, once pious, honest and fearless, had turned, in his words, into a

---

[37] Isabel dos Guimarães Sá shows a parallel case with the Misericórdias in the East, Sá 1997.

[38] Pearson 2001, p. 415.

bunch of shameless deceivers, forgers, envious cowards and other terrible things.[39] The Jesuits who ran the hospital were no better, and their greed was the cause of much evil. Patients under their care were more likely to die than to survive, as the priests were after their goods and belongings—and would auction them, purchase them for next to nothing and re-sell them at a big profit soon after.[40] The five-star reception on arrival experienced by Pyrard was now reported as dreadful by Manucci. The soldiers might well expect to be treated by charitable Jesuits in the hospital, only to find, to their disappointment, that they were to deal with greedy "Canarese or *Topasses* [native or half caste Christians], who frequently demand payment for even the water they [the patients] require."[41] Patients without the means for bribery had to do without the water and food they were entitled to; on top of that, says Manucci, they were treated as if they had chosen to disobey their dietary prescriptions. As a punishment, the deprived patients were put in one of the damp underground cells and, quite likely, died in just a few days. Manucci estimates that only 1/8 of those who got into the hospital would get out alive.[42] In the time he was there, about 25 dead bodies were brought out of the hospital every day, which makes the estimate six times bigger than that of Pyrard.

Manucci had his reasons to be angry. He had been himself confronted by the authorities and put in prison, on the grounds of practicing medicine without a license. Many of his complaints were about the monopolization of healing by the head physicians; he illustrates his points with the tale of a woman who had cured a friar's pains and swollen testicles and, instead of being rewarded, was put in prison.[43] Another story was about a Hindu healer who knew the cure for scrofula; he was jailed as a means to force him to give away his secret—but he preferred to die rather than give it to the Portuguese.[44]

Reading through Manucci's and Tavernier's narratives of decline—which represent the perspective of European travelers—we can envisage that the balance of power between groups within the walls of the hospital was going under a profound change. Tavernier depicts the services

[39] Manucci 1907, Vol. 3, pp. 133–134.
[40] Manucci 1907, Vol. 3, p. 283.
[41] Manucci 1907, Vol. 3, p. 283. Referring to L. F. Thomaz' assertion of Topasses biculturalism, Sanjay Subrahmanyam analyzes their role in society, Subrahmanyam 2009, p. 435.
[42] Manucci 1907, Vol. 3, p. 279.
[43] Manucci 1907, Vol. 3, pp. 135–136.
[44] Manucci 1907, Vol. 3, p. 136.

as lousy; we can add that the hospital was no longer organized around the wellbeing of people like him, and that the first-class services reportedly administered to François Pyrard a few decades earlier, or to Tavernier himself a few years in between, were no longer available to European travelers of old Christian stock. Or, in other words, the hospital had ceased to be a European enclave in the tropics; it did not cater solely to Europeans nor was it run by Europeans alone. An important part of the staff was indigenous, up to the higher ranks. Recent historians report the existence of "black" head physicians in the seventeenth century.[45]

Whether the Royal Hospital went into shambles and became a hunting ground for the greedy, as Manucci suggests, or evolved, silently, as the site where a hybrid medicine matured, as historian Timothy Walker proposes,[46] or was both of them at once, remains a subject for more research. What we know is that the hospital went through profound transformations and that Goa diminished its importance within the scope of the Portuguese imperial and commercial networks, routes and actions. It is likely that by the end of the seventeenth century the hospital was very different from its earlier version. What was it like, then?

We can attempt to answer that question by re-interpreting some of the evidence used in the narratives about European medicine in Goa. There is a widely quoted 1678 memo written by the Portuguese Counselor in India Christovam Sousa Coutinho to his king which has been interpreted by historians of medicine in Goa as the founding moment for the establishment of the teaching of (European) medicine. The governor commented on the lack of physicians and asked the king to send over a couple of teachers who could train the locals, who were talented for medicine. The answer would come slowly, paving the way to the foundation of a local medical School in 1842—such is the master narrative of the Medical School of Goa.[47]

---

[45] Pearson 1996, 2001; Walker 2001.

[46] Walker 2001.

[47] See Correia 1947, pp. 55–56; Figueiredo 1960, p. 74; for a critique, see Bastos 2001, 2002, 2005. A few other streams of tradition contribute to a picture of past glory for Goan medicine: the efforts to promote the teaching of European medicine in India in the early centuries of Portuguese colonization, either linked to Garcia de Orta (d 1568), or the Jesuits; the acknowledgment of the notoriety of Goan physicians outside Goa in later periods, either as scientists in Europe, like Agostinho Vicente Lourenço (1826–1893), or famous specialists in Portugal, like the ophthalmologist Caetano da Gama Pinto (1853–1945) or the surgeon and obstetrician Alfredo da Costa (1859–1910); and the actual contribution of many Goans as the workforce in the colonial health services in Africa. See Costa 1943, and Bastos 2001, 2005, 2007a. For the persistence of that narrative, one can find daily evidence

My suggestion is to reverse that foundational narrative: where the pro-Portuguese authors see the prominence of the colonizers, we can see, precisely, their absence and lack of control regarding the dynamics of healing. The Portuguese staff had diminished dramatically and, on the ground, the Christian native staff that had previously assisted the Portuguese physicians was now in charge of much of the action.

As for the actual building where this action took place, we still know little. We know it was not the palace portrayed in figure 2, with the legend "Hospital Real Militar." That was the Casa da Pólvora (thus named due to its proximity to a gunpowder factory), a palace located in Panelim where the governor resided until 1759 and to where, afterwards, the hospital was temporarily re-located. That relocation happened during a time when the city of Goa, reportedly plagued by fevers, was itself under the process of relocation to "healthier places."[48] The location of the future capital of the state was yet to be decided.

We know that in 1759 the Jesuits who had been running the hospital were expelled from Goa, and that the building was considered as in very bad shape—indeed, in risk of collapsing. Under those circumstances, and because the governor moved his own headquarters to Pangim, further west, the palace of Casa da Pólvora in Panelim became a candidate for hosting the hospital. It had a few annexes that accommodated passing companies of soldiers.[49]

The architect Francisco Tosi Colombina was given the task of planning the conversion of the Casa da Pólvora into a hospital. He expressed his objections about taking care of the sick next to a gunpowder factory and suggested that building a new hospital from scratch in Pangim would be a better and cheaper solution. He also suggested several other possible accommodations for the temporary hospital and referred to the College of S. Roque as a viable one, at no cost. Nonetheless, and referring to

---

in internet posting, such as that who opposed Dr. Nadkumar Kamat to Mr Colaco regarding the glorious past of Goan medicine (see Kamat, N., "Goa's Pathetich Public Health System", *Navhind Times*, April 7, 2003, and http://www.colaco.net/1/nanduGoa'sPatheticPublicHealthSystem.htm, last access in 08/10/2011).

48 Fatima Gracias notes that at that time Old Goa had become a very unhealthy place, in which 7–8 patients died every day in the hospital. Gracias suggests that the option of moving to the hospital to the palace of Casa da Polvora came from the recommendation of the governor Count of Ega, Gracias 1994, p. 126. Although Germano Correia holds to the prevailing notion that the bad airs of Goa would necessarily lead to decay and hence to the transference of the city to healthier places, he also accounts for a parcel of sociological motives—too much ambition, rivalries, envy, competition, see Correia 1941.

49 See Saldanha 1926, and Colombina 1759.

himself as a "poor architect", meaning with it that he could work with small budgets, he used his best skills to draw a map with the minimal and less expensive adaptations possible in the Casa da Pólvora.[50]

Colombina's plan allowed for the accommodation of four hundred and eighty people, and costs would be limited to about 30–40 thousand *xerafins*, as the stones, woods, doors, windows, tiles and other materials (worth about 50 thousand *xerafins*) would be brought from the ruined older hospital. He planned separate rooms for the pharmacy, for the different services, and appropriate infirmaries for the "frenetic insane", for the "*galicados*" (syphilitic), for the sick, for the wounded and for the convalescents.[51]

There are strong indications that even the minimalist plans of Colombina were not followed in full, and not immediately. According to Father Saldanha, the demolishing of the old hospital occurred in 1770 and the patients were temporarily lodged in the college of S. Roque.[52]

Whatever the Royal Hospital might have been like at the time of François Pyrard, in the early seventeenth century, in one and a half centuries it was at the verge of ruin and asking for an urgent re-location. Goa, too, was no longer the shining star within a network of wealthy routes. The riches were gone. The most inexpensive plan for the relocation of the hospital was chosen—it was one that counted on the recycling of the stones, woods and tiles of the old building, and that partially explains why there is so little left of it.

Research on the hospital sources for that period carried by historian Fatima Gracias emphasized a picture of unruly chaos and corruption within the hospital: "mismanaged by the staff appointed by the government", whom channeled to their own pockets the funds of the hospital and indulged in gambling, the hospital had "no trained doctors" and "no discipline was observed". Nurses were incompetent, there was no hygiene. Patients cooked for themselves, ate freely, and walked around in dirty clothes. Visitors brought them alcohol and often spend the night there. Medicines coming from Europe were adulterated. This picture of decay lasted until the turn of the century.[53]

Yet, it was in that shifting scenario that much of the interactions between streams of knowledge had occurred. Both Pearson and Walker

---

50 Colombina 1759.
51 Colombina 1759.
52 Saldanha 1926, p. 191.
53 Gracias 1994, pp. 126–127.

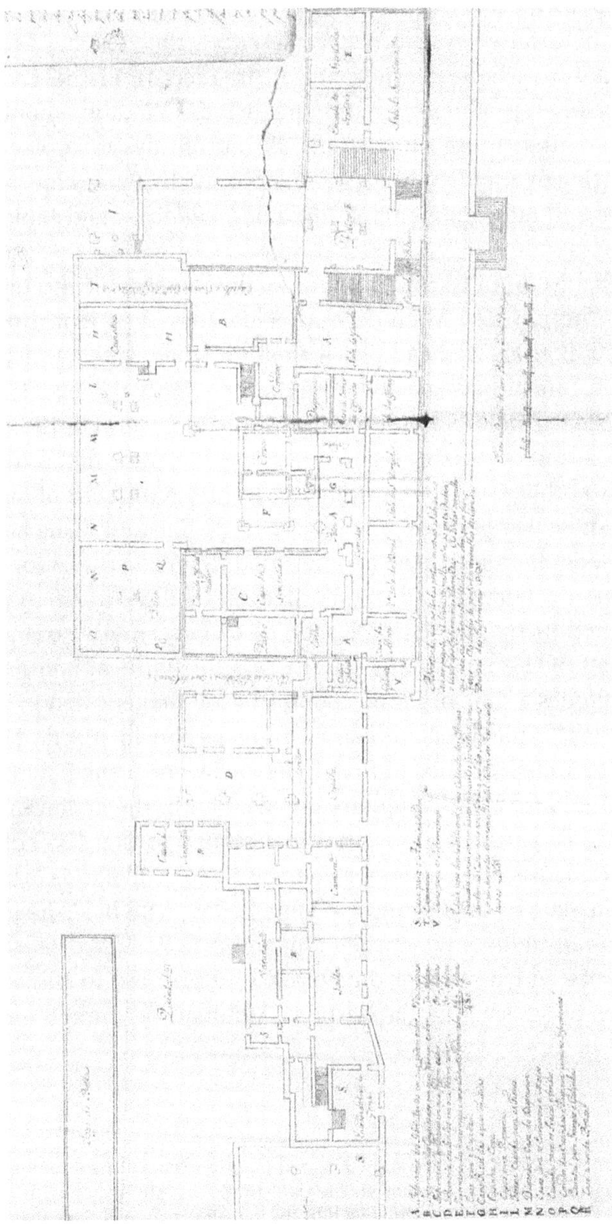

Figure 3. Adaptations to the Casa da Pólvora proposed by Francesco Colombina in 1759, from Carita 1995, p. 29, original at the Biblioteca da Ajuda (see Colombina 1759).

suggest that from the early moments of Portuguese administration in India there was some experimenting with drugs and remedies and some transmission of medical knowledge that went both ways between the Portuguese and the local *vaidyas*.[54] Walker describes the Hospital as a bed of experimentation where pharmaceutical products from the East and West came together, producing a hybrid medicine.[55] What we should add to their views is that those interactions did not always take place in a glamorous setting of grandeur like the one depicted by Pyrard for the earlier period, but, in later moments, in decaying buildings and temporary locations.

It was probably to an unruly hospital in the annexes of the Casa da Pólvora that António José Miranda e Almeida arrived in 1801. Goa had been without a Portuguese head physician for a while, and, according to the chroniclers, much was expected from this one. He had been a lecturer at the University of Coimbra and was in charge of governing the health services in India and organizing regular teaching. We know that things did not flow easily and he tried to return to Portugal from the start of his time in Goa—a wish he was granted only in 1814. In the meantime, he actually trained a few people in medicine and awarded them a certification. That included Bernardo Peres da Silva, who became famous in the political arena and joined the parliament in Lisbon as a representative of India.[56]

The first half of the nineteenth century was for Portugal and most of the related colonies a time of serious political unsettlement that included Napoleonic wars, a move of the capital from Lisbon to Rio de Janeiro (1808–1820), the independence of Brazil, the civil wars in the mainland, a new Constitution and a parliamentary regime. Part of the action in India involved fractions, parties and loyalties that related to that level of politics. Some doctors were relocated for political reasons, like the Goan Bernardo Peres da Silva or the Portuguese Lima Leitão, who held the post of Head Physician in India only between 1819 and 1822.[57]

Macro politics added another dimension of dissention to the already complex micro politics within the hospital. Although we cannot draw the

---

[54] Pearson 1996.

[55] Walker 2001. According to Correia, the hospital practices had suffered too much the influence of indigenous beliefs; this took to the ban on dietary products like meats and broths and the adoption of native remedies like the *panchagavia*, a mix of five liquids (milk, butter, curd and the two excreta) produced from the cow, see Correia 1948.

[56] Gracias 1914.

[57] Figueiredo 1961.

picture in full, we know that the nineteenth century was a time of drastic changes and remodeling within the health services. We also know that we have to read through, and in spite of, some of the narratives written in the twentieth century about those changes. As I showed in other places, it was only at the beginning of the twentieth century that Goa became strategically important to the late imperial moment lived by the Portuguese administration, one in which Africa was the main target. Throughout the nineteenth century, Goa and its hospitals were the setting for a rich dynamics of local life that we can only partially grasp.[58]

In 1841, the capital of *Estado da Índia* moved to Pangim, temporarily renamed Nova Goa, and the military hospital was relocated in the building of the Maquinezes Palace, formerly a part of the Jesuits' estate, by the river Mandovi. It became known as the Military Hospital of Nova Goa. In 1851 it was renamed the Regimental Hospital of Goa. There were other two regimental hospitals in Daman, and Diu, the other territories that composed the *Estado da Índia*.

The military hospitals of the mid-nineteenth century were no longer the multi-function establishments that in the past had provided room, board and symbols of status to the colonizers. They were actual hospitals with the main mission of providing treatment to the soldiers. More importantly, they were no longer catering to the Portuguese alone. The military hospital of Nova Goa was supposed to accommodate far more than a small group of Portuguese, and also beyond the larger group of Christian natives; it was supposed to also welcome the non-Christians who at the time served in the Portuguese army.

The society, the power relationships within it, and the interweaving of groups and their interests had changed dramatically from the setting where the original Royal Hospital existed. Nineteenth-century Goa was no longer a place where the Portuguese went to look for riches and distinguished positions, as in the early centuries of their presence on the subcontinent, but was a site of tensions, dissensions and misunderstandings between different groups who had different shares of power and agency over their own destinies.[59] As far as medical institutions show, Goan politics and society were entirely different in the early seventeenth century, when the great Royal Hospital existed, and in the mid-nineteenth century, when the medical school was founded. In the sixteenth and seventeenth

58 See Bastos 2007a, 2009.

59 Pinto 2007; Bastos 2007b.

centuries, a luxury hospital catered to the Portuguese and excluded the locals (apart from the tasks of servers and assistants); with the decline of the role of Goa within Portuguese colonialism, the relative positions of social groups changed. Local Christians got more control over material and symbolic resources and, in the end, adopted the medical institutions of the Portuguese for their own purposes and with their *sui generis* adaptations.

The health reports coming from Pangim in its two first decades as capital (1840s–50s) are quite revealing of the tensions that existed there. With the help of those reports, together with legislation and assorted memos from the health services of the Portuguese colony *Estado da Índia*, we are in a position not only to move away from the semi-fictional generic representations of Goan colonial hospitals and to break with the lines of continuity that Germano Correia and Pacheco de Figueiredo trivialized.

The testimonies of head physician Francisco Torres, head surgeon José António de Oliveira, and head physician Eduardo de Freitas e Almeida bring us into a reality that contrasts sharply with the oral and written tradition of a generic golden past, with the glow of Pyrard's depictions, or the evil plots portrayed by Manucci; the reports of the directors bring us the real stuff of infirmaries, pharmacies, latrines, kitchens, diseases, patients, bodies, remedies, prices, laws, rules, regulations, order and chaos.

The Portuguese physicians in charge complained about the limitations and malfunctioning of both hospital and medical school. They also provide details and comments that call for further interpretive efforts in the relationship between medicine and colonial politics in the context of Goa. The kind of political interactions revealed by the close analysis of the health services suggests that far from being a colony that carried out the decisions and instructions of a metropolitan center, Goa was, then, a place where local groups had a strong political influence, even when the rule and command seemed to emanate from the Portuguese administration.

## The Nineteenth Century: Diversity Acknowledged, with a Limit

While in the past the hospitals in colonial Goa had mostly catered to the Catholics or aimed to convert those who received treatment, when we get to the mid nineteenth century a different reality emerges. There were soldiers who were not Christian and should be served by the hospital, which had to find ways to attract them. In 1846, the head physician Francisco

Torres expressed his concern with the fact that people from other faiths would not accept the care of the hospital, preferring instead to be treated at home.[60]

European medicine existed amidst a variety of practices; physicians and pharmacists had strong competitors in the *curões* (healers) and *herbolários* (herbalists).[61] The colonial reports did not distinguish the Ayurvedic practitioners (*vaidyas*) from the village folk healers. There were also the assorted services provided by blood-letters, barbers and midwives. In the nineteenth century, Portuguese authorities tried zealously to maintain the supremacy of European-style medicine and, in vain, tried to prosecute its competitors.[62] Authorities acknowledged that most people preferred to go to the local pharmacists and healers, and that sometimes even the physicians would go to the healers, or adopt some of the healers' secret remedies.[63] Moreover, those in charge of arresting and punishing the healers did not engage in the task, for prosecutors and prosecuted were bound together by the ties of kinship, vicinity, reciprocity, and other social obligations.[64] In sum, the picture of a politically imposed supremacy of European medicine annihilating indigenous healing practices and other associated forms of knowledge does not really come across in the sources; reality was far more complex and chaotic, to the despair of some of the directors of the health services.

Amidst such diversity, the military hospital was one of the few bounded enclaves that provided consistent European-style medical care to the soldiers. But while the treatment followed universal principles, its delivery was mediated by the complex rules of segregation. First of all there was a military hierarchy; there were separate wards for the different ranks. Then, more complex and less explicit, there were the issues of religion and caste. Faced with the reluctance of the non-Christian soldiers regarding admission, as the practices of the hospital might jeopardize their ritual principles of separation and religious observance, the Portuguese head physician Francisco Torres tried in the 1840s to implement a religious-sensitive ward policy that segregated different religions and rites.

Francisco Maria da Silva Torres arrived in Goa in 1844 to hold the post of head physician and to face a number of challenges. Upon arrival he

---

60 Torres 1846b.
61 Oliveira 1853; Almeida 1854, 1856a.
62 Almeida 1856b, 1857.
63 Oliveira 1853.
64 Oliveira 1853.

had to respond to outbreaks of cholera and smallpox. He had to organize a hospital where there was medical teaching but no didactic materials like books or scientific instruments, or even corpses for dissection. The hospital building was in dire need of repair. According to his 1846 report, the surgical wards had no ventilation or light; the skin infirmary was in a humid place and a long way from the bath-house; the drug deposit was in a wretched and damp place, causing numerous and costly losses; the pharmacy was a grubby slum; the kitchen in filthy chaos; and the so-called bath-house was a miserable and petty place whose only entitlement to its name was having two copper basins within its walls.[65]

More interesting for our perspective, though, were his comments on the ways the hospital could, or could not, serve those requiring different religious rites. In his perception, the "Gentiles" could not tolerate being inpatients at the hospital. Many things offended their beliefs and practices. And while at certain moments Francisco Torres indulged in elaborating on the backwardness of the natives, when it came to soldiers—who should be in the care of the hospital—he tried to (or he was forced and pressured to) provide equal treatment for all the different groups. In order to treat the "Gentiles" and "Moors", he created separate infirmaries fit to accommodate their ritual needs. Whether this came from his initiative, was inspired elsewhere, or resulted from competent lobbying from the constituency we can only speculate. But it is a fact that he was able to implement a model of segregated infirmaries under the rationale of providing better treatment.

In his words, he was able to accomplish what "had been considered impossible since the beginning of our domain in Asia", that is, to bring the indigenous patients to the infirmaries. As proof, he confirmed that the infirmaries were filled up with non-Christians and that they were quite happy with the strict care and respect for their varied "beliefs and races". In a memo dated 29 October 1845, after a ceremony that included a procession and a visit by the governor-general to the on-going renovation works at the military hospital, he elaborated on the issue.[66] The purpose of the work was to accommodate the "Gentile and Moorish soldiers", who, in spite of the existence of a regular hospital, would stay and treat themselves at home rather than enter a place that could threaten their ritual practices. Torres mentioned how he was sorry for the fact

65 Torres 1846a.
66 Torres 1845b.

that, for religious reasons, some of the patients would go home and be left on their own without the good care that the hospital could provide them, thus putting their health and their very existence at unnecessary risk. For him, appropriate accommodation, cleanliness, ventilation, diet and remedies—just like in the military hospital in Lisbon—had direct effects on the process of healing. Plus, there should be some amenities that could produce peace of mind, which was vital for a thorough healing. Therefore, for the Hindu patients, there was a room where the pavement was properly dunged, where they had leaf-dishes for their meals, where they could find the appropriate equipment for their ablutions, and where each of them could find a nurse of compatible caste. Francisco Torres was even more emphatic with one detail he considered important for the well-being of the patients: that he was planning to hang on the walls "the images of their idols", and that "Brama, Visnu, Sevá and the Ganezes were going to help Medicine with their moral influence."[67]

We don't know whether those pictures were ever hung on the walls. We know that the segregation of Christians and non-Christians prevailed in infirmaries, toilets, kitchens, and prisoner-infirmaries.[68] But the interest in local customs that Torres showed so openly did not have close followers—nor did his optimism regarding reform. When Francisco Torres left India in March 1849, the head surgeon José António de Oliveira took charge and, as early as April 10th, he produced a report that contained pessimistic remarks about the military hospital and the medical school. They contrast in tone with the early years of Francisco Torres in India. Oliveira complained about the lack of resources, the carelessness of the employees, and what may be understood as widespread corruption. As for the hospital pharmacy—about which Torres had been so enthusiastic—Oliveira noted how it was going downhill, with no appropriate personnel, and decreasing demand for its services.

Besides the military hospital, where most of the reported action took place, in the mid nineteenth century there was, just outside Pangim, another hospital that catered to the poor and civilians and was administered by the Misericórdia. As I mentioned above, it had evolved from the merging of several smaller hospitals. According to Torres, in his memo of 12 March, 1846, "If there is in Goa an establishment that is poorly governed, and that fulfills the least of the purposes for which it was created, it is the

67 Torres 1845b.
68 Oliveira 1853.

Hospital of the Poor, run by Santa Casa da Misericórdia."[69] The place was described as worthless and a third of its patients died there—a contrast with what he reported on other occasions for the military hospital, where, in his words, they were fortunate enough to have a very low number of deaths.[70] A few years later, Almeida commented along the lines of Torres about the Hospital of the Poor, which, in his view, should be moved to Pangim and placed next to the Regimental (Military) Hospital. Almeida's arguments added to the previous ones the fact that the students would benefit much from the observation of a more varied kind of patient.[71]

## Conclusions and Perspectives

If the layout of the Royal Hospital of Goa in the early 1600s matched the organization of a colonial society with small European enclaves and a number of connections with the local groups that included using their workforce while excluding them from the healthcare services, the developments and transformations of the health institutions in Goa indicate that the society changed into something entirely different from the early colonial society. When we get to the nineteenth century, the hospitals that inherited the tradition of the Royal Hospital were very different from it. No longer catering for the colonizers alone, they organized the care of the sick and provided a basis for medical teaching that did not reflect the rationale of imperial governance. Portuguese delegates expressed their puzzlement and sometimes impotence regarding the prevailing order—which they saw as lack of order. Something else was at play—a set of local interests that included the learning and use of European medicine in ways that did not exclude local healing knowledge.

We can see the nineteenth century military hospital as a reflection of the colonial order, but not as the ultimate enclave of empire that followed an idealized rationale of European dominance: here, as in the governance of the colony, the materiality of power was one of several streams that did not melt into a single system, whether homogeneous or plural, but coexisted in peculiar arrangements of differences and tensions. Whether we see them as hybrid formations, half-lives, subaltern arrangements, equivocal compatibilities, or institutionalized misunderstandings, they represent

[69] Torres 1846a.
[70] Torres 1845a.
[71] Almeida 1856b.

not the clear-cut picture of a colonial order idealized by historians on both sides, but the more realistic colors of colonial disarray.

## Bibliography


Abreu, Laurinda, 2001. "O papel das Misericórdias dos 'lugares de além-mar' na formação do império português". *História, Ciências Saúde—Manguinhos*, 8, 3, pp. 591–611.

Almeida, Eduardo de Freitas e, 1854, *Oficio de 11-7-1854*, to Ignacio da Fonseca Benevides, Presidente do Conselho da Saúde Naval e Ultramar. Lisbon, Arquivo Histórico Ultramarino, Sala 12, Serviços de Saúde da Índia, Maço 1987.

——, 1856a, *Oficio de 8-2-1856*, to Ignacio da Fonseca Benevides, Presidente do Conselho da Saúde Naval e Ultramar. Lisbon, Arquivo Histórico Ultramarino, Sala 12, Serviços de Saúde da Índia, Maço 1987.

——, 1856b, *Oficio de 24-11-1856*, to Ignacio da Fonseca Benevides, Presidente do Conselho da Saúde Naval e Ultramar. Lisbon, Arquivo Histórico Ultramarino, Sala 12, Serviço de Saúde da Índia, Maço 1987.

——, 1857, *Relatorio pertencente ao anno de 1857*. Lisboa, Arquivo Histórico Ultramarino, Sala 12, Serviço de Saúde da Índia, Maço 1987.

Bastos, Cristiana, 2001, "Doctors for the Empire: The Medical School of Goa and its Narratives". *Identities*, 8, 4, pp. 517–548.

——, 2002, "The inverted mirror: dreams of imperial glory and tales of subalternity from the Medical School of Goa". *Etnográfica*, VI, 2, pp. 59–76.

——, 2005, "Race, medicine and the late Portuguese empire: the role of Goan colonial physicians". *Journal of Romance Studies*, 5, 1, pp. 23–35.

——, 2007a, "Medical Hybridisms and Social Boundaries: Aspects of Portuguese Colonialism in Africa and India and India in the Nineteenth Century". *Journal of Southern African Studies*, 33, 4, pp. 767–782.

——, 2007b, "Medicina, império e processos locais em Goa, século XIX". *Análise Social*, 182, pp. 99–122.

——, 2009, "Borrowing, Adapting and Learning the Practices of Smallpox: Notes from Colonial Goa". *Bulletin of the History of Medicine*, 83, pp. 140–162.

Carita, Hélder, 1995, *Palácios de Goa*. Lisbon, Quetzal.

Colombina, Francesco Tosi, 1759, "Hospital" (Letter to the Governor about the adaptations need to turn the annexes of Casa da Pólvora into a hospital). Ms. Lisbon, Biblioteca da Ajuda, Av. 54–X-20, n.º 64.

Correia, A. Germano da Silva, 1917 *História do Ensino Médico na India Portuguesa*. Nova Goa: Imprensa Nacional.

——, 1941, *O ensino de medicina e cirurgia em Goa nos séculos XVII, XVIII*[e] *XIX: história do ensino médico-cirúrgico no Hospital Real de Goa, antes da fundação da Escola Médico-Cirúrgica de Nova Goa*. Bastorá, Tipografia Rangel.

——, 1948, "O Hospital Real de Goa nos Séculos XVI e XVII", *Arquivos da Escola Médico-Cirúrgica* A, 18, pp. 159–248.

Costa, Pedro Joaquim Peregrino da, 1943, "Médicos da Escola de Goa nos Quadros de Saúde das Colónias (1853–1942)". *Boletim do Instituto Vasco da Gama*, 57, pp. 1–43, 58, pp. 1–66.

——, 1957, "A Escola Médica de Goa e a sua projecção na Índia portuguesa e no Ultramar", in: P. J. P. Costa, ed., *Escola Médico-Cirúrgica de Goa (1842–1957)*. Bastorá, Tipografia Rangel, pp. 19–34.

Dalgado, Sebastião Rodolfo, 1919–1921, *Glossário Luso-Asiático*. Coimbra, Academia das Sciencias.

Figueiredo, João Manuel Pacheco de, 1960, "Escola Médico-Cirúrgica de Goa: esboço histórico". *Arquivos da Escola Médico Cirúrgica de Goa*, A, 33, pp. 119–237.

——, 1961, *A vida acidentada do Físico-mór Lima Leitão, mestre de medicina em Goa e em Lisboa*. Porto, Tipografia Sequeira.

Gracias, Fátima, 1994, *Health and hygiene in colonial Goa (1510–1961)*. New Delhi, Concept Publishing House.

Gracias, José António Ismael, 1914, "Fisicos-Móres da India no Seculo XIX. Memoria historica". *O Oriente Português*, XI, 11–12, pp. 255–278.

Linschoten, Jan Huygen van, 1596, *A ilha e cidade de Goa metropolitana da India e partes orientais que esta en 15 graos da banda do norte*, engraved by Baptista van Doetichum, Amsterdam.

——, 1885, *The voyage of John Huyghen van Linschoten to the East Indies from the old English translation of 1598*. London, Hakluyt Society.

Manucci, Nicolò, 1907, *Storia do Mogor*, English translation: *Moghul India 1653–1708 or Storia do Mogor*, 4 vols., W. Irvine, ed., London, John Murray.

Martins, José F. Ferreira, 1912, *Historia da Misericórdia de Goa 1621–1910*. Nova Goa, Imprensa Nacional, Vol. 2.

Mendes, Lopes, 1886, *A India Portuguesa*. Lisboa, Imprensa Nacional.

Oliveira, José António de, 1853, *Relatório do Estado das Repartições de Saúde do estado da Índia, 11-7-1853*, to Ignacio da Fonseca Benevides, do Conselho de Saúde Naval e Ultramar. Lisbon, Arquivo Histórico Ultramarino, Sala 12, Serviços de Saúde da Índia, Maço 1987.

Pearson, M. N., 1996, "First Contacts Between Indian and European Medical Systems: Goa in the Sixteenth Century", in: D. Arnold, ed., *Warm Climates and Western Medicine*. Amsterdam, Rodopi, pp. 20–41.

——, 2001, "The Portuguese State and Medicine in Sixteenth Century Goa", in: K. S. Mathew—T. R. de Souza—P. Malekandathil, eds., *The Portuguese and the Socio-Cultural Changes in India, 1500–1800*. Tellicherry, Institute for Research in Social Sciences and Humanities, pp. 401–419.

Pinto, Rochelle, 2007, *Between Empires: Print and Politics in Goa*. Delhi, Oxford University Press.

Pyrard, François, 1998, *Voyage de Pyrard de Laval aux Indes orientales, 1601–1611*, 2 vols., G. Bouchon, ed., Paris, Chadeigne.

Sá, Isabel dos Guimarães, 1997, *Quando o rico se faz pobre: misericórdias, caridade e poder no império português 1500–1800*. Lisbon, Comissão Nacional para as Comemorações dos Descobrimentos Portugueses.

Saldanha, M. J. Gabriel de, 1926, *História de Goa, Vol. II, História arqueológica*. Nova Goa, Livraria Coelho.

Santos, Sebastião da Costa, 1925, *A Escola de Cirurgia do Hospital Real de Todos os Santos, 1565–1775*. Lisbon, Faculdade de Medicina.

Silva, Vitor Freire da, 1998, *O Hospital Real de Goa*, tese de mestrado em historia de arte, Lisbon, Faculdade de Letras.

Souza, Teotónio R. de, 1979, *Medieval Goa*. New Delhi, Concept.

Subrahmanyam, Sanjay, 2009. "Between a Rock and a Hard Place: Some Afterthoughts", in: S. Schaffer—L. Roberts—K. Raj—J. Delbourgo, eds., *The Brokered World: Go-Between and Global Intelligence, 1770–1820*. Sagamore Beach, Science History Publications—Uppsala studies in the history of science, 35, pp. 429–440.

Torres, Francisco Maria da Silva, 1845a, *Oficio de 10–7–1845*, Lisbon, Arquivo Histórico Ultramarino, Sala 12, Serviço de Saúde da Índia, Maço nº 1987, Ofícios dos empregados, 1840–1868.

——, 1845b, *Oficio de 29-10-1845*, Lisbon, Arquivo Histórico Ultramarino, Sala 12, Serviço de Saúde da Índia, Maço 1987, Ofícios dos empregados, 1840–1868.

——, 1846a, *Oficio de 12-3-1846*, to Bernardino António Gomes, Presidente do Conselho da Saúde Naval e Ultramar. Lisbon, Arquivo Histórico Ultramarino, Sala 12, Serviço de Saúde da Índia, Maço 1987, Ofícios dos empregados, 1840–1868.

——, 1846b, *Oficio de 21-4-1846*, to Bernardino António Gomes, Presidente do Conselho da Saúde Naval e Ultramar. Lisbon, Arquivo Histórico Ultramarino, Sala 12, Serviços de Saúde da Índia, Maço 1987, Ofícios dos empregados, 1840–1868.

Walker, Timothy, 2001, "Remedies from the *Carreira da Índia*: Asian Influences on Portuguese Medicine during the Age of Enlightenment". *The Portuguese Studies Review*, 9, 1–2, pp. 170–193.

Xavier, Ângela Barreto, 2007, *A Invenção de Goa*. Lisbon, Imprensa de Ciências Sociais.

Županov, Ines G. 1999. *Disputed Mission: Jesuit Experiments and Brahmanical Knowledge in Seventeenth-century India*. New Delhi, Oxford University Press.

——, 2008, "Conversion, Illness and Possession: Catholic Missionary Healing in Early Modern South Asia", *Divins remèdes. Médecine et religion en Asie du sud*. Paris, collection *Purusartha*, 27, Editions de l'Ecole des Hautes Etudes en Sciences Sociales, pp. 263–300.

# TRADITION ET RÉFORME DU *DĀR AL-ŠIFĀ* AU DECCAN

Fabrizio Speziale

## Introduction : Hôpitaux et institutions musulmanes dans la société du Deccan

Cet article examine la fondation de deux hôpitaux (*dār al-šifā, šifā-ḫāna*) dédiés à la médecine avicennienne, appelée *yūnānī ṭibb* en Inde[1], et qui furent établis dans la ville de Hyderabad. Le premier *dār al-šifā* fut institué à la fin du XVIe siècle, sous le sultan Muḥammad Qulī Quṭb Šāh (m. 1612), le fondateur de Hyderabad. Le second, le Niẓāmiya ṣadr šifā-ḫāna, fut établi à l'époque coloniale sous le dernier Niẓām, Mīr 'Uṯmān 'Alī Ḫān (r. 1911–1948). Le premier établissement incarne le modèle type de l'hôpital traditionnel du monde musulman selon lequel le *dār al-šifā* faisait partie d'un complexe incluant d'autres établissements, tels la mosquée et la madrasa. Le second présente d'importants nouveaux éléments s'éloignant du modèle ancien et qui reflètent les tendances réformistes et d'ouverture vers le savoir scientifique colonial, qui à cette époque s'affirmèrent parmi les médecins *yūnānī*.

Les musulmans introduisirent dans le monde scientifique indien une nouvelle école médicale dont l'hôpital comptait parmi les institutions typiques. L'établissement des hôpitaux découlait essentiellement des activités et donations des souverains et des nobles dont le mécénat alimentait également la production d'ouvrages médicaux et scientifiques ainsi que la fondation d'autres institutions et établissements typiques des villes musulmanes, tels les mosquées, madrasas, sanctuaires (*dargāh*), hammams, caravansérails. Comme ces établissements, les hôpitaux pouvaient être fondés ou financés grâce à des *waqf* (fondation de mainmorte) et des *jāgīr* (revenus de terres et de villages), constitués par les sultans et les nobles.

D'importantes considérations à propos des hôpitaux établis au Deccan découlent de l'analyse de leur rôle vis-à-vis de celui d'autres institutions musulmanes, notamment de celles qui se trouvaient également liées à la

[1] Sur le terme *yūnānī ṭibb* (médecine grecque) cf. Speziale 2005.

pratique et à la transmission de la médecine (*ṭibb*). Si on les compare à d'autres institutions, les hôpitaux se développèrent plus tardivement au Deccan et demeurèrent toujours beaucoup moins nombreux que les établissements comme les madrasas, les *dargāh* ou les hammams. Les conditions nécessaires à la création d'hôpitaux au Deccan ne purent être réunies qu'une fois le pouvoir politique et le milieu scientifique musulmans solidement implantés. Lorsque des hôpitaux furent édifiés à Bidar et à Hyderabad, ces villes comptaient parmi les principaux centres d'études musulmanes de la région. Ainsi, ces hôpitaux, au contraire d'autres établissements, furent uniquement établis au cours des phases d'affirmation du pouvoir de certaines dynasties et de développement urbain de leur capitale. Il faut comparer en particulier le rôle des hôpitaux à celui des familles. Les familles de médecins, au sein desquelles le savoir était transmis de père en fils, constituaient l'institution médicale musulmane la plus importante au Deccan. Avant le XX^e^ siècle, l'hôpital détenait une importance infiniment plus modeste que les cabinets des médecins et leurs lignées, qu'il s'agisse de l'assistance aux malades ou de l'enseignement médical. Les familles conservaient évidement des formes beaucoup plus durables de transmission de la pratique, tandis que les hôpitaux ne constituaient pas des institutions permanentes au Deccan. Les hôpitaux, et les *waqf* constitués pour les financer, ne survivaient que rarement aux changements de pouvoir et de dynasties. Par exemple, le *dār al-šifā* édifié par le sultan Muḥammad Qulī ne demeura vraisemblablement pas en activité à l'époque des Niẓāms (1720–1948). Durant de longues périodes, il ne se trouvait donc pas d'hôpitaux opérant au Deccan. Les *waqf* constitués pour financer les institutions telles que les madrasas[2] et les *dargāh*[3], également actives dans l'enseignement médical et l'assistance aux malades,

[2] À l'époque d'Akbar (r. 1556–1605) la médecine fut incluse dans le programme de cours des madrasas de l'empire moghol, cf. Abū al-Fażl, 2001, vol. 1, p. 289. Le *dars-i niẓāmī*, le programme qui s'impose dans les madrasas indiennes dès le XVIII^e^ siècle, n'inclut pas, au début, la médecine, qui sera ajoutée plus tard. Sayyid Aḥmad Ḫān (m. 1898) rapporte qu'à son époque le *dars-i niẓāmī* incluait six textes de médecine, qui étaient surtout des abrégés ou commentaires du *Qānūn* d'Avicenne (m. 1037), cf. Sufi 1941, pp. 120, 124. A la fin du XIX^e^ siècle, la médecine est insérée dans le cours de la madrasa de Deoband, l'une des écoles religieuses islamiques les plus importantes du sous-continent.

[3] Plusieurs hospices et sanctuaires soufis offraient – et ils offrent encore aujourd'hui – assistance à malades et sans-logis. Les cultes de guérison des saints musulmans attiraient des nombreux malades, également parmi les hindous, et certains sanctuaires en particulier devinrent célèbres pour leurs rituels de guérison, cf. Speziale 2008, 2010a.

étaient en revanche beaucoup plus durables que les *waqf* constitués pour les hôpitaux.

Avant l'époque coloniale, la place de l'hôpital dans l'instruction médicale au Deccan resta également fort limitée. Dans ce domaine, le rôle joué par l'enseignement privé et les familles était incomparablement plus important. C'est seulement à partir des dernières années du XIXe siècle, que la nouvelle école étatique de médecine *yūnānī* de Hyderabad – ensuite englobée dans l'hôpital – commença à acquérir une certaine importance. À cette époque, une partie considérable des professeurs, étudiants et médecins de l'école, de l'hôpital et des dispensaires établis par les derniers Niẓāms étaient constituée par les membres des familles de médecins.

Si ces remarques indiquent que l'hôpital ne fut certainement pas l'institution médicale musulmane la plus importante du Deccan, son développement dans cette région détient néanmoins une place considérable pour l'histoire tardive de cette institution au sein du monde musulman. Ce fut en effet à Hyderabad que fut établi l'un des hôpitaux de médecine avicennienne parmi les plus importants de l'Inde et de l'ensemble du monde musulman du XXe siècle, alors même que dans les pays islamiques, la médecine avicennienne était en fort déclin. Les sources nous offrent des descriptions assez lacunaires des plus anciennes de ces institutions au Deccan, dont on sait très peu regardant les médecins qui y étaient employés. Les sources concernant l'hôpital et les dispensaires étatiques établis à l'époque des derniers Niẓāms sont en revanche beaucoup plus détaillées, alors que furent également composés d'importants ouvrages en ourdou décrivant le milieu médical *yūnānī* de Hyderabad à cette époque.

## Les premiers hôpitaux

La culture scientifique musulmane s'implanta plus solidement dans le Deccan avec la dynastie des sultans Bahmanī, fondée en 748/1347, dont la capitale fut Gulbarga, puis Bidar. Les capitales des Bahmanī, et plus tard, celles des sultanats du Deccan qui surgirent avec le déclin des Bahmanī, devinrent des centres capables d'attirer de nombreux savants musulmans sunnites et chiites d'Iran et des pays arabes, comme de l'Inde du Nord. Ainsi, la communauté des étrangers (*āfāqī*) allait occuper un rôle important dans la vie politique, scientifique et culturelle des sultanats du Deccan.

Un *dār al-šifā* fut établi à Bidar sous ʿAlāʾ al-Dīn II (r. 1435–1457), le deuxième sultan bahmanide à régner dans cette ville. L'hôpital était probablement situé entre la madrasa de Maḥmūd Gāwān et le fort de Bidar[4]. L'Iranien Muḥammad Qāsim Hindūšāh Firišta (né vers 978/1570), qui était également médecin et auteur d'un traité persan sur la médecine indienne[5], mentionne l'hôpital dans son histoire des royaumes indo-musulmans, *Gulšan-i Ibrāhīmī*[6]. Firišta écrit que ʿAlāʾ al-Dīn II constitua en *waqf* les revenus (*maḥṣūl*) des quelques villages pour les dépenses en médicaments (*adwiya*) et nourriture (*aġḏiya*) de l'hôpital[7]. La même information est donnée par Sayyid ʿAlī Ṭabāṭabāʾī, un historien irakien contemporain de Firišta qui fut au service des sultans de Golconde et d'Ahmadnagar. Il cite plus spécifiquement « deux » villages, dont les revenus furent constitués en *waqf*[8]. En sus, Firišta écrit qu'au *dār al-šifā* de Bidar on employait soit des médecins musulmans soit des médecins hindous[9]. Selon une autre source, citée par Rahbar Fārūqī, auteur de la première histoire en ourdou de la médecine *yūnānī* en Inde[10], tous les types de diètes y étaient dispensés gratuitement, ce qui indique peut-être qu'une alimentation différente était préparée, selon que les patients étaient hindous ou musulmans[11].

On peut supposer que cet hôpital était encore en fonction au début du XVIe siècle. Il est improbable que l'hôpital ne soit pas resté ouvert à l'époque de l'apogée du pouvoir bahmanide, sous le vizir Maḥmūd Gāwān (m. 1481), un Iranien originaire du Gilan qui établit une importante madrasa à Bidar et était lui-même un savant en médecine[12]. On ne retrouve pas de références sur la condition de cet hôpital à l'époque de la dynastie des Barīd Šāh, qui régna sur Bidar de 1528 à 1619.

Avec le déclin bahmanide, on vit au Deccan la création de cinq sultanats dont les trois plus importants, Ahmadnagar (1490–1633), Bijapur

---

4 Voir le plan de la ville dans Yazdani 1995, troisième de couverture. A l'époque des Niẓāms, le *civil dispensary* de Bidar se trouvait à proximité de cet endroit de la ville, cf. Framurz Jung 1894, p. 9.

5 Intitulé *Dastūr al-aṭibbā*, cf. Speziale 2010b, pp. 418, 420–421.

6 Firišta avait migré d'Astarabad (Iran) au Deccan, où il entra au service des cours des sultans d'Ahmadnagar et de Bijapur, il inclut dans son *Gulšan-i Ibrāhīmī* (appelé aussi *Tārīḫ-i Firišta*) des descriptions d'autres hôpitaux établis sous des souverains musulmans en Inde.

7 Firišta 1290/1874, p. 333.

8 Ṭabāṭabāʾī 1355/1936, p. 87.

9 Firišta 1290/1874, p. 333.

10 L'ouvrage fut publié à Hyderabad en 1937, cf. Fārūqī 1356/1937.

11 Fārūqī 1356/1937, p. 136. La source citée par Fārūqī est le *Tārīḫ-i Rašīd al-Dīn Ḫānī*, un ouvrage historique en ourdou composé au XIXe siècle par Ġulām Imām Ḫān.

12 Cf. Ḥasanī 1408/1988, vol. 3, p. 123.

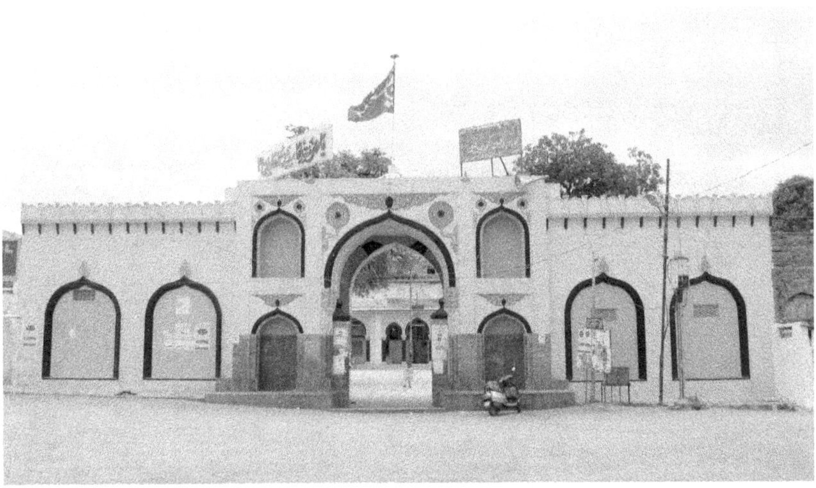

Figure 1. Portail du *dār al-šifā* de Hyderarabd (1595–96).

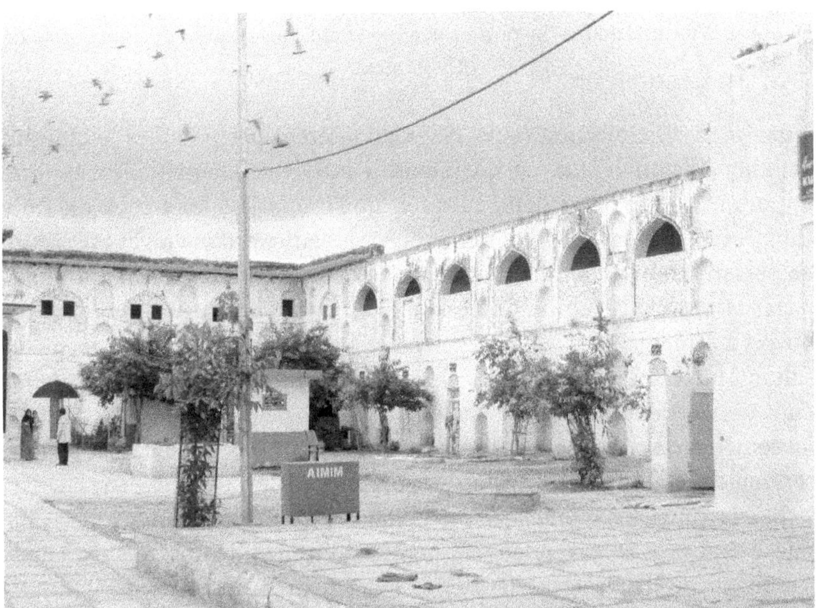


Figure 2. Vue de la cour intérieure du *dār al-šifā* de Hyderabad.

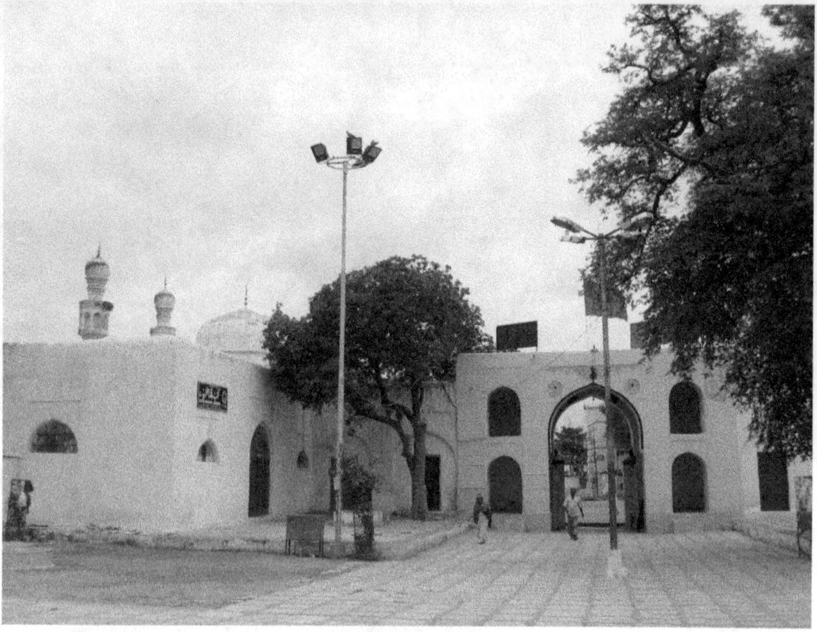

Figure 3. Vue intérieure du portail avec au fond la mosquée du *dār al-šifā* de Hyderabad.

(1490–1686) et Golconde (1518–1687), adoptèrent par périodes le chiisme comme religion d'État, ce qui favorisa le développement de rapports importants entre les milieux culturels de l'Iran safavide et ceux du Deccan. Des médecins d'origine iranienne et des auteurs d'ouvrages médicaux en persan furent notamment attachés aux cours des Niẓām Šāh d'Ahmadnagar et des Quṭb Šāh de Golconde. Fārūqī rapporte qu'un *šifā-ḫāna* fut ouvert à Ahmadnagar par le médecin Zayn al-Dīn Simānī, sous le règne du sultan Murtażā I (r. 1565–1588). Cependant, on ne sait pas si ce *šifā-ḫāna* était un véritable hôpital ou seulement un dispensaire. Fārūqī écrit que les remèdes qui y étaient préparés étaient vendus, ce qui peut faire supposer que cet établissement n'était pas financé grâce à un *waqf*[13].

Par la suite, un *dār al-šifā* fut établi à Hyderabad, la nouvelle capitale des Quṭb Šāh, fondée en 999/1590–01. Les Quṭb Šāh régnaient sur un territoire vaste et fertile, et leur capitale devint une ville opulente, leur sultanat étant le principal centre mondial pour l'extraction des diamants. Le cinquième sultan de la dynastie, Muḥammad Qulī

[13] Fārūqī 1356/1937, p. 141.

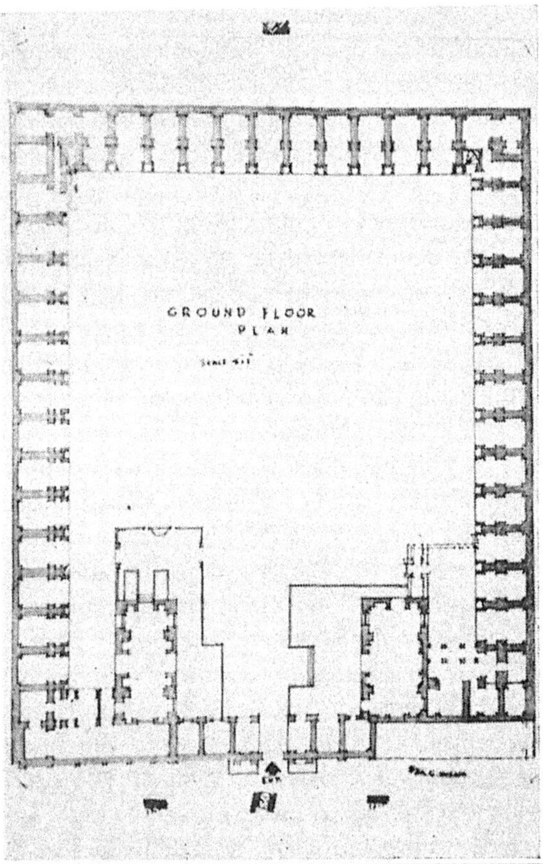


Plan 1. Plan du premier étage du *dār al-šifā* de Hyderabad, d'après Reddy 1957.

(r. 1580–1612), abandonna la forteresse surpeuplée de Golconde et non loin de cette-ci, à l'est, fonda Hyderabad. La ville fut planifiée à la période hautement symbolique du passage du premier au deuxième millénaire de l'hégire (l'année 1000 tomba en 1591–92). Muḥammad Qulī était un contemporain du moghol Akbar (r. 1556–1605) et du safavide Šāh ʿAbbās (r. 1588–1629), et comme ces souverains il fit édifier un hôpital dans sa nouvelle capitale. Les villes majeures du royaume safavide disposaient à cette époque d'hôpitaux[14] et d'Iran arrivaient d'éminents médecins qui furent attachés à la cour des Quṭb Šāh. Parmi les Quṭb Šāh, Muḥammad

14 Voir les articles de Hasan Tadjbakhsh et de Willem Floor dans ce volume.

Qulī fut le plus important mécène des études médicales, et l'un des plus importants de l'Inde de son époque, considérant que quatre traités médicaux en persan furent composés pour lui[15]. L'établissement de l'hôpital de Hyderabad se situe donc à une époque caractérisée par un grand développement urbain et architectural, qui correspond à la phase majeure du mécénat de la littérature médicale à la cour, alors même que le *pīšwā* du sultanat, l'Iranien Mīr Mu'min, était un savant en médecine.

Le *dār al-šifā* de Hyderabad fut édifié en 1004/1595–96[16]. L'hôpital faisait partie d'un complexe qui comprenait un hammam, un caravansérail, une mosquée et une madrasa. Le *dār al-šifā* fut placé à proximité de la rive sud du fleuve Musi, vers le nord-est de la ville, en un point éloigné du centre. À son côté se trouvait le jardin Bāġ-i Muḥammad Šāhī, dont la beauté fut célébrée par le même sultan Muḥammad Qulī dans un de ses poèmes[17]. Un bref portrait de l'hôpital, deux décennies environ après son établissement, est donné dans le *Tārīḫ-i Muḥammad Quṭb Šāh* (1026/1617), une histoire anonyme des Quṭb Šāh. Ce texte rapporte que dans le *dār al-šifā* étaient employés des médecins experts – dotés du « souffle qui rend la vie aux mourants » (*masiḥā-nafas*) –, il mentionne la pharmacie (*dārū-ḫāna*) de l'hôpital et la présence d'oulémas et d'étudiants. Il parle également du hammam situé à côté du *dār al-šifā* et en admire le bâtiment, remarquant que même un peintre dans son atelier n'aurait pu le concevoir[18]. Selon le *Mah-nāma* (1229/1814), un ouvrage historique plus tardif de Ġulām Ḥusayn Ḫān, un savant qui écrivit également sur la médecine, l'hôpital pouvait accueillir environ quatre mille malades[19]. Cette information se retrouve parfois citée à propos du *dār al-šifā* de Hyderabad[20]. Cependant, ce chiffre paraît très exagéré et il est raisonnable de penser à une erreur de transcription ; il s'agissait peut-être de quatre cents, ce qui reste un chiffre assez élevé par rapport au nombre de chambres du bâtiment. Le chiffre de quatre cents pouvait éventuellement se référer au complexe entier du *dār al-šifā*, qui incluait un caravansérail, dont le bâtiment n'a cependant pas été conservé.

---

15 Cf. Speziale 2009a.
16 Cf. Bilgrāmī 1342/1924, pp. 13–15 ; Sherwani 1974, p. 314.
17 Sur le Bāġ-i Muḥammad Šāhī cf. Husain 2000, p. 36.
18 *Tārīḫ-i Muḥammad Quṭb Šāhī*, f. 189v.
19 Ḫān, *Mah-nāma*, p. 352.
20 Cf. pour exemple Jaggi 1977, p. 127.

Ce *dār al-šifā* compte parmi les vestiges les plus anciens d'hôpitaux indiens de l'époque musulmane conservé jusqu'à nos jours[21]. Le bâtiment compte environ quatre-vingts chambres situées au sein de quatre ailes, sur deux étages, et disposées autour d'une grande cour (fig. 2). L'entrée de l'hôpital est orientée vers le nord, elle est constituée par un portail dont la façade extérieure comporte quatre niches, deux de chaque côté, et est ornée de médaillons et décorations de stuc à motifs floraux dont le style est conforme à celui d'autres constructions d'époque qutbšahide (fig. 1). Les arches et les niches sont en pointe, comme celles du Čār Mīnār (1591). Les niches situées à coté du portail sont surmontées par des *ʿalam* (étendards) de stuc, symboles de la foi chiite du sultan. Des niches et des décorations de stuc, de petits médaillons, *ʿalam* et plumets, apparaissent également sur la façade de la porte sud et sur les ailes du bâtiment donnant sur la cour. L'aile nord, qui inclut le portail, loge huit chambres à chaque étage. Les trois autres ailes logent douze ou treize chambres par étage (voir plan 1), tandis que des escaliers conduisent du deuxième étage à la terrasse. Quelques chambres de l'aile sud sont munies de niches et d'armoires[22].

On ne retrouve que des indications limitées à propos des médecins qui travaillaient dans ce *dār al-šifā*. Mīr Muḥammad Mu'min Astarābādī (m. 1034/1625 environ), savant chiite et premier ministre (*pīšwā*) du sultanat, fut probablement celui qui décida de l'emplacement de l'hôpital[23]. Il était également un savant en médecine et composa pour Muḥammad Qulī un traité sur la pharmacopée intitulé *Iḫtiyārāt-i Quṭb Šāhī*, un commentaire de l'*Iḫtiyārāt-i Badīʿī* de Zayn al-Dīn al-Anṣārī (m. 806/1403) de Chiraz[24]. Mīr Mu'min joua vraisemblablement un rôle important dans la conception du plan urbain de Hyderabad et la disposition des principales

21 Le bâtiment du *dār al-šifā* se trouve aujourd'hui dans un état d'abandon. Pour les autres édifices du complexe, le hammam n'existe plus, et les ruines du caravansérail ont été englobées par de laides habitations abusives, cf. Sherwani 1974, p. 315. Il reste seulement la mosquée, édifiée par Muḥammad Qulī en face de l'entrée de l'hôpital (fig. 3).

22 Sur le bâtiment cf. Reddy 1961, p. 23 ; Sherwani 1974, p. 314.

23 Mīr Mu'min favorisa grandement l'influence d'éléments iraniens et la diffusion du chiisme dans la ville, essayant de faire de Hyderabad une nouvelle Ispahan, cf. Zūr 1941, pp. 113–115. En Iran, il avait été attaché à la cour du safavide Šāh Ṭahmāsp (r. 1524–1576), en tant que tuteur de son fils Ḥaydar. Mīr Mu'min arriva à Golconde peu après la mort du sultan Ibrāhīm Quṭb Šāh (m. 988/1580) et quelques années plus tard Muḥammad Qulī le nomma *pīšwā*, charge à laquelle il fut maintenu durant le règne de Muḥamamd Quṭb Šāh (r. 1612–1626). Sur Mīr Mu'min cf. en particulier la biographie de Zūr 1941.

24 Il composa également la *Risāla-yi miqdāriya*, un traité sur les mesures et les poids, incluant ceux utilisés en médecine.

constructions, dont l'hôpital, qui se trouvait proche de sa résidence[25]. En 1014/1605, il fait édifier à Sayyidābād[26] une mosquée qui se différencie d'autres mosquées érigées à la même période par son plan qui reprend, à moindre échelle, le modèle du *dār al-šifā* de Hyderabad[27]. Selon une note d'Aṣġar Bilgrāmī, l'hôpital fut placé sous la direction de Ṣafī al-Dīn Muḥammad Ṭabīb Gīlānī[28]. Ce nom suggère que ce médecin, ou sa famille, étaient originaires du Gilan (Iran), on ne possède cependant pas de détails biographiques précis sur sa vie. On sait qu'il était en activité à l'époque de Muḥammad Qulī, à sa cour probablement, et qu'il composa deux textes en persan : le *Taḏkira al-šahwāt fī tabṣirat al-laḏḏāt*, un traité sur la sexologie, et le *Dastūr al-ṭibb*, un dictionnaire des termes médicaux[29].

Certaines sources font mention que des salaires élevés furent assignés par le gouvernement aux médecins employés dans cet hôpital. Le *Hadīqat al-ʿālam*, ouvrage attribué à Mīr ʿĀlam (m. 1223/1808), explique que le but en cela était que les médecins soient satisfaits, afin qu'ils se consacrent entièrement à leur emploie au *dār al-šifā*[30]. Il est vraisemblable que cette mesure ait visé à encourager les médecins qualifiés à y travailler, au lieu de se cantonner à l'activité privée et au service des nobles, dont les profits considérables comptaient parmi les principales raisons poussant à cette époque les médecins musulmans étrangers à émigrer vers les villes indiennes. Cependant, on ignore ce que fut l'efficacité de cette mesure, ni si d'autres médecins connus pour avoir été attachés aux cours de Muḥammad Qulī et de ses successeurs, furent également associés au *dār al-šifā*.

Le *dār al-šifā* et sa madrasa ont souvent été présentés comme étant un centre dédié à l'enseignement médical[31]. Celui-ci constituerait un cas très rare pour cette époque, considérant que l'on ne connaît pas de madrasas qui aient été exclusivement consacrées à l'enseignement médical, ni d'écoles médicales fonctionnant à l'intérieur d'hôpitaux, en activité dans

---

[25] Cf. le plan de la ville donné par Sherwani 1968, p. 12.

[26] Localité située à quelques kilomètres de Hyderabad.

[27] La mosquée de Sayyidābād incluait en sus un caravansérail ou une école, cf. Zūr 1941: 47–53, 65–85 ; Sherwani 1974, pp. 316–317.

[28] Cette note de Bilgrāmī, l'auteur du *Ma'ātir-i Dakan* (cf. Bilgrāmī 1342/1924), est donnée sous la forme d'une communication personnelle adressée par Bilgrāmī à Subba Reddy, dans l'article de Reddy 1962, p. 28.

[29] Le premier fut composé en 987/1579, cf. Munzawī 1362/1983, p. 564 ; 1382/2003, pp. 3356, 3453.

[30] Mīr ʿĀlam 1309/1892, vol. 1, p. 217, cf. également Fārūqī 1356/1937, p. 142.

[31] Cf. par exemple Reddy 1961, p. 24 ; Reddy 1962, p. 22 ; Sherwani 1968, p. 30, 1974, p. 314 ; Jaggi 1977, p. 127 ; Bari 1986–1987, p. 136 ; Azmi 2004, p. 26.

les villes de l'Inde moghole ou de l'Iran safavide. À notre avis, il est plus vraisemblable de supposer que la madrasa du *dār al-šifā* de Hyderabad était une madrasa traditionnelle, où étaient enseignées les disciplines religieuses et scientifiques – y compris la médecine – faisant partie du cursus d'études des madrasas indiennes. On ne dispose pas de détails précis sur le cursus utilisé dans les madrasas de la période quṭbšahide, on sait cependant qu'à la même époque, la médecine faisait partie de celui des madrasas de l'empire moghol[32]. Comme nous l'avons déjà précisé, plusieurs hôpitaux faisaient partie de complexes incluant d'autres institutions ; des complexes comprenant un hôpital et une madrasa se retrouvent à l'époque safavide dans les villes d'Ispahan, Tabriz et Chiraz. Le seul enseignant dont on connaît la présence à cette époque à la madrasa du *dār al-šifā* de Hyderabad est Mullā Ḫalqī Šūstarī, lui aussi un savant d'origine iranienne ayant émigré vers le Deccan. Ḫalqī Šūstarī n'était pas un médecin, Niẓām al-Dīn Aḥmad, un historien du règne du sultan ʿAbd Allāh Quṭb Šāh (r. 1626–1672), et contemporain de Šustarī, le décrit en tant que poète et savant du *ʿilm-i jafr* et rapporte qu'à l'époque de ʿAbd Allāh, il enseignait les sciences rationnelles et traditionnelles (*ʿulūm-i maʿqūl wa manqūl*) ainsi que les disciplines mathématiques (*funūn-i riyāẓī*)[33]. Le fait que quelques sources y mentionnent l'activité de *ʿulamā*, à commencer par la plus ancienne, le *Tārīḫ-i Muḥammad Quṭb Šāhī*[34], fait là aussi supposer que l'école du *dār al-šifā* était une madrasa traditionnelle et non un centre consacré à l'enseignement de la médecine[35].

Les voyageurs européens qui visitèrent Hyderabad à l'époque des deux derniers sultans quṭbšāhides, ʿAbd Allāh et Abū al-Ḥasan (r. 1672–1687), ne mentionnent pas l'hôpital[36]. Un événement situé à l'époque moghole paraît cependant indiquer que le *dār al-šifā* était encore ouvert à l'époque d'Awrangzīb (r. 1658–1707), qui conquit Hyderabad en 1098/1687. Le

32 Cf. note 2.

33 Niẓām al-Dīn Aḥmad 1961, pp. 210–111.

34 *Tārīḫ-i Muḥammad Quṭb Šāhī*, f. 189v ; cf. aussi Mīr ʿĀlam 1309/1892, vol. 1, p. 217.

35 Qādir Ḫān, un historien de la première moitié du XIXe siècle, rapporte que des formes d'allocation (*maʿāš*) étaient assignées par le gouvernement aux étudiants de la madrasa, Qādir Ḫān 1306/1889, pp. 16–17.

36 Jean-Baptiste Tavernier (m. 1689), qui visita la ville à l'époque du sultan ʿAbd Allāh, rapporte que dans les royaumes de Vijayanagar, de Golconde et de Bijapur il n'y avait guère de médecins que pour les rois et les princes. Peu après, Tavernier ajoute cependant que dans les bonnes villes il y avait quelques hommes qui tâtaient le pouls des malades en donnant potions et emplâtres, pour lesquels ils ne prenaient que la valeur de deux liards, Tavernier 1676, vol. 2, pp. 189–190.

sunnite Awrangzīb ordonna de fermer tous les *ʿāšūr-ḫāna*[37] de la ville, sauf les lieux où l'on conservait une relique ou un *ʿalam* étant à l'origine de quelques miracles. Cela était le cas d'une relique de l'Imam Zayn al-ʿAbidīn (m. 94/712) qui avait été apportée de Syrie à l'époque des Quṭb Šāh, et qu'Awrangzīb commanda de transférer au *dār al-šifā*, de sorte à ce que les malades puissent bénéficier de sa bénédiction. Dans un *farmān* daté du mois de *rajab* 1110/janvier 1699, Awrangzīb ordonna également qu'une certaine quantité d'argent soit prélevée du budget de l'hôpital et assignée à l'achat de fleurs et d'encens utilisés pour honorer la relique[38]. A l'époque moghole, un hôpital existait également à Awrangabad, dont Muḥibb ʿAlī ibn ʿAbd al-Mahdī fut le surintendant (*dāroġa*) sous Šāh Jahān (r. 1628–1658)[39]. Muḥammad Zamān fut ensuite le *dāroġa* de cet hôpital sous Awrangzīb, il recevait un salaire mensuel de 136 roupies, bien que selon un récépissé (*qabż al-wāṣil*) de son salaire, il était dispensé (*muʿāf*) d'être présent à l'hôpital[40].

## La réforme du *dār al-šifā* : le Niẓāmiya Ṣadr Šifā-ḫāna

Le contrôle des Moghols fut suivi par l'arrivée au pouvoir des Niẓāms qui régnèrent sur Hyderabad de 1724 environ à 1948. Durant le XIXe siècle et la première moitié du XXe, Hyderabad devint avec Delhi, Lucknow et Bhopal, l'un des centres de la dernière époque de la littérature médicale indo-persane, du développement de la littérature médicale ourdoue et de nouvelles institutions visant à adapter la tradition *yūnānī* aux conditions scientifiques de l'Inde coloniale, marquées par la suprématie de la science occidentale. Le projet du nouvel hôpital *yūnānī* de Hyderabad, comme celui d'autres institutions *yūnānī* créées vers la même époque, était étroitement lié aux instances du mouvement de réforme de la médecine *yūnānī* qui s'affirma à la période coloniale. L'hôpital *yūnānī* de Hyderabad et son collège résultèrent ainsi d'une nouvelle conception de l'hôpital avicennien, qui sous plusieurs aspects se détachait du modèle traditionnel du

37 Les *ʿāšūr-ḫāna* sont des lieux de culte chiites dans lesquels sont conservées les *ʿalam* (étendards) dédiés aux martyres de Karbala, qui sont portées en procession pendant le mois de *muḥarram*.

38 Cf. Rizvi 1986, vol. 2, p. 340, et aussi Bilgrāmī 1342/1924, pp. 14–15. La relique était conservée dans une aile de l'hôpital, mais a été déplacée dans un édifice récent bâti au centre de la cour.

39 Yahya 1950, pp. 211–212.

40 Khan 1958, pp. 122–123.

*dār al-šifā*, assimilant en revanche des éléments des institutions médicales coloniales. A l'époque des Niẓāms, le milieu scientifique de la ville changea profondément, la classe de savants étrangers disparut et la ville attira à l'inverse de nombreux médecins *yūnānī* venus d'autres villes indiennes. Les descriptions du *dār al-šifā* que l'on retrouve dans les ouvrages historiques composés à l'époque des Niẓāms ne font pas supposer que l'ancien hôpital ait encore fonctionné à cette époque[41].

Après la chute du dernier Moghol en 1857, le vaste État des Niẓāms devint le plus grand État princier musulman de l'Inde. L'époque des Niẓāms, comme celle des Qajars (1794–1925) en Iran, fut marquée par la modernisation scientifique et médicale, et en 1846, cinq ans avant l'ouverture de l'école polytechnique (*dār al-funūn*) de Téhéran, fut instituée la première école médicale moderne de Hyderabad[42]. Le soutien à la médecine occidentale augmenta au cours du règne d'Afżal al-Dawla (r. 1857–1869), lorsque fut ouvert le premier hôpital moderne de la ville, à Afżal Ganj. Des médecins musulmans formés à l'école *yūnānī* commencèrent à étudier également la médecine allopathique[43]. C'est à la fin du XIX^e^ siècle, que la médecine *yūnānī* fut intégrée au système de santé de l'État de Hyderabad. Cela conduisit à l'établissement de plusieurs dispensaires publics, dans la capitale et dans les villes du Deccan, sous le contrôle des Niẓāms. Ce programme de réformes visant à doter la médecine *yūnānī* d'institutions plus modernes, sous le contrôle de l'État, culmina avec l'édification d'un grand hôpital au centre de Hyderabad, le Niẓāmiya ṣadr šifā-ḫāna.

Les premières institutions étatiques dédiées à la médecine *yūnānī* furent établies à l'époque du sixième Niẓām, Mīr Maḥbūb ʿAlī Ḫān (r. 1869–1911). Dans un discours adressé aux médecins *yūnānī* de la ville en 1317/1900, à l'occasion de son anniversaire, Maḥbūb ʿAlī Ḫān se déclara favorable à une combinaison entre les médecines orientale et occidentale[44]. Entre 1889 et 1891 furent établis dans la ville de Hyderabad un département de médecine *yūnānī* (*sar-rišta-yi ṭibābat-i yūnānī*), la Madrasa-yi ṭibbiya pour l'enseignement médical, et trois dispensaires (*šifā-ḫāna*) d'État. Dès 1306 f.[45]/1896

---

[41] Cf. Mīr ʿĀlam 1309/1892, vol. 1, p. 217 ; Qādir Ḫān 1306/1889, pp. 16–17 ; Ġulām Ḥusayn Ḫān 1308/1891, p. 25 ; Fārūqī 1356/1937, pp. 141–142.

[42] Jusqu'en 1884, les classes de la Hyderabad Medical School étaient données en ourdou et la plupart des premiers diplômés de l'école étaient des musulmans, cf. Reddy 1961, pp. 46–57.

[43] Fārūqī 1356/1937, pp. 171, 176.

[44] Fārūqī 1356/1937, pp. 180–181.

[45] Le calendrier *faṣlī* (abrégé en f.), utilisé sous les Niẓāms, avait été introduit au Deccan à la période moghole.

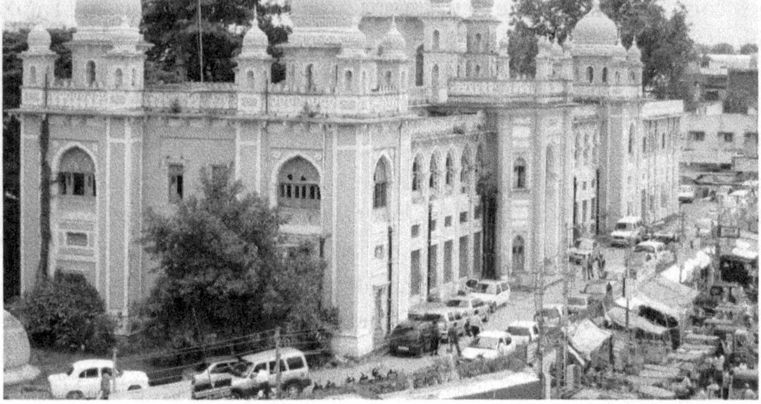

Figure 4. Bâtiment principal du Niẓāmiya ṣadr šifā-ḫāna (1926–1939) vu du Čār Mīnār.

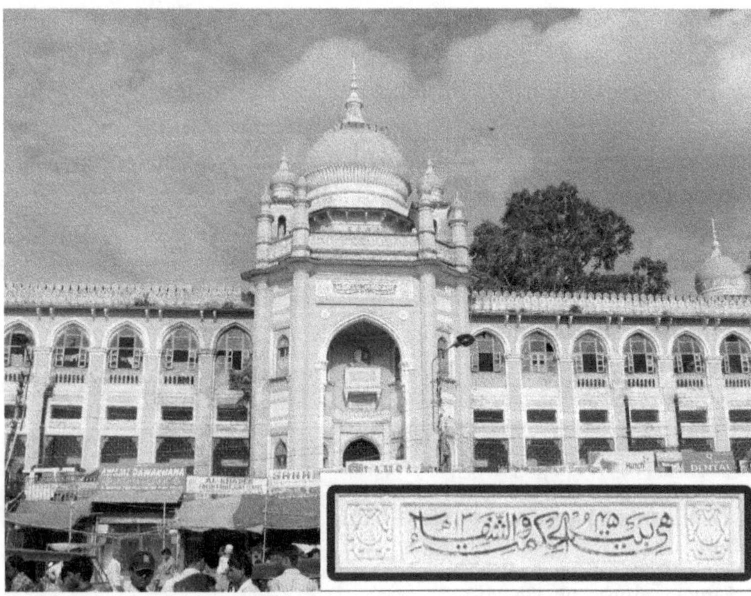

Figure 5. Portail du Niẓāmiya ṣadr šifā-ḫāna avec le chronogramme : *hiya al-bayt al-ḥikma wa al-šifā*, « Ceci est la maison de la sagesse et de la guérison ».

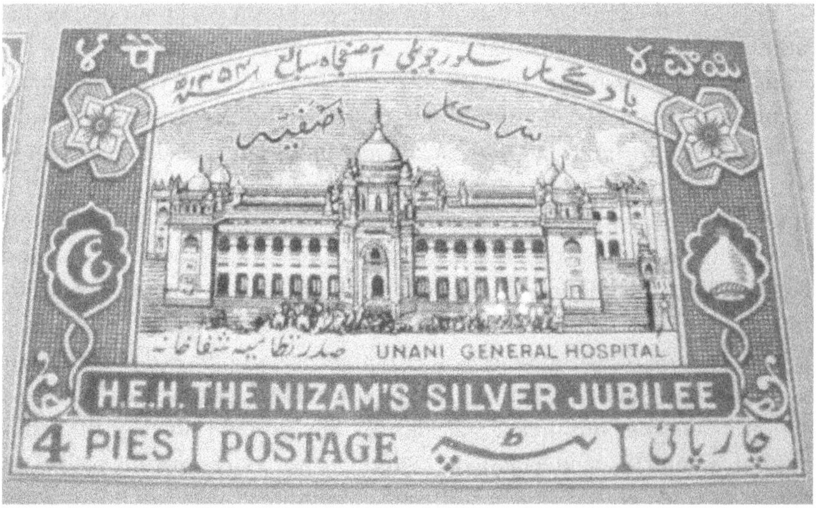


Figure 6. Timbre commémoratif du Niẓāmiya ṣadr šifā-ḫāna émis pour l'anniversaire des vingt-cinq années du règne de Mīr ʿUṯmān ʿAlī Ḫān.

la direction de tout le département fut placée sous le contrôle de l'*afsar al-aṭibbā* (chef des médecins)[46]. Selon les rapports officiels, en 1308 f./1898, les *šifā-ḫāna* de la ville eurent 116 298 patients sous traitement[47], alors qu'en 1319 f./1910 leur nombre avait atteint 817 967[48]. Nombreux étaient les cas d'accouchement traités dans ces *šifā-ḫāna*, cela montrant la méfiance des femmes musulmanes envers le nouveau service allopathique[49]. Jusqu'au début du XXe siècle, le département *yūnānī* demeura cependant de dimensions assez modestes. Au début des années 1920, la capacité des hôpitaux allopathiques de Hyderabad restait également assez limitée, sachant que

46 Fārūqī 1356/1937, pp. 177–178.

47 *Report on the Administration* 1308–1312 f. [1898–1903], p. 329.

48 *Report on the Administration* 1316–1319 f. [1906–1910], p. 89.

49 Durant les trois années 1903–1906 le département des femmes (*zanāna*) de l'hôpital Afżal Ganj eut 297 patientes hospitalisées, dont environ la moitié étaient constituée par les cas d'accouchement, alors qu'en 1315 f./1906, les dispensaires *yūnānī* traitèrent 20 333 cas d'accouchement, *Report on the Administration* 1313–1315 f. [1903–1906], pp. 172–173, 175, cf. aussi Attewell 2007, pp. 117–118.

selon l'étude de Rehman, il y avait en tout 338 lits en 1923 pour une population urbaine de plus de quatre cent mille habitants[50].

Le programme de réforme étatique de la médecine *yūnānī* connut sa phase majeure à l'époque du dernier Niẓām, Mīr ʿUṯmān ʿAlī Ḫān (r. 1911–1948). Un nouveau plan (*iskīm jadīd*) fut lancé et financé dans le but de réorganiser et de renforcer le département *yūnānī*. A partir des années 1920, quelques dispensaires ayurvédiques se mirent également à recevoir un soutien de l'État[51]. En 1344 f./1934–35, lorsque les travaux pour la construction du nouvel hôpital *yūnānī* étaient en cours, il se trouvait dans la zone urbaine de Hyderabad 10 *šifā-ḫāna* d'État et 18 privés subventionnés, dont 2 étaient ayurvédiques[52]. Des bourses d'étude furent assignées aux étudiants de la Madrasa-yi ṭibbiya[53]. Les postes qui furent créés dans les dispensaires d'État, dans la Madrasa-yi ṭibbiya, puis à l'hôpital attiraient les médecins *yūnānī* venus d'autres régions du pays. Des revues et ouvrages médicaux sortirent en ourdou et en 1330f./1920–21 on fonda l'association des médecins *yūnānī* de la ville (Anjuman-i aṭibbā-yi yūnānī). En 1937, Rahbar Fārūqī publia à Hyderabad la première histoire en ourdou de la médecine *yūnānī*, qui comprend des descriptions de la plupart des hôpitaux établis par les musulmans en Inde[54].

Le projet pour la construction du Niẓāmiya ṣadr šifā-ḫāna fut annoncé dans un *farmān*, daté du 27 *jamādī al-ṯānī* 1344/12 janvier 1926[55], avisant de l'édification d'un bâtiment magnifique (*ʿālī-šān ʿimārat*) au coût de 500 000 roupies[56]. La première pierre de l'hôpital fut posée par le même Mīr ʿUṯmān ʿAlī Ḫān, l'année lunaire suivante[57]. Le projet d'hôpital fut lié à celui visant à réformer la Madrasa-yi ṭibbiya. Toujours en 1336 f./1926,

---

50 Rehman 1990, p. 130.

51 En 1346–47 f./1936–38, une section ayurvédique attachée au département *yūnānī* fut instituée et un financement de 35 000 roupies fut assigné à la médecine ayurvédique, *Report on the Administration* 1346 f. [1936–1937], p. 143 ; *Report on the Administration* 1347 f. [1937–1938], p. 157.

52 Alors que dans les districts du Deccan fonctionnaient 78 dispensaires d'État et 37 subventionnés, *Report on the Administration* 1344 f. [1934–1935], p. 99.

53 En 1343 f./1933–34, étaient attribuées 12 bourses d'étude allant de 8 à 20 roupies par mois, *Report on the Administration* 1343 f. [1933–1934], p. 91.

54 Fārūqī 1356/1937.

55 Soit peu de temps après la fin de la construction du nouvel hôpital allopathique Osmania.

56 Le texte de ce *farmān* est rapporté par Fārūqī 1356/1937, p. 199, et dans le *Dastūr al-ʿamal Niẓāmiya ṭibbī kālij*, p. 3.

57 Selon le *Dastūr al-ʿamal Niẓāmiya ṭibbī kālij*, p. 4, la première pierre fut posée le 14 *rabīʿ al-ṯānī* 1345/22 octobre 1926, or selon Fārūqī cela se passa trois jours après, le 17 de *rabīʿ al-ṯānī*, Fārūqī 1356/1937, p. 199.

fut émis un autre *farmān* sollicitant la présentation d'un schéma (*iskīm*) pour la réorganisation des charges des médecins et de l'enseignement à la Madrasa-yi ṭibbiya[58], pour laquelle avait été également proposée une affiliation à l'université Osmania[59], or elle fut finalement transformée en un collège attaché à l'hôpital, le Niẓāmiya ṭibbī kālij.

Il apparaît que le bâtiment de l'hôpital était déjà presque terminé en 1350/1931–32[60], cinq ans après le début des travaux, or l'ouverture de la section pour les malades hospitalisés n'eut lieu que plusieurs années après. Ces retards étaient liés à la question plus vaste concernant la réorganisation de l'ensemble du département *yūnānī* et de la Madrasa-yi ṭibbiya. Cela indique que le fonctionnement du département n'était probablement pas considéré comme très satisfaisant et suffisamment systématique[61]. En 1344 f./1934–35, le budget du département fut réduit à 126 533 roupies contre les 154 226 de 1341 f./1931–32[62]. La question des fonds nécessaires à la réforme du département *yūnānī* se débloqua seulement après 1345 f./1936, lorsque fut nommé un comité d'experts venant de différentes parties de l'Inde, lequel se réunit à Hyderabad pour évaluer le projet de réorganisation du département[63]. L'année suivante, il fut enfin décidé d'allouer la somme de 150 615 roupies – à utiliser sur trois ans – pour la réorganisation des départements *yūnānī* et ayurvédique[64]. Cette décision coïncida avec un autre événement important : les célébrations données en grande pompe, en 1937, pour l'anniversaire des vingt-cinq années de règne de Mīr ʿUṯmān ʿAlī Ḫān. À cette occasion, un timbre commémoratif de l'hôpital fut émis (fig. 6) et le département de médecine *yūnānī* offrit au Niẓām une boîte à courrier en argent comportant l'image gravée de l'hôpital[65], soit un échange d'amabilités à interpréter comme des signaux indiquant que son ouverture était enfin proche.

58 *Dastūr al-ʿamal Niẓāmiya ṭibbī kālij*, p. 2.

59 Cf. Fārūqī 1356/1937, p. 201.

60 Cela est rapporté soit par Fārūqī 1356/1937, p. 199, soit par le *Report on the Administration* 1341 f. [1931–1932], p. 79.

61 Par exemple, en 1347 f./1937–38, peu avant l'ouverture de l'hôpital, les dispensaires subventionnés dans les districts n'avaient pas envoyé leurs rapports au département, *Report on the Administration* 1347 f. [1937–1938], p. 158.

62 *Report on the Administration* 1341 f. [1931–1932], p. 79 ; *Report on the Administration* 1344 f. [1934–1935], p. 99.

63 *Report on the Administration* 1345 f. [1935–1936], p. 122.

64 *Report on the Administration* 1346 f. [1936–1937], p. 143 ; *Report on the Administration* 1347 f. [1937–1938], p. 157 ; sur la section ayurvédique du département cf. note 51.

65 Conservé au Nizam's Museum de Hyderabad, acc. n. 58.

Le Niẓāmiya ṣadr šifā-ẖāna fut inauguré par Mīr ʿUṯmān ʿAlī Ḫān le 7 *šawwāl* 1358/20 novembre 1939[66]. Le coût du bâtiment de l'hôpital et du collège s'éleva finalement à un million de roupies environ[67]. Il s'agissait alors d'une des institutions *yūnānī* les plus grandes et les plus modernes du sous-continent, dotée de l'électricité, d'ampoules et de ventilateurs. Le bâtiment principal de l'hôpital, de style indo-sarrasin, est remarquable et constitue un important exemple d'architecture publique de l'époque des Niẓāms (fig. 4). Dans le Niẓāmiya ṣadr šifā-ẖāna se mêlent des éléments de l'architecture moghole comme le *pīšṭāq*, le portail monumental (fig. 5), et des interprétations modernes. L'usage du dôme dans l'architecture laïque – qui se retrouve dans d'autres bâtiments édifiés peu avant, tels la Cour suprême et en particulier l'hôpital Osmania – dénote notamment l'influence des modèles coloniaux[68].

Le Niẓāmiya ṣadr šifā-ẖāna et son collège incluaient un dispensaire, une section pour visiter les patients non résidents, une pharmacie, une bibliothèque, une salle anatomique pour la dissection (*dār al-tašrīḥ*) et un laboratoire d'analyses[69]. Le laboratoire d'analyses fut ouvert en 1359 f./1940–41, lorsque l'hôpital fut également doté d'un hammam médical (*ṭibbī ḥammām*). En outre, il fut décidé d'employer des infirmiers, au lieu d'infirmières, pour lesquels des classes commencèrent la même année[70]. Cela était nécessaire car la majorité des patients hospitalisés étaient des hommes. Le département *zanāna*, pour les femmes, fut ouvert une année après seulement, en 1351 f./1941–42, et était doté de 21 lits[71].

Le Niẓāmiya ṣadr šifā-ẖāna comptait au total presque 150 lits[72], soit environ la même capacité que l'ancien hôpital allopathique Afżal Ganj, avant l'ouverture du nouvel Osmania. En 1942–43, le Niẓāmiya ṣadr šifā-ẖāna était le troisième hôpital de la ville par le nombre de lits, après l'Osmania, qui en comptait 749, et le Victoria Zanana Hospital, réservé aux femmes, qui comptait 300 lits[73]. Cependant, par rapport au nombre de

---

66 Au Nizam's Museum de Hyderabad sont conservés les ciseaux et l'assiette en argent (acc. n. 60) utilisés pour la cérémonie inaugurale.

67 *Dastūr al-ʿamal Niẓāmiya ṭibbī kālij*, p. 19. Le terrain avait coûté 230 494 roupies, cf. Fārūqī 1356/1937, p. 199.

68 Auparavant les dômes étaient réservés aux édifices religieux, dans lesquels ils symbolisaient la voûte du ciel, cf. Vaughan 2001, p. 474.

69 Cf. *Dastūr al-ʿamal Niẓāmiya ṭibbī kālij*, pp. 21–22, 31.

70 *Report on the Administration* 1350 f. [1940–1941], p. 154.

71 *Report on the Administration* 1351 f. [1941–1942], p. 138.

72 Bien qu'au moment de son inauguration seuls 50 lits étaient en fonctionnement, *Dastūr al-ʿamal Niẓāmiya ṭibbī kālij*, p. 7.

73 Pour les statistiques sur les hôpitaux allopathiques de la ville cf. Rehman 1990, pp. 130–134.

patients hospitalisés, il était le deuxième, en cela proche de l'activité du même Osmania, au moins selon les rapports officiels. Dans sa première année d'activité, le Niẓāmiya ṣadr šifā-ḫāna traita 14 934 patients hospitalisés[74], contre 15 756 pour l'Osmania en 1942–43[75]. Il est probable qu'une partie des malades hospitalisés au Niẓāmiya ṣadr šifā-ḫāna étaient des pauvres, et il s'agit vraisemblablement de l'une des raisons principales pour laquelle furent prévues des chambres particulières destinées à être louées aux patients aisés[76]. En 1951–52, 22 lits du Niẓāmiya ṣadr šifā-ḫāna furent assignés à la section ayurvédique[77].

Tableau A. Nombre des patients traités et budget du Niẓāmiya ṣadr šifā-ḫāna et du collège dans la période 1939–1951 (nd = non disponible)

| | 1939–octobre 1940 | octobre 1940–octobre 1941 | octobre 1941–octobre 1942 | septembre 1948–mars 1950 | avril 1950–mars 1951 |
|---|---|---|---|---|---|
| atients hospitalisés | 14 934 | nd | nd | 61 023 | 44 382 |
| atients non hospitalisés | 446 940 | nd | nd | 644 500 | 510 450 |
| otal des patients traités | 461 874 | 434 540 | 416 931 | 705 523 | 554 832 |
| épense de l'hôpital en roupies | 39 569 | 86 053 | 79 804 | nd | 213 508 |
| épenses du collège en roupies | 39 659 | 43 408 | 39 981 | nd | nd |

ources: *Report on the Administration* 1349 f. [1939–1940], p. 142 ; 1350 f. [1940–1941], pp. 145–155 ; 351 f. [1941–1942], pp. 138–139 ; *Report on the Administration of Hyderabad State, September 1948-Iarch 1950*, pp. 106–107 ; *Hyderabad Administration Report, April 1950–March 1951*, pp. 148–149.

Il faut souligner certains aspects du programme de réforme de la médecine *yūnānī* à Hyderabad, lequel mena à l'ouverture du Niẓāmiya ṣadr šifā-ḫāna. On observe là des différences importantes par rapport au mouvement qui à l'époque coloniale conduisit à l'établissement de nouvelles institutions *yūnānī* à Delhi et à Lucknow, villes qui étaient sous le contrôle

74 *Report on the Administration* 1349 f. [1939–1940], p. 142.
75 Rehman 1990, p. 134.
76 Cf. Fārūqī 1356/1937, p. 200.
77 *Hyderabad Administration Report, April 1951–March 1952*, p. 98.

britannique. Dans ces deux villes, les institutions *yūnānī* qui furent créées pour adapter la tradition au contexte colonial étaient essentiellement liées aux efforts de médecins privés et de leurs familles, comme dans le cas des Šarīfī et de l'Hamdard à Delhi[78], ainsi que des 'Azīzī à Lucknow. L'établissement de nouvelles institutions *yūnānī* à Hyderabad et à Bhopal[79], villes gouvernées par des souverains musulmans, restait en revanche très lié au patronage royal et à la politique sanitaire étatique.

Il se trouve peu d'indications sur ce que fut la position, ou les positions, des médecins de Hyderabad vis-à-vis du projet d'hôpital. Il est indubitable qu'une partie de l'Anjuman-i aṭibbā-yi yūnānī a soutenu le projet tandis que le premier secrétaire de l'association, Ḥakīm Maqṣūd 'Alī Ḫān, devint le directeur du collège de l'hôpital. Cependant, l'établissement d'un hôpital ne faisait apparemment pas partie des objectifs premiers de l'Anjuman-i aṭibbā-yi yūnānī, à sa fondation[80]. Il est possible que certains médecins *yūnānī* aient au contraire perçu le projet d'un grand hôpital public comme une menace pour l'activité de leurs cabinets et dispensaires. Maqṣūd 'Alī Ḫān et Rahbar Fārūqī, tous deux favorables au programme étatique de réforme, se lamentaient notamment de l'inertie des médecins *yūnānī* de la ville[81]. Le plus important narrateur contemporain de ces événements fut Rahbar Fārūqī, qui dans le paragraphe consacré à l'époque du dernier Niẓām, n'hésite pas à attribuer la décadence de la tradition à la négligence de ses pratiquants, célébrant en revanche pompeusement sa revivification grâce à l'œuvre du Sulṭān al-'ulūm (Roi des sciences), Mīr 'Uṯmān 'Alī Ḫān[82]. Le même Mīr 'Uṯmān 'Alī Ḫān, à l'occasion de l'inauguration du dispensaire *yūnānī* Majīdiya à Hyderabad, en 1346 f./1936, réprimanda les médecins *yūnānī* pour la carence d'attention portée à la recherche, soulignant en même temps que l'établissement du nouvel hôpital devait servir non seulement à traiter les malades, mais également à promouvoir les études et les recherches des médecins *yūnānī*[83].

Le Niẓāmiya ṣadr šifā-ḫāna paraît donc davantage constituer le résultat d'un programme étatique de réformes visant à créer des institutions

[78] Sur l'Hamdard cf. l'article d'Anna Vanzan dans ce volume.

[79] Sur Bhopal cf. l'article de Claudia Preckel dans ce volume.

[80] Cf. Attewell 2007, pp. 121–122.

[81] Fārūqī 1356/1937, pp. 190, 195 ; sur Maqṣūd 'Alī Ḫān cf. Attewell 2007, p. 121. Attewell mentionne également l'existence de contrastes parmi des membres de l'Anjuman et son secrétaire.

[82] Fārūqī décrit avec le même style pompeux la fondation et le bâtiment de l'hôpital, en attente d'inauguration, Fārūqī 1356/1937, pp. 190, 198–201.

[83] Le dispensaire était dédié au prince Majīdī Pāšā ; le discours du Niẓām, prononcé pendant la cérémonie d'ouverture, est rapporté par Fārūqī 1356/1937, pp. 203–204.

médicales modernes sous le contrôle de l'État, qu'un projet alimenté par les requêtes de la majorité des médecins *yūnānī* de la ville. Le soutien à la médecine *yūnānī* constituait un élément de la politique culturelle de Mīr ʿUṯmān ʿAlī Ḫān. L'étude de Pernau a notamment montré comment la politique culturelle du Niẓām se liait à la recherche de légitimation de son pouvoir et aux ambitions consistant à se présenter comme le leader des musulmans indiens[84]. Les Niẓāms avaient été des continuateurs de la tradition moghole du mécénat dans les sciences musulmanes et indiennes, et Mīr ʿUṯmān ʿAlī Ḫān pouvait se présenter comme étant l'un des derniers souverains musulmans dont le projet culturel incluait un vaste soutien à l'ancienne médecine avicennienne, l'un des derniers symboles encore vivants de l'école scientifique musulmane. De plus, comme d'autres sultans musulmans avant lui, tel le troisième Niẓām Sikandar Jāh (r. 1803–1829)[85], il patronna la médecine ayurvédique. Son fils, le prince Aʿẓam Jāh Bahadur inaugura une importante institution *yūnānī* de l'Inde du nord, où se trouvait également un hôpital, le Ṭibbiya College de l'Aligarh Muslim University, ainsi que le dispensaire ayurvédique Niẓām (Ṣadr dawā-ḫāna Niẓām āyurvēdik) à Hyderabad en 1935[86].

Le choix de l'emplacement du Niẓāmiya ṣadr šifā-ḫāna, dont le bâtiment imposant fut édifié dans un lieu très symbolique de la ville, est significatif à ce titre. Au début, il avait été projeté de placer l'hôpital à proximité du fleuve Musi[87], or il fut finalement choisi de le bâtir en face de la mosquée de la Mecque et du Čār Mīnār, le monument le plus important de Hyderabad, marquant le centre de la vieille ville. Pour commémorer la fondation de l'hôpital, Mīr ʿUṯmān ʿAlī Ḫān composa un chronogramme indiquant l'année (1345 h.q./1926), et déclarant : *hiya al-bayt al-ḥikma wa al-šifā*, « Ceci est la maison de la sagesse et de la guérison ». Ce verset, qui fut inscrit sur le portail monumental de l'hôpital (fig. 5), évoquait évidemment le *Bayt al-ḥikma* établi à Bagdad sous le califat abbasside, l'une des institutions les plus glorieuses et anciennes de la tradition scientifique musulmane. Ces activités eurent vraisemblablement une résonance en dehors du sous-continent également, et peu après l'ouverture de l'hôpital, Muḥammad Sayyid Muṣṭafā, ex-directeur

---

[84] Pernau 2000, pp. 96–114.
[85] Cf. Speziale 2010b, pp. 408, 436.
[86] Fārūqī 1356/1937, pp. 204–205.
[87] Fārūqī 1356/1937, p. 199. L'hôpital allopathique Osmania se trouvait déjà sur le fleuve Musi.

de l'hôpital de Médine, fut envoyé par les Saoudiens à Hyderabad pour examiner les institutions *yūnānī* locales[88].

Bien que le soutien à la médecine *yūnānī*, sous les derniers Niẓāms, s'inscrivait dans la tradition de mécénat des grands souverains musulmans, tels les Moghols, les nouvelles institutions qui furent crées, dont le Niẓāmiya ṣadr šifā-ḫāna, se différenciaient à plusieurs égards des anciennes formes de mécenat. La fondation et le financement de l'hôpital ne dépendaient plus de la constitution d'un *waqf* ou d'un *jāgīr*[89]. L'hôpital faisait partie d'un nouveau département qui, au moins en principe, avait été institué pour se conformer aux caractéristiques saillantes de l'organisation des départements et des institutions médicales occidentales. Le Niẓāmiya ṣadr šifā-ḫāna était en effet un établissent différent de l'ancien modèle du *dār al-šifā*. Il n'était plus une partie d'un complexe incluant d'autres établissements musulmans comme la mosquée ou le hammam. Le hammam médical du Niẓāmiya ṣadr šifā-ḫāna était en revanche pensé comme un instrument moderne destiné au traitement de certaines pathologies. À la disparition de ces éléments s'ajoutait l'incorporation de caractéristiques marquant la nécessité de conformer le Niẓāmiya ṣadr šifā-ḫāna et son école aux hôpitaux et collèges allopathiques, tels la salle anatomique, le laboratoire d'analyses, et l'enseignement de matières issues de la médicine occidentale. Farūqī remarque notamment les efforts employés ici pour développer la médecine *yūnānī* sur des « principes absolument modernes » (*bi'l-kull jadīd uṣūl*)[90]. Cependant, l'on ne possède pas de données détaillées permettant d'évaluer exactement dans quelle mesure ces efforts destinés à la modernisation se répercutèrent – surtout au début – sur la pratique des médecins *yūnānī* à l'intérieur de l'hôpital.

Bien que le Niẓāmiya ṣadr šifā-ḫāna ait symboliquement aspiré à imiter les grandes institutions scientifiques musulmanes du passé, il répondait donc d'abord à une logique visant à doter la médecine *yūnānī* de structures analogues à celles de la médecine allopathique. Le *farmān* du 12 janvier 1926, annonçant la construction de l'hôpital, le justifie en remarquant que dès lors qu'un bâtiment grandiose (*ša'n-dār*) avait été construit pour l'Afżal Ganj il fallait faire un bâtiment similaire pour le traitement *yūnānī*[91]. Il est également surprenant que le discours lu aux médecins

---

[88] Hussain 1977, p. 157.

[89] En Iran, jusqu'au début du XX^e^ siècle, plusieurs hôpitaux étaient encore fondés grâce à des *waqf*, cf. à ce sujet l'article d'Omid Rezai dans ce volume.

[90] Farūqī 1356/1937, p. 199.

[91] *Dastūr al-ʿamal Niẓāmiya ṭibbī kālij*, p. 3.

*yūnānī* par Mīr ʿUṯmān ʿAlī Ḫān, à l'occasion de l'inauguration de l'hôpital, bien qu'évoquant le thème récurrent de l'ancienne origine de la tradition *yūnānī*, ne comprenne en revanche aucun passage célébrant le rôle des anciens hôpitaux musulmans, pas même celui établi par les Quṭb Šāh[92] ! Le Niẓāmiya ṣadr šifā-ḫāna n'avait pas été conçu pour constituer la réplique d'un ancien *dār al-šifā*, mais pour réformer cette institution en l'adaptant aux conditions scientifiques de l'époque coloniale.

## Le collège de l'hôpital

Ces tendances se répercutèrent notamment sur le projet du nouveau collège *yūnānī* attaché à l'hôpital. Comme on l'a déjà souligné, le projet du Niẓāmiya ṣadr šifā-ḫāna se lia à celui de réorganiser la méthode d'enseignement de la Madrasa-yi ṭibbiya. Comme l'indique Guy Attewell dans son ouvrage, l'enseignement de la Madrasa-yi ṭibbiya de Hyderabad, avec ses classes en persan et en arabe uniquement, avait fait l'objet de critiques[93]. L'une des fonctions de l'hôpital devait être justement d'offrir davantage d'opportunités au niveau de la formation pratique des étudiants du collège. En effet, en 1345 f./1935–36, le nombre d'étudiants de la Madrasa-yi ṭibbiya, dont le cursus menant au diplôme durait trois ans, était tombé à 50, puis à 40 l'année suivante, tandis qu'en 1338 f./1928–29 il y avait 220 étudiants[94]. Le modèle musulman de la madrasa fut ainsi abandonné pour adopter l'idée moderne du collège, et le nouveau Niẓāmiya ṭibbī kālij fut inauguré avec l'hôpital.

Le nouveau collège véhiculait d'importants changements visant à standardiser et à moderniser la formation des médecins *yūnānī*. La réforme didactique s'incarna en premier lieu à travers le changement des langues d'instruction. Les langues utilisées à la Madrasa-yi ṭibbiya étaient le persan et l'arabe, limitant donc essentiellement l'accès à ceux qui faisaient des études traditionnelles musulmanes. La langue principale du Niẓāmiya ṭibbī kālij devint l'ourdou ; l'arabe restant, avec l'ourdou, uniquement au

---

92 *Dastūr al-ʿamal Niẓāmiya ṭibbī kālij*, pp. 6–9.

93 Déjà en 1895, soit peu après sa fondation, la méthode traditionnelle d'instruction employée à la Madrasa-yi ṭibbiya fut critiquée dans un courrier officiel, à cause du manque de règles précises dans l'enseignement et pour la carence regardant la formation pratique des étudiants, Attewell 2007, p. 128.

94 Dont 180 dans les classes en persan et seulement 40 dans les classes en arabe, cf. *Report on the Administration* 1338 f. [1928–1929], p. 69 ; *Report on the Administration* 1345 f. [1935–1936], p. 122 ; *Report on the Administration* 1346 f. [1936–1937], p. 143.

titre de langue d'enseignement utilisée lors des deux dernières années de spécialisation permettant de devenir médecin *māhir*. Ce projet se rapportait évidemment à celui qui avait inspiré l'université Osmania, dans laquelle tous les cours sur les sciences occidentales étaient en ourdou[95], et dont le bâtiment principal, celui de l'Arts College, fut inauguré par le Niẓām un mois après celui du Niẓāmiya ṭibbī kālij. Cela signifiait le passage à la langue musulmane dans laquelle circulaient le plus en Inde les idées de la médecine occidentale, et en même temps la possibilité de véhiculer les études *yūnānī* à travers une langue plus populaire, au lieu des langues aristocratiques comme le persan et l'arabe. Il faut remarquer que l'arabe fut choisi au titre de deuxième langue d'enseignement, alors même que son rôle dans le milieu indo-musulman était notamment promu par les mouvements religieux réformistes de l'époque coloniale. Le persan ne fut pas retenu, bien qu'il ait été la langue la plus importante de la littérature médicale indo-musulmane, et bien que les classes en persan de la Madrasa-yi ṭibbiya aient toujours compté plus d'étudiants que celles en arabe.

La transformation en collège impliquait l'augmentation des années d'études et le renforcement de l'instruction des matières modernes. Le cursus du Niẓāmiya ṭibbī kālij était divisé en deux niveaux de diplôme (*sanad*), celui de trois ans, uniquement en ourdou, pour le grade de *ṭabīb mustanad*, équivalent au *sanad* de l'ancienne madrasa, et celui de cinq ans pour le grade de *ṭabīb māhir* (médecin expert). Pour ce qui concerne les textes d'étude, le passage à l'ourdou excluait de l'enseignement les textes de la tradition persane[96], et l'instruction était centrée sur les traductions ourdoues du *Qānūn* d'Avicenne (m. 429/1037) et sur ses commentaires, ainsi que sur les manuels et les traductions en ourdou de Ḥakīm Kabīr al-Dīn, le vice-directeur du collège. L'instruction dans les disciplines traditionnelles musulmanes comptait en tout un cours de langue et un de littérature arabe la première année, et un cours sur la philosophie et la logique la deuxième année, basé sur le *Hidāya al-ḥikma* d'Aṯīr al-Dīn al-Abharī (m. 663/1264)[97].

---

95 Cf. Pernau 2000, pp. 104–112.

96 Les traductions en ourdou de quelques textes indo-persans furent cependant insérées plus tard, tels le *Qarābādīn-i qādirī* d'Akbar Arzānī et l'*Iksīr-i Aʿẓam* d'Aʿẓam Ḫān, *Čār sālah niṣāb*, p. 50.

97 Ouvrage qui connut une diffusion considérable en Inde surtout à travers le commentaire de Mullā Ṣadrā (m. 1636).

L'importance donnée à l'enseignement des matières occidentales augmenta. L'instruction en chirurgie fut cependant limitée à un seul cours, la troisième année, et était basée sur deux textes de Ḥakīm Kabīr al-Dīn, plus une partie pratique[98]. L'enseignement de l'anatomie, divisé en deux cours situés les deux premières années, se basait au début sur un seul livre, le *Tašrīḥ-i Kabīr* (en deux volumes) de Ḥakīm Kabīr al-Dīn. Les deux dernières années du diplôme de *ṭabīb māhir* incluaient un cours de chimie (*kīmiyā*) et deux cours de recherche comparative en médecine ancienne et moderne (*taḥqīq wa taṭbīq-i ṭibb-i qadīm wa jadīd*). D'autres matières telles l'hygiène (*ḥifẓ-i ṣiḥḥat*), la toxicologie (*ʿilm al-sumūm*) et le *fann-i wilādat*[99], étaient également en partie basées sur le savoir occidental moderne[100].

Des efforts furent destinés au recrutement des enseignants. Au début, le collège comptait six professeurs, dont la plupart étaient également membres du comité pédagogique (*majlis-i taʿlīmī*) du collège[101], trois professeurs assistants (*madad-gār*) et des chargés d'enseignement. Les postes attribués aux médecins formés en dehors de la ville montrent de façon très évidente la volonté d'ouvrir le collège aux tendances plus réformistes venant des villes de l'Inde du nord, et notamment du milieu de Delhi. Le premier directeur (*ṣadr*) de l'école fut Ḥakīm Maqṣūd ʿAlī Ḫān (n. 1886–87), qui était le fils d'un autre médecin éminent, Manṣūr ʿAlī Ḫān (m. 1337/1919, La Mecque), qui migra à Hyderabad où il devint le directeur de la Madrasa-yi ṭibbiya[102]. Maqṣūd ʿAlī Ḫān était comme son père originaire de Muradabad, il reçut une formation traditionnelle, ayant étudié les sciences religieuses, la philosophie et la médecine. À Hyderabad, il fut au début assistant de son père à la Madrasa-yi ṭibbiya, puis il eut une brillante carrière dans le système *yūnānī* étatique, travaillant comme surintendant (*muhtamim*) de différents dispensaires de la ville. En 1355/1936, lorsque l'ouverture de l'hôpital était dans l'impasse, il fut nommé *ṣadr muhtamim-i ṭibābat-i yūnānī*, au nouveau poste de direction du département *yūnānī*. Le Niẓām exprima dans un *farmān* le souhait que la désignation de Maqṣūd ʿAlī Ḫān puisse servir à réformer rapidement le

98 *Dastūr al-ʿamal Niẓāmiya ṭibbī kālij*, p. 41.

99 Le cours de *fann-i wilādat* (lit. science de la génération) traitait de différentes questions comme l'embryologie, la gestation et la néonatologie, *Čār sālah niṣāb*, pp. 31–32.

100 *Dastūr al-ʿamal Niẓāmiya ṭibbī kālij*, pp. 36–45.

101 Qui incluait aussi Ḥakīm Muʿīn al-Dīn Jhajjarī et Ḥakīm Hibat Allāh, *Dastūr al-ʿamal Niẓāmiya ṭibbī kālij*, pp. 12–13.

102 Manṣūr ʿAlī Ḫān étudia à Deoband et fut un disciple de Rašīd Aḥmad Gangohī, Nāṣir 1944, pp. 11–14 ; Šifā-yi Ḥaydarābādī 1952, pp. 147–151.

département *yūnānī*[103]. En effet, ce fut sous sa direction que la question complexe de la réorganisation du département et de l'ouverture de l'hôpital et de son collège, se débloquèrent enfin. Ḥakīm Šifā-yi Ḥaydarābādī[104] souligne son habilité administrative, la place de ses efforts dans l'achèvement du projet de l'hôpital et de son collège, et rapporte qu'il encouragea l'arrivée au collège et à l'hôpital de médecins éminents venant d'autres villes indiennes[105].

Le plus important de ces médecins était Ḥakīm Kabīr al-Dīn (m. 1976), qui avait longtemps enseigné à l'Ayurvedic and Yūnānī Ṭibbiya College établi à Delhi par Ajmal Ḫān (1863–1927)[106]. Il fut nommé vice-directeur du Niẓāmiya ṭibbī kālij, où il enseigna neuf ans. Son arrivée épousait parfaitement le projet de réforme linguistique du collège, Kabīr al-Dīn étant l'un des plus prolifiques auteurs et traducteurs de livres médicaux en ourdou, dont plusieurs furent adoptés dans le cursus du collège. Comme Ajmal Ḫān, il était favorable à la réforme de la tradition *yūnānī* à travers l'assimilation d'éléments de la médecine moderne, et à Hyderabad, il enseigna justement le cours sur la recherche comparative en médecine ancienne et moderne, en plus du cours de pharmacologie[107]. C'est également de Delhi que venait Fażl al-Raḥmān Ḫān, qui en 1935 avait fondé avec Kabīr al-Dīn la Jāmiʿa ṭibbiya[108], une autre école *yūnānī* de Delhi[109]. Sayyid ʿAlī Āšufta venait de Lucknow, où étudia Mawalwī Muḥammad Ibrāhīm, qui fut également formé à l'Ayurvedic and Yūnānī Ṭibbiya College de Delhi et enseigna l'anatomie à la Madrasa-yi ṭibbiya puis la philosophie et la logique au Niẓāmiya ṭibbī kālij[110]. Mawalwī Ḥakīm Muʿīn al-Dīn Jhajjarī[111], Mawalwī

---

103 Fārūqī 1356/1937, p. 186.

104 Un médecin de l'époque du dernier Niẓām qui fut l'auteur d'un important ouvrage biographique sur les médecins *yūnānī* du Deccan, ses contemporains, cf. Šifā-yi Ḥaydarābādī 1952.

105 Šifā-yi Ḥaydarābādī 1952, p. 153 ; Nāṣir 1944, pp. 15–17.

106 Ajmal Ḫān, un médecin et homme politique issu de la famille Šarīfī de Delhi, il fut l'un des plus influents médecins *yūnānī* de l'époque coloniale, cf. Speziale 2009b.

107 Šifā-yi Ḥaydarābādī 1952, pp. 250–262 ; Ẓill al-Raḥmān 1995, pp. 319–322 ; *Dastūr al-ʿamal Niẓāmiya ṭibbī kālij*, p. 10.

108 Šifā-yi Ḥaydarābādī 1952, p. 258.

109 Deux textes en ourdou de Fażl al-Raḥmān Ḫān furent inclus dans le cursus du Niẓāmiya ṭibbī kālij, cf. *Dastūr al-ʿamal Niẓāmiya ṭibbī kālij*, p. 40.

110 Muḥammad Ibrāhīm était originaire de la région de Muradabad et commença à travailler à Hyderabad en 1913–14, Šifā-yi Ḥaydarābādī 1952, pp. 213–214.

111 Originaire de Jhajjar, proche de Delhi, il arriva avec son père à Hyderabad en 1913 et y étudia à la Madrasa-yi ṭibbiya avant de se rendre à Delhi ; au Niẓāmiya ṭibbī kālij, il enseignait les cours d'hygiène et de toxicologie, Šifā-yi Ḥaydarābādī 1952, pp. 172–174 ; *Dastūr al-ʿamal Niẓāmiya ṭibbī kālij*, p. 10.

Ḥakīm Hibat Allāh[112] et Mawalwī Ilyāsīn Ḫān, qui furent engagés comme professeurs assistants, avaient étudié à l'Ayurvedic and Yūnānī Ṭibbiya College de Delhi. Parmi les professeurs se trouvait le docteur allopathique Mirzā Ḥamīd Allāh, qui enseignait la chirurgie, et pour le cours de chimie on appela Mawalwī ʿAbd al-Ḥayy de l'université Osmania[113].

Le passage à l'ourdou et la présence de médecins éminents engendrèrent une augmentation du nombre d'étudiants et de diplômés, qui cependant ne fut pas très élevée, si l'on considère que l'instruction était gratuite et qu'il y avait également des bourses d'études[114]. La première année de son existence le collège eut 78 étudiants. L'effectif chuta à 64 l'année suivante, pour remonter à 72 en 1351 f./1941–42, ce qui constituait moins de la moitié du nombre d'étudiants de la Madrasa-yi ṭibbiya à la fin des années 1920. Le budget du collège était la première année le même que celui de l'hôpital, mais l'année suivante il ne représenta plus que sa moitié (cf. tableau A). Dix ans après son ouverture, 80 médecins *mustanad* étaient sortis du collège, pour seulement 18 *māhir*[115]. La Madrasa-yi ṭibbiya, et le collège qui lui succéda affaiblissaient le rôle pédagogique des familles et de l'instruction privée, cependant ces écoles ne furent pas capables à cette époque de les remplacer entièrement. Les fils des médecins commencèrent à étudier à la Madrasa-yi ṭibbiya, travaillant ensuite dans les *šifā-ḫāna* de la ville ; le *sanad* de la Madrasa-yi ṭibbiya était utile quant au recrutement pour les postes d'État, mais n'était pas indispensable. L'instruction privée ne disparut pas, mais bénéficia au contraire des lacunes du nouveau système éducatif. Comme le montrent les biographies des médecins *yūnānī* composées à cette époque à Hyderabad, les diplômés de la Madrasa-yi ṭibbiya complétaient souvent leur formation chez les enseignants privés de la ville[116].

---

112 Né à Hyderabad en 1310f./1900–01, il étudia au début à la Madrasa-yi ṭibbiya, puis à Delhi où il travailla également au *šifā-ḫāna* de l'Ayurvedic and Yūnānī Ṭibbiya College ; il fut l'auteur de quelques textes médicaux et enseigna l'anatomie à la Madrasa-yi ṭibbiya puis au Niẓāmiya ṭibbī kālij, Šifā-yi Ḥaydarābādī 1952, pp. 200–204.

113 Un autre docteur allopathique fut également chargé de l'enseignement de la médecine légale (*ṭibb-i qānūnī*), cf. *Dastūr al-ʿamal Niẓāmiya ṭibbī kālij*, pp. 10–11.

114 Allant de 20 à 30 roupies par mois.

115 *Report on the Administration of Hyderabad State, September 1948–March 1950*, p. 106.

116 Cf. Nāṣir 1944 ; Šifā-yi Ḥaydarābādī 1952.

## Conclusion

On a examiné dans cet article les hôpitaux de médecine *yūnānī* établis au Deccan à différentes époques, en analysant notamment l'évolution de cette institution au cours du passage de la première modernité à l'époque coloniale. Le *dār al-šifā* édifié à Hyderabad à la fin du XVI^e^ siècle était basé sur le modèle traditionnel musulman, selon lequel l'hôpital faisait partie d'un complexe incluant une mosquée et d'autres établissements typiques des villes musulmanes, un modèle qui avait été introduit en Inde à partir du monde iranien et arabe. Parmi les anciens établissements de ce type fondés par les musulmans en Inde, le bâtiment du *dār al-šifā* de Hyderabad est probablement le plus important à s'être bien conservé jusqu'à aujourd'hui. Cependant, les sources décrivant cet hôpital et son activité sont peu détaillées. Les rares savants signalés pour avoir été associés à l'époque quṭbšahide au *dār al-šifā*, et à sa madrasa, étaient d'origine iranienne.

L'adaptation au milieu scientifique de l'époque coloniale fut l'événement qui détermina les plus grands changements de cette institution en Inde. Le projet du Niẓāmiya ṣadr šifā-ḫāna ne se basait alors plus sur le modèle du *dār al-šifā*, et son école abandonna définitivement le style d'enseignement de la madrasa. Le Niẓāmiya ṣadr šifā-ḫāna était un produit, et un instrument, du plan de réforme de la tradition *yūnānī*, et son projet était influencé par les institutions de la médecine occidentale moderne. Ce fut sous cette forme hybride, incorporant des éléments de la médecine allopathique, que des hôpitaux de médecine *yūnānī* demeurèrent encore en activité au XX^e^ siècle au sous-continent. La fondation du Niẓāmiya ṣadr šifā-ḫāna s'inséra à l'intérieur du programme de réformes des institutions *yūnānī* lancé par l'État de Hyderabad, qui atteignit son apogée sous le dernier Niẓām. Ce programme de réformes, qui dura environ un demi-siècle[117], constitua l'un des premiers plans importants d'un État contemporain du sous-continent visant à réglementer et moderniser les médecines traditionnelles locales, anticipant de plusieurs décades la politique analogue des États postcoloniaux. L'hôpital Niẓāmiya et son collège sont encore en activité aujourd'hui. Ils ont été incorporés dans le nouveau département d'État pour les médecines traditionnelles créé après l'indépendance, et restent parmi les principales institutions *yūnānī* de l'Inde.

---

[117] Les dominions des Niẓāms furent annexés à l'union indienne en 1948.

## Bibliographie

### A. *Sources primaires*

Abū al-Fażl, ʿAllāmī, 2001, *Āʾīn-i Akbarī*, traduction anglaise : *The Ā-īn-i Akbarī*, 3 vols., H. Blochmann ; H. S. Jarrett, éds., Delhi, Low Price Publications, (1er éd. Calcutta, 1868–1894).

Bilgrāmī, Sayyid ʿAlī Aṣġar, 1342/1924, *Maʾāṯir-i Dakan*. Hyderabad.

Fārūqī, Qāżī Muʿīn al-Dīn Rahbar, 1356/1937, *Islāmī ṭibb šāhānah sarparastiyūn men*. Hyderabad (réédition : Hyderabad, Maktaba-yi ʿAīn al-ʿUlūm, 1420/1999).

Firišta, Muḥammad Qāsim, 1290/1874, *Tārīḫ-i Firišta*, 2 vols., Kanpur.

Ġulām Ḥusayn Ḫān, 1308/1891, *Tārīḫ-i gulzār-i Āṣafiya*. Hyderabad.

Ḫān, Ġulām Ḥusayn Jawhar, *Mah-nāma*, ms. pers. Hyderabad, Salar Jung Museum and Library, *tārīḫ* 364.

Ḥasanī, ʿAbd al-Ḥayy ibn Faḫr al-Dīn, 1408/1988, *Nuzhat al-ḫawāṭir wa bahjat al-masāmiʿ wa al-nawāẓir*. Hyderabad, Dāʾirat al-Maʿārif, vol. 3 (3e éd.).

Mīr ʿĀlam, Abū al-Qāsim, 1309/1892, *Hadīqat al-ʿālam*, 2 vols., Hyderabad.

Nāṣir, Ḥakīm Ẓafar al-Dīn Muḥammad, 1944, *Tīr ba-hadaf*. Hyderabad, Maktaba-yi Ḥakīm-i Dakan (1er éd. 1941).

Niẓām al-Dīn Aḥmad, ibn ʿAbd Allāh Ṣāʿidī Šīrāzī, 1961, *Ḥadīqat al-salāṭīn*, S. ʿAlī Aṣġar Bilgrāmī, éd., Hyderabad, Idāra-yi adabiyāt-i urdū.

Qādir Ḫān, Munšī Bīdarī, 1306/1889, *Tārīḫ-i Quṭb Šāhī*. Hyderabad, Burhāniya.

Šifā-yi Ḥaydarābādī, Ḥakīm, 1952, *Taḏkira-yi aṭibbā-yi ʿahd-i ʿUṯmānī*, Maqṣūd ʿAlī Ḫān, éd., Hyderabad.

Ṭabāṭabāʾī, Sayyid ʿAlī, *Burhān-i maʾāṯir*, 1355/1936. Delhi.

*Tārīḫ-i Muḥammad Quṭb Šāhī*, ms. Paris, Bibliothèque Nationale, supplément persan 1809.

Zūr Qādirī, Muḥī al-Dīn, 1941, *Ḥayāt awr kār nāma-yi Mīr Muḥammad Muʾmin*. Hyderabad.

### B. *Rapports et documents*

*Čār sālah niṣāb*. Hyderabad, Government Niẓāmiya ṭibbī kālij, s.d.

*Dastūr al-ʿamal Niẓāmiya ṭibbī kālij*. Hyderabad, 1348 f./1939.

*Hyderabad Administration Report, April 1950–March 1951*. Hyderabad, 1951.

*Hyderabad Administration Report, April 1951–March 1952*. Hyderabad.

Khan, Yusuf Husain, ed., 1958, *Selected Documents of Aurangzeb's Reign*. Hyderabad, Central Records Office.

*Report on the Administration* = *Report on the Administration of His Highness The Nizam's Dominions for the years* : 1308–1312 f. [1898–1903], Hyderabad, 1907 ; 1313–1315 f. [1903–1906], Hyderabad, 1910 ; 1316–1319 f. [1906–1910], Madras, 1913 ; 1338 f. [1928–1929], Hyderabad, 1932 ; 1341 f. [1931–1932], Hyderabad, 1933 ; 1343 f. [1933–1934], Hyderabad, 1937 ; 1344 f. [1934–1935], Hyderabad, 1938 ; 1345 f. [1935–1936], Hyderabad, 1938 ; 1346 f. [1936–1937], Hyderabad, 1939 ; 1347 f. [1937–1938], Hyderabad, 1940 ; 1349 f. [1939–1940], Hyderabad, 1942 ; 1350 f. [1940–1941], Hyderabad, 1943 ; 1351 f. [1941–1942], Hyderabad, 1945.

*Report on the Administration of Hyderabad State, September 1948–March 1950*. Hyderabad.

Yahya, Y. H., ed., 1950, *Selected Documents of Shāh Jahān's Reign – Muntaḥab-i kāġazāt-i ʿahd-i Šāh Jahān*. Hyderabad, Daftar-i Dīwānī.

### C. *Sources secondaires*

Attewell, Guy, 2007, *Refiguring Unani Tibb. Plural Healing in Late Colonial India*, Orient Longman, Delhi.

Azmi, Altaf Ahmad, 2004, *History of Unani Medicine in India*. Delhi, Jamia Hamdard.

Bari, Abdul, 1986–1987, « Unānī Medicine during the Reign of Quṭb Shāhī Dynasty ». *Studies in History of Medicine and Science*, X–XI, pp. 135–147.

Framurz Jung, 1894, *A Guide to Beder with Historical Notes*. Madras, Lawrence Asylum Press.

Husain, Ali Akbar, 2000, *Scent in the Islamic Garden. A study of Deccani Urdu Literary Sources*. Karachi, Oxford University Press.

Hussain, S. A. 1977, « Unani Medicine during Nizam Dynasty ». *Bulletin of the Indian Institute of History of Medicine*, VII, 3–4, pp. 154–160.

Jaggi, O. P., 1977, *Medicine in Medieval India*. Delhi, Atma Ram.

Munzawī, Aḥmad, 1362 h. š./1983, *Fihrist-i muštarak-i nusḫahā-yi ḫaṭṭī-i fārsī-i Pākistān*. Islamabad, Iran Pakistan Institute of Persian Studies, vol. 1.

——, 1382 h. š./2003, *Fihristwāra-i kitābhā-yi fārsī*. Téhéran, vol. 5.

Pernau, Margrit, 2000, *The Passing of Patrimonialism : Politics and Political Culture in Hyderabad 1911–1948*, Manohar, Delhi.

Quraishi, Salim al-Din, 1991, *Catalogue of the Urdu Books in the India Office Library (1800–1920)*. London (1er éd. 1982).

Reddy, Subba D. V., 1957, « Dar-us-Shifa (House of Cures) Built by Sultan Muhammad Quli in 1595 A. D. ». *Indian Journal of the History of Medicine*, 2, December 1957, pp. 102–105.

——, 1961, *Glimpses of Medical Heritage of Deccan. Proceedings of the Academy of Medical Sciences*, III, 4, Hyderabad.

——, 1962, « Mohammad Quli's interest in People's Health and Medical Aid », in : M. Qadiri Zūr, éd., *Qutb Shahi Sultans and Andhra Samskriti*. Hyderabad, Idara-e adabiyat-e urdu, pp. 15–27.

Rehman, Aijaz ur-, 1990, « Growth of the Hospital System in Hyderabad – Historical and Demographic Aspects : 1880's–1950's ». *Bulletin of the Indian Institute of History of Medicine*, XX, 2, pp. 123–139.

Rizvi, Athar Abbas, 1986, *A Socio-Intellectual History of the Isnā 'Asharī Shī'is in India*, 2 vols., Canberra.

Sherwani, Haroon Khan, 1968, *Muḥammad-Qulī Quṭb Shāh Founder of Haidarabad*. New York, Asia Publishing House.

——, 1974, *History of the Quṭb Shāhī Dynasty*. Delhi, Munshiram.

Speziale, Fabrizio, 2005, « Linguistic strategies of de-Islamisation and Colonial science: Indo-Muslim physicians and the yūnānī denomination ». *International Institute for Asian Studies Newsletter*, 37, p. 18.

(version en ligne : http://www.iias.nl/nl/37/IIAS_NL37_18.pdf).

——, 2008, « Le médecin des rêves. Culte des saints et guérison onirique chez les musulmans du Deccan », in : I. Zupanov – C. Guenzi, éds., *Divins remèdes, Médecine et religion en Asie du Sud*, collection *Purusartha*, 27. Paris, Editions de l'École des Hautes Études en Sciences Sociales, pp. 163–190.

——, 2009a, « India xxxiii. Indo-Muslim Physicians ». *Encyclopaedia Iranica*, (version en ligne : www.iranica.com).

——, 2009b, « Ajmal Khan ». *Encyclopaedia of Islam*, Third Edition, 2009–1, Leiden, E. J. Brill, p. 56.

——, 2010a, *Soufisme, religion et médecine en Islam indien*. Paris, Karthala.

——, 2010b, « Les traités persans sur les sciences indiennes : médecine, zoologie, alchimie » in : D. Hermann – F. Speziale, éds., *Muslim Cultures in the Indo-Iranian World during the Early-Modern and Modern Periods*. Berlin, Institut Français de Recherche en Iran – Klaus Schwarz Verlag, pp. 403–447.

Sufi, G. M. D., 1941, *Al-Minhāj: Being the Evolution of the Curriculum in the Muslim Educational Institutions of India*. Lahore.

Tavernier, Jean-Baptiste, 1676, *Les six voyages de Jean-Baptiste Tavernier,... qu'il a fait en Turquie, en Perse, et aux Indes,... Seconde partie, Où il est parlé des Indes, et des Iles voisines*. Paris, G. Clouzier et C. Barbin.

Vaughan, Philippa, 2001, « Il subcontinente indiano : da sultananto a impero moghul », in : M. Hattstein – P. Delius, éds., *Islam. Arte e Architettura*. Köln, Könemann (éd. or. *Islam : Kunst und Architektur*, Köln, 2000).

Yazdani, Ghulam, 1995, *Bidar : its History and Monuments*. Delhi (1er éd. London, 1947).

Ẓill al-Raḥmān, Sayyid Ḥakīm, 1995, *Dillī awr ṭibb-i yūnānī*. Delhi, Urdu Academy.

# HEALING THE PEOPLE AND THE PRINCES: HOSPITALS, ḤAKĪMS AND DOCTORS IN BHOPAL

Claudia Preckel

## Introduction: The Begums of Bhopal

Founded in the 18th century by Dūst Muḥammad H̱ān (d. 1728), a Pashtun adventurer, the princely state of Bhopal was ruled by four women for more than one century. These women, called the Begums of Bhopal, enacted a number of reforms, especially in the fields of religious education and the infrastructure of the state. This article shows how the Begums constructed and upheld Bhopal's health system by founding hospitals and dispensaries. The Begums supported the establishment of hospitals and medical services of Western modern medicine, however, they also supported the Muslim physicians who practiced the old Graeco-Arab medical tradition based on the teachings of Avicenna (Ibn Sīnā, d. 1037), which was called *yūnānī ṭibb* (Greek medicine) in India.[1] During the colonial period, the Begums of Bhopal were among the Indian Muslim rulers who most supported the establishment of new *yūnānī* institutions, especially of State run dispensaries, and the same ruling family used to be treated by *yūnānī* physicians. This however did non not lead to the creation of *yūnānī* hospitals. All the hospitals established in Bhopal during the Begums' rule provided western medical treatment and their activity was partially supported by the British. Two of the Begums, Šāh Jahān Begum (r. 1868–1901) and Sulṭān Jahān Begum (r. 1901–1926), were particularly active in the field of promoting women's education and women's healthcare. In addition, a hospital for women, where female doctors were employed, was established in Bhopal in the 1880s.[2] Indian woman, especially at the start of the spread of medical colonial establishments, were particularly unwilling to go to Western-style general hospitals or to be examined by a male doctor. The same Begums represent an important example of this attitude:

[1] On *yūnānī* medicine in India see Quaiser 2004; Attewell 2007; Speziale 2009a; Speziale 2010.

[2] On the reforms concerning women health in Bhopal state see also Lambert-Hurley 2007b.

they were very reluctant to allow their bodies to be examined and, as was the case with other members of the ruling family, they were not treated at hospitals in case of illness. As we will see, the Begum's views about women's health and education promoted modernization while relying on Muslim tenets, and they were inspired by the Muslim reformist movements of colonial India.

When Qudsiya Begum (r. 1818–1837) became ruler of Bhopal, she was a widow of only nineteen years of age. She used to be in *parda*, but immediately after her accession to the throne, she publicly abandoned the veil. Particularly to the British, she appeared as an Amazon warrior. Although the British were extremely doubtful about female rule, they could not find any male alternative and they finally decided to support Qudsiya's claims. Very little is known about the health system under Qudsiya Begum's reign. One of the main achievements of this period was the construction of the Bhopal waterworks and the laying of water pipelines throughout the state.[3] During her reign the Jāmiʿ Masjid (Friday mosque) was also erected and given a large endowment (*waqf*). It is possible that a dispensary for the poor was attached to the Jāmiʿ Masjid, as part of its *waqf*, or to another mosque of the city. Qudsiya Begum (d. 1881) had to step down from power in favor of her son-in-law Jahāngīr Muḥammad Ḫān (r. 1837–1844) who had married Qudsiya's daughter and only child, Sikandar Begum. Nawāb Jahāngīr Muḥammad Ḫān had at his service Muḥammad Aʿẓam Ḫān, an eminent Muslim traditional physician of Rampur who was the author of famous medical texts in Persian, such as the *Iksīr-i Aʿẓam*, on therapeutics, the *Muḥīṭ-i Aʿẓam*, on the *materia medica*, and the *Qarābādīn-i Aʿẓam*, a pharmacopoeia.[4]

More is known about the medical system under Sikandar Begum's rule (r. 1844–1868). During Sikandar's reign, Bhopal was still an Afghan military principality,[5] and the state administration concentrated on warfare.[6] Sikandar Begum received military education and, as her mother, she did not wear the *parda*. In 1854, Sikandar Begum founded the Medical Department of Bhopal. Although the majority of Bhopal's population was

[3] Sulṭān Jahān Begum 1918, pp. 68–70.

[4] See Siddiqi 1980.

[5] For Sikandar's reign see Preckel 2000, pp. 47–104; Khan 2000, pp. 90–118.

[6] According to the treaty of 1819 with the British, the Begum had to provide troops to support the British fight against the Marathas. Qudsiya Begum increased the expenditure of the Bhopal Contingent to 200,000 rupees, and Sikandar Begum added a further sum to this. The Bhopal Contingent hence could be equipped with additional staff and a surgeon, Preckel 2000, p. 51.

Hindu, the Medical Department was organized along the lines of *yūnānī* medicine. After the establishment of the Central India Agency in 1854, the Agency Hospital for the soldiers and the members of the British administration was erected in Sehore, around 20 miles from Bhopal. This hospital was under the supervision of the Agency Surgeon, who treated also the ruling family. In 1857, when the Mutiny against the British took place, Sikandar Begum did not side with the rebellion and was able to control the anti-British riots in Bhopal. To reward her loyalty, the British awarded the Begum with the Order of the Star of India.

## Medical Reforms under Šāh Jahān Begum (1868–1901)

Immediately after Sikandar's death, her daughter Šāh Jahān Begum succeeded her to the throne. Šāh Jahān's reign differed very much from that of her mother as Šāh Jahān did not show as much interest in military capabilities and physical education as her mother did. Šāh Jahān has been often described as having a delicate and feminine character and the focus of her reign shifted to poetry, architecture and literature. Therefore during Šāh Jahān's rule the military lost its dominant role in the affairs of the Bhopal state. What emerged was a new focus on Islamic education and re-interpretation of religious texts, especially in the fields of Islamic law (*fiqh*) and prophetic traditions (*ḥadīṯ*), and also proper female behavior.

Important medical reforms were enacted during Šāh Jahān's reign, such as vaccination campaigns and regulations for lepers. Šāh Jahān supported both Western medicine and native *yūnānī* physicians and during her reign the number of dispensaries—either *yūnānī* or allopathic—in the Bhopal Agency rose to seven.[7] The Begums of Bhopal were among those Indian rulers who vigorously promoted the vaccination of their subjects. Šāh Jahān's daughter, Sulṭān Jahān Begum, wrote in the biography of her mother that,

> Nothing has proved more efficacious in the prevention of small-pox than vaccination; and now the rich and the poor alike have come to realize its usefulness. But thirty, or more, years ago people were much afraid of being vaccinated. Great difficulty used to be experienced everywhere in getting vaccinated. Her Highness [Šāh Jahān] was however convinced of its utility and forthwith opened a Vaccination Department in Bhopal, and got her own grandson Nawab Mohammad Nasrulllah Khan [...] vaccinated first. As

[7] Sulṭān Jahān Begum 1926, p. 69.

a further incentive she also appointed a special reward for each child that was vaccinated.[8]

Šāh Jahān's faith in vaccination was criticized by Sir William Tebb (d. 1917), a British social reformer and fierce opponent of vaccination campaigns. In his book titled *The Recrudescence of Leprosy and its Causation*, he held vaccination responsible for the spread of leprosy in India. Concerning Šāh Jahān's efforts to establish the Leper Asylum of Sehore, Tebb wrote:

> This benevolent lady, the Begum of Bhopal, Nawab Shahjehan, has been persuaded to extend vaccinations in her province, upon which she spends 5000 rupees yearly, employing 35 vaccinators [...] thus unwittingly spreading the foul disease at the point of the lancet, and helping to fill the wards of the hospital which her benevolence has established.[9]

Šāh Jahān was even able to convince the practitioners of *yūnānī* medicine, the *ḥakīms*, to vaccinate the people. The *ḥakīms* were employed by the Vaccination Department, which was not under the supervision of the Agency Surgeon. Sulṭān Jahān reported in her autobiography that it was due to the will of her stepfather Ṣiddīq Ḥasan Ḫān that a *ḥakīm*, namely Munšī Rajab ʿAlī Ḫān, was appointed as officer in charge of the Vaccination Department.[10] Apparently, 14,440 vaccinations were performed by the *ḥakīms* in 1885.[11] However, at the same time (1884–1885), the Agency Surgeon Dr. Dane reported only 7,240 vaccinations in his area of responsibility, which was an increase compared to the years before, but only half the rate reported by the *ḥakīms*.[12]

## The Prince of Wales' Hospital

Two years after her accession to the throne Šāh Jahān established a first small allopathic hospital in Bhopal. The hospital was classified as III-A, meaning that it was supported by private individuals.[13] It might be assumed that the majority of these funds came from the ruling family as well as

8 Sulṭān Jahān Begum 1926, pp. 71–72.

9 Tebb 1893, p. 333.

10 Sulṭān Jahān Begum 1922, pp. 90–91.

11 *Report on the Political Administration of the Territories within the Central India Agency (1883–84)*, 1885, p. 119.

12 *Selections from the Records of the Government of India, Foreign Department* 1886, p. 117.

13 The following classes were attributed to hospitals and dispensaries in the Central Indian Agency: Class I, supported by the British Government of India; Class II, Supported by local bodies; Class III-A, supported by private individuals; Class III-B, supported partly by private individuals and partly by the state, see Roberts 1904, p. 7.

from other members of the Bhopal gentry. The next and most important step concerning the establishment of hospital services in Bhopal city was the construction of the Prince of Wales' Hospital, which was inaugurated in 1878. The Hospital was built in memory of the Prince of Wales' visit to India in 1875–76. During his visit, the Prince of Wales, later King Edward VII (r. 1901–1910), had visited several already existing hospitals such as those in Calcutta. In other cities, the local rulers had announced the foundation of a hospital to be named after the Prince of Wales: the Raja of Kolhapur (Maharashtra), for example, assigned 20,000 British pounds to the founding of the Prince of Wales' Hospital in Kolhapur.[14]

The Prince of Wales' Hospital of Bhopal followed modern colonial medicine and it was put under the supervision of the Agency Surgeon Dr. Dane, though the Hospital Assistant Walī Muḥammad, a Muslim allopathic physician, was put in charge of it. Walī Muḥammad later became one of Sulṭān Jahān's secretaries and served as a doctor to the ruling family.[15] When it was opened the hospital had 26 beds for inpatients, the half of those available at the Agency Hospital of Sehore which was reserved to the soldiers and the colonial elite. At the end of Šāh Jahān's rule in 1901, Bhopal city had a population of 77,023 while the whole Bhopal State counted 665,961 inhabitants,[16] meaning that one eighth of the population was residing in the capital where the only civil hospitals were located. Apparently, the year it was inaugurated, the Prince of Wales' had a daily average attendance of 93 patients,[17] which rose to 143.8 (inpatients and outpatients) in 1883, which meant more than 52,000 for the year.[18] But according to another source, 51,208 patients (inpatients and outpatients) underwent medical treatment in the hospital and the other seven dispensaries of the Bhopal Agency in 1884–85, whereas there were only 39,061 in 1883. The same source records that in 1884–85 at the Prince of Wales' Hospital 859 minor operations were performed, but only 60 major ones,

---

14 Hopkins 1910, p. 142.

15 Sulṭān Jahān Begum 1912, p. 279–280. Walī Muḥammad is described by the British sources as a skilful physician "doing a good job, and giving satisfaction to the State", *Report on the Political Administration of the Territories within the Central India Agency (1881–82)*, 1883, p. 144.

16 See *Imperial Gazetteer of India*, 1908, pp. 125, 133; Luard 1908, p. 95, 98. The population of the Bhopal State fell from 952,486 in 1891 to 665,961 in 1901; this decline was caused by heavy rainfalls during the monsoon period 1899–1900, which was further responsible for a famine.

17 "Medical Progress in Bhopal" 1927, p. 1241.

18 *Report on the Political Administration of the Territories within the Central India Agency (1881–82)*, 1883, p. 140.

while the previous year there were 12 major and 297 minor operations performed.[19]

During the epoch of Sulṭān Jahān Begum (r. 1901–1925) the Prince of Wales' Hospital was expanded. Steps were taken to improve the condition of the hospital which, according to the official records, during the first decade of the 20th century had shown a decrease in the number of patients visited. In 1911, the Prince of Wales' treated almost 400 inpatients and more than 29,000 outpatients, meaning an attendance of about 80 patients for day, i.e. less than the rate of 1878. These data show also that many persons received medical care as outpatients whereas only a relatively small number of them were hospitalized as inpatients. The prevailing diseases recorded were malarial fevers, rheumatic afflictions, eye diseases, disorders of the digestive system, ulcers and diseases of the skin, which seems to indicate that major surgical operations were not many.[20]

During the last years of Sulṭān Jahān's reign, the construction of a new red sandstone building was begun. On October 31st 1927 the new building of the Prince of Wales' Hospital was opened by the Begum accompanied by her son Ḥamīd Allāh Ḫān (r. 1926–1949), to whom she had abdicated the year before. By the late 1920's the initial distrust of the locals seems to have been largely overcome and the year the new building was inaugurated the hospital had an average daily attendance of 500 patients. The Begum contributed generously towards the provision of the new building which was erected by the Public Works Department at a cost of about 30,000 British Pounds. The new building included a modern operating theatre, new wards for patients, an x-ray plant and modern laboratories. During the opening ceremony Nawāb Ḥamīd Allāh Ḫān referred particularly the need of providing a separate ward for paying patients, a measure that obviously aimed to make hospital services more attractive to the wealthier classes, who usually preferred to be treated at home.[21] The improvements made are testified to by the American traveler Alexander Powell who was there in the late 1920s:

> I might mention that the *Prince of Wales' Hospital* in Bhopal, built and maintained by members of the reigning family, is one of the finest institutions of this kind in India, as up-to-date in its methods and equipment as any in the United States. I know, because I went there daily.[22]

---

[19] *Selections from the Records of the Government of India, Foreign Department* 1886, p. 83.
[20] Roberts 1912, p. 8.
[21] See "Medical Progress in Bhopal" 1927, p. 1241.
[22] Powell 1929, p. 274.

The Prince of Wales' Hospital was originally designed only for the treatment of male patients, but this changed slowly. In 1903, 14 women were also treated as inpatients,[23] though female patients were given the opportunity to be treated at the Lady Lansdowne Hospital for women, where there were facilities for Muslim women wearing *parda*. After Indian Independence, the Prince of Wales' Hospital was renamed King George's Hospital and then Hamidia Hospital.[24] It is nowadays the main government hospital of the city and gained international attention in 1984, when it treated thousands of patients after the Bhopal chemical disaster.

## The Agency Hospital and the Leper Asylum in Sehore

As Sehore was the place where the Bhopal Battalion was stationed, it was decided that the Agency Hospital was to be erected there. The Agency Hospital was established in the 1850's and had accommodation for 50 resident patients. The Agency Surgeon, who was also the Medical Officer of the 9th Bhopal Infantry, was in charge of this hospital. It was the only hospital in Bhopal State that was a Class I institution, meaning that it was mainly funded by an Imperial grant. Other funds came from the Bhopal State and from other states of the Bhopal Agency. Šāh Jahān Begum contributed to the support of this hospital and private donations arrived also from other local nobles.[25]

After the establishment of Bhopal railway system during Šāh Jahān's reign, a small Station Hospital and dispensary was built at Sehore. It was part of the Great Indian Peninsula Railway built by the British and had five beds for men and one for the treatment of women. In 1903, according to the reports of the British administration, this hospital was "in need of much improvement in respect both of accommodation and equipment".[26] In the same year, 53 male patients, but only 4 women, were treated as inpatients, and almost 2000 outpatients were treated in the dispensary.[27]

New regulations concerning people suffering from leprosy (*kuṛh*) were passed in the early 1890's. Previously, people suffering from this disease were ordered to leave Bhopal City; they were housed elsewhere and food

23 *Selections from the Records of the Government of India, Foreign Department* 1904 p. 13.

24 In 1957, a new 180 beds' wing for women was opened, *The Eleventh Year of Freedom, 1957–58*, 1959, p. 417.

25 Šāh Jahān Begum 1876, p. 143.

26 Roberts 1904, p. 8.

27 Roberts 1904, p. 47.

was supplied to them by the State Poor House.[28] It was only during the last decade of Šāh Jahān's rule that this policy changed and the Leper Asylum in Sehore was founded. The activity of the Sehore Leper Asylum was closely connected to the Christian missionary efforts in Bhopal. The plan of establishing a leper asylum was backed by Colonel Wylie, the then Political Agent, who invited members of the Friends' Foreign Mission Association[29] to work in the asylum. Wylie solicited the help of Šāh Jahān who granted land for the asylum and agreed to make an annual grant of 4,500 rupees for maintenance expenses.[30] This initiative coincided with the activities of the Leprosy Commission for India (1889). With the Lepers' Act of 1898, leper asylums were recognized as sites for medical treatment and confinement: the Government of British India put leprosy under the category of contagious diseases and campaigned for the segregation of lepers.[31]

The Leper Asylum of Sehore was opened on July 17th, 1891, and the newly erected building could accommodate 160 lepers. It seems that in the beginning the new regulations concerning the segregation of lepers in asylums were not applied so strictly in Bhopal. During the year 1903, the average number of inmates of the Leper Asylum of Sehore was merely 44.8, meaning that only a quarter of the places were actually occupied.[32] It was also clear that those working in the leper asylum did not believe in healing the disease. The Agency Surgeon Dr. Dane at the opening ceremony of the Sehore Leper Asylum said, "We do not expect to cure these unfortunate people, as, notwithstanding the praises which are repeatedly being bestowed on [...] 'certain cures', there is no doubt that a cure for leprosy has still to be discovered."[33]

Although the Sehore asylum was under the supervision of Dr. Dane, members of the Friends' Mission were working there. The British backed the idea of having lepers medically treated as well as religiously taught by Christian missionaries. It seems that in the beginning Šāh Jahān tolerated the Friends' Mission's work in Sehore despite the fact that one of the main objectives of the missionaries' work in the leper asylums was of a religious

---

[28] Sulṭān Jahān Begum 1926, p. 68.

[29] The members of the Religious Society of Friends are commonly known as Quakers. For the efforts of the Quaker missionaries in Bhopal see Lambert-Hurley 2006. For a report of their activities in India and Bhopal see The Society of Friends 1897, pp. 111–117.

[30] Tebb 1893, p. 333, quoting the *Bombay Gazette* of 17th July, 1891.

[31] See Kakar 2006, p. 192.

[32] Roberts 1910, pp. 13, 47.

[33] Tebb 1893, p. 333.

nature. Christian missionaries believed that leprosy was a disease of the soul and that physical deformities were a manifestation of sin. On the basis of this believe, they favored the separation of lepers from patients with other diseases.[34] As leprosy was seen as a sign of impurity of the soul, the teaching of the gospels and Christian education played a main role in the treatment. Some missionary reports considered such work in Leper Asylums as quite successful as several conversions to Christianity were reported among the patients in leper asylums. In Tara Taran (Panjab), for example, the daily evangelism seemed to result in the conversion of almost a quarter of the inmates of the local leper asylum.[35]

Having gained an entry into the Sehore Cantonment by taking charge of the Leper Asylum, the Friends' Mission could establish two bungalows in Sehore—used as a base for their missionary activities—and a resident mission in Bhopal city. They also sent two female missionaries to Bhopal city to work with Muslim women. These activities however were not further encouraged by Šāh Jahān during the last years of her reign and finally Sulṭān Jahān restricted them. Street-preaching, open-air services, dispensary and hospital work were prohibited in Bhopal and the missionaries were forbidden to evangelize in the *zanāna* (women apartments).[36] Only female missionaries were allowed to work in Bhopal city, as tutors of daughters and wives of court officials and nobles, whereas the male Friends' Mission's activities were reduced to the work in the Sehore Leper Asylum until the 1930s, when the Quakers finally left Bhopal.[37]

## *Tahḏīb al-niswān* and Female Health

Three years after her enthronement, Šāh Jahān Begum married the Islamic scholar Sayyid Ṣiddīq Ḥasan Ḫān al-Qannawjī (1832–1890).[38] Ṣiddīq Ḥasan Ḫān was one of the main figures of the *Ahl-i ḥadīṯ*, an influential Islamic reformist movement that emerged in colonial India.[39] The Begum and her husband intended to introduce in Bhopal an Islamic rule based on

[34] See Kakar 2006.
[35] Harding 2008, pp. 105 ff.
[36] Lambert-Hurley 2006, p. 257.
[37] On the difficulties encountered by the Quakers in Bhopal see also The Society of Friends 1897, pp. 112, 114–115.
[38] Preckel 2008, pp. 167–170.
[39] The *Ahl-i ḥadīṯ* did not accept the *taqlīd* and aimed to back each legal decision with the Quran and the *ḥadīṯ* (traditions) of the Prophet, see Preckel 2007.

the *šarīʿa* law. However, in Šāh Jahān's view this did not meant to cease the co-operation with the British authorities, which on their hand were critical of Šāh Jahān's decision to appear always veiled in public after her second marriage with Ṣiddīq Ḥasan Ḫān. Unlike other Muslim reformist movements of the 19th century, the *Ahl-i ḥadīt* strictly upheld the *parda* system. In Šāh Jahān's view, wearing the veil was a way to enable Muslim women to take part in the social activities outside the walls of the *zanāna*. For this sake she also created a special bazaar, where *parda* women could earn their living by selling goods and homemade food.

Šāh Jahān also wrote a book in Urdu for the education of the Muslim women entitled *Tahḏīb al-niswān wa tarbiyat al-insān* (Cultivation of women and education of mankind).[40] The book was first published in 1881, and has been republished several times. *Tahḏīb al-niswān* belongs to the first generation of female practical guidebooks in Urdu, focusing on moral, religious and health instruction. The Begum mentioned relevant *ḥadīṯ* and Quranic quotations concerning female life in society and proper female behavior. She stressed that either health or disease came from God alone and that the hour of death is determined by Allāh's will. The book followed the principles of *yūnānī* medicine and the Begum recommended treatment by a qualified *ḥakīm*. Šāh Jahān described the female body during pregnancy and admonished women to exercise caution (*iḥtiyāṭ*) in order to avoid abortion. The instructions of medical character given in the text include the descriptions of dietary rules to be followed during pregnancy and after birth and various advices for curing child diseases and female disorders.[41]

## The Lady Lansdowne Hospital for Women

Šāh Jahān was particularly concerned about women's healthcare and the provision of medical treatment for women in *parda*. Due to their seclusion, women were often unable to see a physician. In the 1880s, Šāh Jahān opened a small *zanāna* hospital in Bhopal, where veiled women could be treated by women physicians and nurses.[42] However, this hospital had

---

[40] Šāh Jahān Begum 1970; see also Preckel 2004; Pernau 2008, pp. 297–299.

[41] Šāh Jahān Begum 1970, pp. 19–22 (female disorders and their treatment), 31–42 (proper female behaviour and diseases during pregnancy), 43–118 (recommendations for child rearing and cure of child diseases).

[42] Sulṭān Jahān Begum 1912, pp. 152, 155.

very limited facilities. To create a bigger hospital Šāh Jahān looked for support from the British. In 1891, the Viceroy of India Lord Lansdowne (d. 1927)[43] and his wife visited Bhopal and Lady Lansdowne agreed to support Šāh Jahān's plan for creating a bigger women's hospital in Bhopal. It was decided to make extensive additions to the already existing building and to name the new institution the Lady Lansdowne Hospital. The hospital was located at the Lower Lake of Bhopal city, on the road leading to the Bhopal railway station and it is known nowadays as Sultania Zanana Hospital.

The new wings were built quite rapidly and the Lady Lansdowne Hospital was inaugurated the following year, on 24th May 1892. This date was chosen by Šāh Jahān as it was Queen Victoria's birthday. Among the guests of the function were Major M. B. Meade, the Political Agent, other members of the British administration and local authorities. In her speech Šāh Jahān praised the work carried out by the Lady Doctor and emphasize the role that this institution should play in the training of midwives:

> I am glad to say that the Lady Doctor has carried out her preliminary duties of fitting up the hospital in a very creditable manner. I trust that the institution will continue to prove its utility under her charge, and the midwives trained by her in this institution, will prove themselves highly useful for our beloved subjects.[44]

The Lady Lansdowne Hospital was partly funded by the National Association for Supplying Female Medical Aid to the Women of India, known also as the Dufferin Fund. The Dufferin Fund provided in particular the Lady Doctors who actually run the Lady Lansdowne Hospital. Lady Dufferin (d. 1936), wife of the Viceroy in India, had established the fund in 1885 for the provision of medical care to Indian women.[45] The Dufferin Fund became the most important medical institution of this kind in colonial India. Although Lady Dufferin held the *parda* system responsible for the

---

43 Several hospitals were named after him throughout India, e.g. the Lansdowne Hospital of Nabha (Panjab) and the Lansdowne Hospital of Calcutta.

44 Sulṭān Jahān Begum 1912, pp. 154–155.

45 The Lady Dufferin Fund followed three main aims: "Firstly—To provide medical tuition for native female students. Secondly—Medical relief, by establishing female hospitals and dispensaries, and the placing of Lady Doctors in different towns or districts. Thirdly—Supplying trained nurses and *accoucheuses* [midwifes] for women and children in hospitals and private houses", see "Lady Dufferin and the Women of India", 1891, p. 460; see also Lal 1994. For natives critiques of the Dufferin's Fund and the British debates on Christian evangelical mission and medical support to women in the *zanāna* see Burton 1996, p. 369.

lack of female education and reduced access to the health system, she supported hospitals for *parda* ladies throughout India.[46] One of the main reasons for this compromise with the local social codes was the effort to promote the acceptance of British medical women among the locals. The Begums of Bhopal, on their hand, wanted Muslim women to be treated by female doctors and to develop socials spaces and health services for *parda* women.

The delicacy of the matter of the examination of the female body can be clearly inferred by the attitude shown by the same Begums towards having their own bodies medically examined. As with many other Indian noblemen, the Begums and the members of their family did not go to hospitals when they were ill, but they were treated at home by private physicians. The Begums had at their service both allopathic and *yūnānī* physicians. Several of the allopathic physicians who worked at the hospitals of Bhopal, including the Lady Doctors of the Lansdowne Hospital, treated members of the ruling family at their homes. After her pilgrimage to Mecca and several trips in India Sikandar Begum fell ill and died soon after in November 1868. On this occasion she was visited both by *yūnānī* and English physicians but she strictly refused to be examined, either in hospital or in her palace.[47] In all likelihood, she refused the examination of the body and relied only on the traditional diagnostics of *yūnānī* medicine, such as examination of the pulse (*nabż*) and the urine (*bawl*), which did not involve physical inspection. Sulṭān Jahān died of cancer in 1930 and when she fell ill she was very reluctant to be operated and did not wish to have her body examined. Finally, an operation room was prepared in her palace and the Begum wept constantly while being taken there.[48]

## Medicine and Politics during Sulṭān Jahān Begum's rule (1901–1925)

During the epoch of Sulṭān Jahān the emphasis on female health and *yūnānī* medicine increased. Sulṭān Jahān was a firm believer in the efficacy of *yūnānī* remedies and was convinced that many Indians still had confidence in it. Sulṭān Jahān's granddaughter writes that the Begum "had always more faith and confidence in *hakeems* because their remedies

---

[46] Lal 1994, p. 42.
[47] Šāh Jahān Begum 1876, p. 119; Abida Sultaan 2004, p. 89.
[48] Abida Sultaan 2004, pp. 89–90.

were closer to nature than the doctors".[49] When she was ill, eminent *yūnānī* physicians came to treat her from other Indian cities. Among these were Ḥakīm Ajmal Ḫān of Delhi (see below) and Ḥakīm ʿAbd al-ʿAzīz (m. 1911) of Lucknow, the leaders of the two most renowned families of *yūnānī* physicians of the Colonial period, the Šarīfī of Delhi and the ʿAzīzī of Lucknow.[50] The Begum's faith in *yūnānī* physicians faded probably only once, after the early death of her second daughter Āṣaf Jahān's in 1894, which followed the death of her elder daughter Bilqīs Jahān in 1887.

Sulṭān Jahān opened new dispensaries throughout the state and most of these were *yūnānī* ones. Until the beginning of the 20th century the number of State run dispensaries remained considerably small as there were only seven dispensaries in the whole Bhopal Agency, of which some were offering *yūnānī* treatment. Immediately after Sulṭān Jahān's arrival to the throne the number of *yūnānī* dispensaries (*dawā-ḫāna*) became significantly higher than that of allopathic ones. In 1902–03 there were two hospitals and six allopathic dispensaries which had in all a daily average attendance of 486 patients, while the *yūnānī* dispensaries were thirty-two and had a daily average attendance of 1,380 patients.[51] After few years the number of *yūnānī dawā-ḫāna* increased to thirty-six.[52] It is possible that the bigger ones of these *yūnānī* dispensaries were equipped with a few beds. However, despite the growing emphasis on *yūnānī* medicine which characterized the rule of Sulṭān Jahān, this did not lead to the establishment in Bhopal of a hospital intended only for the *yūnānī* treatment. It was through the creation of new dispensaries, and not of hospitals, that the Bhopal State tried to develop the accessibility of *yūnānī* medicine.

Sulṭān Jahān also backed the project of establishing a new institution for *yūnānī* teaching, on the lines of the others *yūnānī* schools which were founded around the same period in Delhi, Lucknow and Hyderabad. In 1903, the Madrasa-yi Āṣafiya was founded in Bhopal in order to improve and regulate the training of local *yūnānī* physicians. The Āṣafiya Zanāna Dawā-Ḫāna, for the *yūnānī* treatment of women was established next to the Madrasa. These dispensaries were under the supervision of Ḥakīm Nūr al-Ḥasan al-Dihlawī (d. 1912), the *Raʾīs al-aṭṭibā* (Chief physician) of

---

49 Abida Sultaan 2004, p. 90.

50 Sulṭān Jahān wrote in her autobiography that "I may say that it is due to the efforts and skill of two of these physicians, Hakim Ajmal Khan Sahib and Hakim Abdul Aziz Khan Sahib, that I myself am alive at the present day", Sulṭān Jahān Begum 1912, p. 318.

51 *Imperial Gazetteer of India*, 1908, p. 142.

52 Mittal 1990, p. 79.

the State.[53] As with other *yūnānī* physicians of the colonial period, Nūr al-Ḥasan was favorable to the integration of elements of Western medicine as a means to revive the *yūnānī* tradition, as he stressed in the speech given at the opening ceremony of the Madrasa-yi Āṣafiya:

> It is not so very long ago, that the Yunani medical system was in a highly flourishing state. Today, we see its prestige rapidly and steadily declining [...] There are, however, many people who still have faith in the Yunani treatment [...] If we wish to revive this valuable science and bring its methods up to date [...] our object must be not only to teach students the use and effect of medicines peculiar to the Yunani system, but to familiarize them with the many appliances which modern research has placed at the doctor's disposal.[54]

Sulṭān Jahān had close contacts with Ḥakīm Ajmal Ḫān (d. 1927) of Delhi, the most distinguished *yūnānī* physician of the British period.[55] Ajmal Ḫān came from a distinguished family of *ḥakīm*s of Delhi and was one of the main authors of the modernizing reforms of *yūnānī* medicine which were realized during the colonial period. In the early 20th century he founded the Hindustānī Dawā-Ḫāna of Delhi, for the large-scale manufacturing of *yūnānī* drugs. In 1921, he opened the Ayurvedic and Yūnānī Ṭibbiya College, where it was also a hospital ward, and which aimed to upgrade and modernize the instruction in *yūnānī* medicine. With a sum of 25,000 rupees and an annual grant of 150 rupees, Sulṭān Jahān was among the main donors for this institution.[56] Ajmal Ḫān visited Bhopal several times. He treated Sulṭān Jahān and supported her efforts to promote and institutionalize *yūnānī* medicine in Bhopal. Ajmal Ḫān was also a Muslim political leader and most probably Sulṭān Jahān sympathized with his ideas of a strong Muslim community in India.

Other important Muslim figures and movements of colonial India tied connections with Bhopal and the Begum. The Aligarh movement of Sir Sayyid Aḥmad Ḫān (1817–1898) had an important influence on the Muslim culture of colonial India. It was especially Aḥmad Ḫān's wish to promote female education, which found Sulṭān Jahān's support. In 1920, Sulṭān Jahān became the founding Chancellor of the Aligarh Muslim University,

---

[53] Nūr al-Ḥasan practiced as a physicians in Delhi and in his youth had studied in Bhopal with Ḥasanī Faḫr al-Dīn Ḥasanī (d. 1908), who was a physician and the father of the famous scholar ʿAbd al-Ḥayy Ḥasanī (d. 1923), see Ḥasanī 1402/1981, p. 505.

[54] Sulṭān Jahān Begum 1912, pp. 319–20.

[55] On Ajmal Ḫān see Metcalf 1985a; Ibid. 1985b; Pernau 2008, pp. 251–260; Speziale 2009b.

[56] Abdur Razzack 1987, p. 32.

a position that no other woman has held after her. Ten years before, she had enrolled her favorite son and heir Ḥamīd Allāh Ḫān in the Muhammadan Anglo-Oriental College of Aligarh. In Aligarh Ḥamīd Allāh made the acquaintance of several Muslims who later became political leaders and made their way to Bhopal. One of the most important of them was Dr. Muḫtār Aḥmad Anṣārī (1880–1936), who was a friend and political associate of Ajmal Ḫān[57] and took service in Bhopal in the team of doctors responsible for the members of the ruling family. Anṣārī was educated in Hyderabad and at the Madras Medical College. Then he moved to England and worked as a surgeon at the Charing Cross Hospital of London, where a ward has been called Ansari Ward after him. Anṣārī was among the early supporters of the Ḫilāfat Movement (1919–1924). This movement, backed especially by Indian Muslims, aimed to revive the links with the Ottoman Sultan, who was regarded as the leader (*ḫalīfa*) of all Muslims.[58] When World War I broke out, Dr. Anṣārī's organized a medical mission to Turkey. The mission consisted of twenty-two doctors and male nurses and lasted for about eight months. The same Ottoman Sultan praised the mission's efforts to render medical services to the Turkish soldiers. Ḥamīd Allāh was quite supportive of the Ḫilāfat Movement and often invited its leaders to Bhopal. British authorities did not view Ḥamīd Allāh's pan-Islamic activities with favor and gave some delicate warnings to the Begum.[59]

The Begum found herself torn between her loyalty to the British and her feelings of solidarity to the Ottoman ruler which were backed by her son's pan-Islamic ideals. Finally, she gave troops and arms to the British forces with the condition that these were not to be used against Turkish soldiers, and donated thousands of copies of the Quran to the Muslims joining the British troops. Sulṭān Jahān gave also 5,000 rupees to the St. John's Ambulance Service and 3,000 rupees to the British Women's Hospital of London. She supported in particular the project and the maintenance of the hospital ship *Loyalty*, to which the Begum contributed with 200,088 rupees. The idea of buying a ship for hospital services had originated from the Maharaja of Gwalior, Mādhav Rāo Scindia (1886–1925). The ship was the *Empress of India*, a Royal Mail ship which had been plying between North Pacific and South-East Asian ports for more than twenty years. The Maharaja of Gwalior bought it on December 1914 and renamed it *Loyalty*.

---

57 Both Ajmal Ḫān and Anṣārī were members of the Indian National Congress, of the Muslim League and took part in the Ḫilāfat Movement.

58 See Minault 1982; Qureshi 1999.

59 Khan 2000, p. 182.

The *Loyalty* was equipped with operating rooms and more than 500 beds; it carried more than 15,000 war patients and the staff on board included around 80 Indians, among them doctors and assistants.[60]

## The Lady Lansdowne Hospital and Female Healthcare in the Early 20th Century

Other local rulers in the Central India Agency followed the Begums' example and created facilities for the treatment of women, such as the Vikram Hospital For Females, which was opened in 1911 in Narsingarh, ruled by Rāja Sir Arjun Singhjī (r. 1895–1924). Most of these hospitals were not big establishments. In the first decades of the 20th century the staff of the Lansdowne Hospital of Bhopal, which was one of the main cities of the Central India Agency, consisted in all of a Matron and eight local nurses, besides a Lady Doctor in charge of the hospital. At the turn of the century the Lansdowne Hospital had 23 beds. During the year 1903, only 200 women and 67 children were treated as inpatients; in addition, 3561 women, 3273 children and 65 men were treated as outpatients.[61] These data suggest that until the beginning of the 20th century local people were not so prone to have women hospitalized as inpatients. A new wing was added to the Lansdowne Hospital in 1911, containing operation and labor rooms, and quarters for the House Surgeon.[62] The presence of a male House Surgeon seems to indicate that the Lady Doctor was not intended to perform major surgical operations.

In India, qualified women were normally required to work as hospital assistants of male doctors, while in some *zanāna* hospitals, such as the one of Bhopal, they could be put in charge of the hospital. As mentioned above, the Lady Doctors who were in charge of the Lansdowne Hospital worked for the Dufferin Fund, which recruited women doctors from Great Britain. Practicing in India gave British female doctors the opportunity to gain experience and many of them would have hoped to obtain a better post in Britain after a period in India.[63] The women who entered the Dufferin Fund received a little more pay than men, but they had neither pension nor a regularly increasing salary. The Lady Doctors who were

60 Playne 2006, p. 248.
61 Roberts 1904, p. 12.
62 Roberts 1912, p. 9.
63 See Forbes 2005, pp. 121 ff.

brought from England received "in addition to their passage and an allowance for outfit, Rs. 300 per month, with quarters, and they are allowed to have a private practice as well."[64]

They were often recent medical graduates and unmarried women who entered the Dufferin Fund and some of them had also follow some courses in tropical medicine. For instance, Miss Adeline Rubins, who was a Lady Doctor at the Lansdowne Hospital of Bhopal in the 1920s, held a Medical Baccalaureate and a Diploma in Tropical Medicine and Hygiene. During the period she worked at the Lansdowne Hospital she also published a case study which appeared in 1926 in the *British Medical Journal*.[65] An earlier woman doctor in charge of the Lansdowne Hospital had been Miss Ada Neibel.[66] She had entered the Dufferin Fund in 1889 immediately after her medical graduation.[67] Sulṭān Jahān was not satisfied with the services of Miss Neibel and the Begum's disappointment grew especially after the death of her second daughter Āṣaf Jahān, which had been visited by Miss Neibel. Sulṭān Jahān reports this event in her autobiography remarking that Miss Neibel:

> Was neither courteous in her manner nor attentive in her treatment. The disease steadily advanced, and for a week Asif Jahan Begam took no nourishment, any attempt to do so being followed by violent sickness. When Miss Neibel's opinion was asked, she said that she could discover no specific disease from which my daughter was suffering, and, as far as she could see, there was nothing serious the matter.[68]

Sulṭān Jahān was particularly satisfied with the work done at the Lansdowne Hospital by Miss L. Blong. She had graduated from Calcutta Medical College in 1893, the same year entered the Lady Dufferin Fund and took service in Barabanki (Uttar Pradesh) and then moved to Bhopal.[69] During the period she worked at the Lansdowne Hospital Miss Blong also treated members of the Begum family. In her autobiography, Sulṭān Jahān praised Miss Blong's character and ability and emphasized the improvements made at the hospital under her direction:

> She knew my family well, and her kindness had gained her the affection of all classes of the people. She was a noble-minded and sweet-tempered lady,

---

64 "Lady Dufferin and the Women of India", 1891, p. 459.
65 Rubins 1926.
66 Sometimes called Niebel.
67 Forbes 2005, p. 120.
68 Sulṭān Jahān Begum 1912, pp. 164–165.
69 Forbes 2005, p. 120.

> and by her tact and ability had done more to improve the Lady Lansdowne Hospital than any of those who had preceded her.[70]

In addition to the work at the hospital, the Lady Doctor gave classes in nursing and midwifery. During the colonial period the quality of nursing in India had been the object of strong criticism. The image of traditional midwives (*dā'ī*) was even worse than that of nurses, as they were openly regarded as incompetent and dangerous.[71] An emblematic example is given in a report on nursing in India published in 1908 in *The British Journal of Nursing*:

> In Europe nursing has, in recent years, developed into quite a science, and is now chiefly in the hands of highly educated ladies [...] the women of this country [India] have no conception of nursing in the proper sense of the word, and until a radical change takes place in their habits and customs and feelings, and until they are better educated, our difficulties will not be overcome. They would neither subject themselves to the necessary training, nor, on account of their ingrained prejudices, will they fulfill the functions daily performed by a European nurse.[72]

Similar views were held by the Indian elites acquainted with Western culture. In 1909, few years before the inauguration of the Lady Minto Nursing School (see below), Sulṭān Jahān remarked that:

> I know from my own experience how much patients suffer in this country in consequence of the ignorance which prevails of the art of nursing. In Europe, many women receive expert training in this art, which they practice as a profession. They are ready for service not only in hospitals and nursing homes, but in private houses. [...] In India, unhappily, the reverse is the case. It is surely, therefore, a matter of the utmost importance that the steps should be taken to train Indian women as nurses, so that the people in every grade of society may be able to obtain the assistance, they so urgently need.[73]

Various efforts were attempted in this period to improve and regulate the training of midwives. Sulṭān Jahān looked with great interest at Ajmal Ḫān efforts,[74] who in 1909 established in Delhi the Madrasa Ṭibbiya Zanāna and Šifā-Ḫāna (Women Medical School and Dispensary). The Madrasa Ṭibbiya Zanāna aimed to institutionalize the training of midwives and

---

70 Sulṭān Jahān Begum 1912, p. 204.
71 Van Hollen 2003, p. 47; Forbes 2005, pp. 91 ff.
72 "Nursing in India", 1908, pp. 287–288.
73 Quoted in Mittal 1990, p. 80.
74 Ḫān 2002, p. 74.

was inaugurated by the wife of the Lieutenant Governor of Panjab, Lady Dane.[75] Later on it was shifted to the new Ayurvedic and Yūnānī Ṭibbiya College. However, such efforts did not produce the expected results. In 1921, in his speech at the opening of the Ayurvedic and Yūnānī Ṭibbiya College, Ajmal Ḫān complained that the number of girl students in the Madrasa Ṭibbiya Zanāna remained low and that in the previous three years the school had an average of no more than 13 students.[76]

In the same year in which Ajmal Ḫān opened the Madrasa Ṭibbiya Zanāna, Sulṭān Jahān introduced in Bhopal rules for education and certification for both nurses and midwives.[77] The certificate was issued after the completion of a training, which was imparted at the Lady Lansdowne Hospital. Since the profession of *dā'ī* was hereditary, the Begum ordered that the daughters of traditional midwives should be trained by the Lady Doctor before being allowed to practice. The courses at the Lady Lansdowne Hospital were supported by the Dufferin Fund and by the Victoria Memorial Scholarship Fund. The Victoria Fund had been established in 1903, a year after the passing of the first Midwives Act in Great Britain, and aimed to train traditional *dā'ī* throughout India. Sulṭān Jahān Begum contributed between 420 and 488 rupees per annum to the Victoria Fund. In the Central India Agency, other institutions in Gwalior and Indore hosted courses and students of either midwifery or nursing sponsored by the Victoria Fund.

In 1911–12, new facilities for teaching were added to the Lady Lansdowne Hospital of Bhopal. The school was officially named Lady Minto Nursing School and contained quarters for twelve students. As in the case of the Madrasa Ṭibbiya Zanāna of Ajmal Ḫān, in the first years of their existence these courses did not register a growth in the number of students enrolled. In 1909, there were 38 students at Gwalior, 16 at Indore and 39 at Bhopal. Two years later these numbers decreased to 24 students at Gwalior and 31 at Bhopal, while it remained almost unchanged at Indore with 17 students.[78] The same Begum observed that in the beginnings it was not easy to find pupils for this school and it was only after the promise of scholarships that a class was got together.[79]

[75] Ali 1997, p. 16.
[76] Abdur Razzack 1987, p. 25.
[77] "Registration of midwives in Bhopal", p. 56.
[78] Roberts 1912, p. 12.
[79] Mittal 1990, p. 81.

Sulṭān Jahān took particular interest in the education of women and mothers in the fields of first aid, hygiene and child diseases. She wrote two books in Urdu on these topics, the first was *Baččūn kī parwariš,* on child education and childcare which was printed in 1913.[80] A few years later *Ḫānadārī kā dūsrā ḥiṣṣa,*[81] on housekeeping and house hygiene, appeared. Both these texts meant in particular to promote the knowledge of hygienic rules and hygienic products among Indian women, and especially among those living in the *zanāna* apartments. Most of the recommendations on hygiene given in these books follow Western ideas, and the Begum often uses English terms, such as for names of chemical substances. In order to enable women to use these preparations at home—such as those for cleaning the houses—the Begum only mentioned substances used in Europe which were are also available in India and gave either their Urdu or English names.

Sulṭān Jahān used the staff of the Lady Lansdowne Hospital to promote her view of bringing healthcare to women in accordance with the local social codes. The Begum ordered the staff of the hospital to visit regularly the *zanāna* apartments of the city to provide basic hygienic training and medical care for women in *parda* and for children living with them. Sulṭān Jahān wished that the Lady Doctor and the Matron visited personally some of the most important houses of the city, as Indian women of the upper classes were the most reluctant to go to doctors and hospitals. On these occasions, the Matron used to take one of the nurses to instruct her, until the nurse was capable of carrying out an examination herself. Sulṭān Jahān gave several instructions concerning the inspection of the *zanāna* apartments. The hospital staff had to evaluate and give advice to women on topics such as personal cleanliness, especially of the head, the cleaning of clothes, bedding and rooms, ventilation of rooms, defective sanitary arrangements, the removal of refuse, collections of waters which breed mosquitoes, nutrition and hygiene during pregnancy, childbirth and the post-natal period, the storage of food, especially milk, and how to boil and filter water. The Begum considered these visits as an "excellent training" for the local native nurses, whereas *The British Journal of Nursing* regarded them quite skeptically as "a heavy burden" for the Matron in addition to hospital work.[82]

80 Sulṭān Jahān Begum 1913.
81 Sulṭān Jahān Begum 1916.
82 "Nursing in India", 1908, p. 288.

Other initiatives took place in this period to promote childcare. Baby Shows, in which mothers presented their children to a jury who judged their health, were organized in many parts of India. The first Baby Show of the Bhopal Agency was held in Sehore in 1923, where Miss Rubins presented a lecture. In Bhopal city the first of these shows took place during the same year, as part of the Baby Week initiative instigated by Lady Reading, the wife of the Viceroy of India. The event in Bhopal was promoted by the Lady Doctor of the Lady Lansdowne Hospital and by some members of the ruling family like Maimūna Sulṭān Begum, Ḥamīd Allāh's wife.[83]

## Conclusion

This article has explored the role that the establishment of hospitals has played in the medical reforms undertaken in the princely state of Bhopal during the last part of 19th century and the first decades of the 20th century. Before the 1870's there were no civil hospitals in the Bhopal state as the only hospital established in the 1950's in Sehore was reserved for soldiers and the colonial elite. This situation changed under the rule of Šāh Jahān when two hospitals—one for men and one for women—were established in Bhopal city and a Leper Asylum was opened in Sehore. Following the Islamisation of certain fields of the Bhopal administration, like the education section, Šāh Jahān and her daughter Sulṭān Jahān tried to combine Muslim views with a modernization of Bhopal infrastructures along colonial models. Their efforts to combine Muslim and Western elements can be clearly seen in the reforms they promoted in the medical field. On one hand the Begums supported the establishments of modern medical services, on the other they backed the efforts to reform *yūnānī* institutions and when they were sick were often treated by traditional *yūnānī* physicians and never went to modern hospitals. Another important element of this reformist trend was the attention paid to women's healthcare, which again shows the Begums' attitude to reconcile modernization with Muslim principles.

However, despite the support given to *yūnānī* medicine, more expensive projects such as the construction of hospital buildings were realized only for allopathic services, which also received financial support from colonial institutions. The patronage of *yūnānī* medicine resulted in the

[83] Forbes 2005, p. 93.

opening of new dispensaries and of a new school, whereas hospitals, as in other Indian cities, became main symbols of the hegemonic role acquired in colonial India by western medicine over native ones. Anyhow, the efforts made by the Begums to promote medical modernization did not immediately produce the expected results. If we look at the number of the inpatients admitted in Bhopal hospitals during the early decades of their activity we can deduce that at the turn of century there were still many locals—and not just the aristocrats—who avoided being hospitalized as inpatients. Likewise, from 1909 the Lady Lansdowne Hospital became the center of the efforts aiming to modernize women's medical education, however traditional *dā'ī* in the beginning were reluctant to be trained at the hospital. The visits—ordered by Sulṭān Jahān—that the hospital staff had to carry in the *zanāna* apartments can be seen as a clear intention to further accommodate such services with the social codes that discouraged women to be treated outside home.

## Bibliography


Abdur Razzack, H. M., 1987, *Hakim Ajmal Khan: The Versatile Genius*. New Delhi, Central Council for Research in Unani Medicine.

Abida Sultaan, 2004, *Memoirs of a Rebel Princess*. Oxford, Oxford University Press.

Alavi, Seema, 2008, *Islam and Healing: Loss and Recovery of an Indo-Muslim Medical Tradition*. New York, Palgrave Macmillan.

Ali, Azra Asghar, 1997, "Muslim Women and the Beginning of Health Care Culture in British India 1857–1947". *Pakistan Journal of Women's Studies: Alam-e Niswan*, 4, 1, pp. 13–24.

Attewell, Guy, 2007, *Refiguring Unani Tibb: Plural Healing in Late Colonial India*. New Delhi, Orient Longman.

A'ẓam Ḫān, Muḥammad, s.d., *Iksīr-i A'ẓam*. Lahore, Maktaba-yi Daniyāl.

Burton, Antoinette, 1996, "Contesting the Zenana: The Mission to Make 'Lady Doctors for India,' 1874–1885". *Journal of British Studies*, 35, 3, pp. 368–397.

*Census of India*, 1902, vol. XIX-A. Central India. Part II. Tables. Lucknow.

Dufferin and Ava, Harriot Georgina Blackwood Marchioness of, 1889, *Our vice regal life in India: selections from my journal, 1884–1888*. London, Murray.

*The Eleventh Year of Freedom, 1957–58*, 1959, New Delhi, Indian National Congress—All India Congress Committee.

Ernst, Waltraud—Pati, Biswamoy, eds., 2007, *India's Princely States: People, Princes and Colonialism*. London, Routledge.

Forbes, Geraldine H., 2005, *Women in Colonial India: Essays on Politics, Medicine, and Historiography*. New Delhi, Chronicle Books.

Ḫān, Rašīd Aḥmad, 2002, *Ḥayāt-i Ajmal*, Delhi (1st ed. 1937).

Harding, Christopher, 2008, *Religious Transformation in South Asia: the Meanings of Conversion in Colonial Punjab*. Oxford, Oxford University Press.

Hasan, Mushirul—Jalil, Rakhshanda, 2006, *Partners in Freedom: Jamia Millia Islamia*. New Delhi, Niyogi Books.

Ḥasanī, 'Abd al-Ḥayy ibn Faḫr al-Dīn, 1402/1981, *Nuzhat al-ḫawāṭir wa bahjat al-masāmi' wa al-nawāẓir*. Hyderabad, Dā'irat al-Ma'ārif, vol. 8, completed by Abū al-Ḥasan 'Alī Nadwī (2nd ed.).

Hopkins, John Castell, 1910, *The Life of King Edward VII*. Toronto, Skull.
*Imperial Gazetteer of India*, 1908, vol. VIII, Oxford, Clarendon Press, new edition.
"Infant Welfare in India", 1928, *British Medical Journal*, 1, 3520, June 23, p. 1082.
Kakar, Sanjiv, 1996, "Leprosy in British India, 1860–1940: Colonial Politics and Missionary Medicine". *Medical History*, 40, pp. 215–230.
——, 2006, "Medical Developments and Patient Unrest in the Leprosy Asylum, 1860 to 1940", in: B. Pati—M. Harrison, eds., *Health, Medicine and Empire: Perspectives on Colonial India*. New Delhi, Orient Longman, pp. 188–216.
Khan, Shaharyar, 2000, *The Begums of Bhopal: a Dynasty of Women Rulers in Raj India*. London, I. B. Tauris.
"Lady Dufferin and the Women of India", 1891, *Strand Magazine*, 2, July, pp. 459–461.
Lal, Maneesha, 1994, "The Politics of Gender and Medicine in Colonial India: the Countess of Dufferin's Fund, 1885–1888". *Bulletin of the History of Medicine*, 68, 1, pp. 29–66.
Lambert-Hurley, Siobhan, 2006, "An Embassy of Equality? Quaker Missionaries in Bhopal State, 1890–1930", in: A. A. Powell-S. Lambert-Hurley, eds., *Rhetoric and Reality: Gender and the Colonial Experience in South Asia*. New Delhi, Oxford University Press.
——, 2007a, *Muslim Women, Reform and Princely Patronage: Nawab Sultan Jahan Begam of Bhopal*. London, Routledge.
——, 2007b, "Subtle Subversions and Presumptuous Interventions: Reforming Women's Health in Bhopal State", in: A. Ghosh, ed., *Behind the Veil: Resistance, Women and the Everyday in Colonial South Asia*. New Delhi, Permanent Black.
Lelyveld, David, 2003, *Aligarh's First Generation: Muslim Solidarity in British India*. New Delhi, Oxford University Press (1st ed. Princeton, 1978).
Luard, Charles Eckford, 1908, *Bhopal State Gazetteer*, Vol. 3, Calcutta, Superintendent Government Press.
"Medical Progress in Bhopal", 1927, *The British Medical Journal*, 2, 3495, December 31, pp. 1241–1242.
Metcalf, Barbara, 1985a, "Nationalist Muslims in British India: The Case of Hakim Ajmal Khan". *Modern Asian Studies*, 19, 1, pp. 1–28.
——, 1985b, "Hakim Ajmal Khan: Rais of Delhi and Muslim 'Leader' ", in: R. Frykenberg, ed., *Delhi Through the Ages*. New Delhi, Oxford University Press, pp. 299–315.
Minault, Gail, 1982, *The Khilafat Movement: Religious Symbolism and Political Mobilization in India*. New York, Columbia University Press.
Mittal, Kamla, 1990, *History of Bhopal State: Development of Constitution, Administration and National Awakening, 1901–1949*. New Delhi, Munshiram Manoharlal.
"Nursing in India", 1908, *The British Journal of Nursing*, Vol. 41, October 10, pp. 287–88.
Pernau, Margrit, 2008, *Bürger mit Turban: Muslime in Delhi im 19. Jahrhundert*. Göttingen, Vandenhoeck & Ruprecht.
Playne, Somerset, 2006, *Indian States: a Biographical, Historical, and Administrative Survey*. New Delhi, Asian Educational Services (1st ed. 1921).
Powell, Alexander, 1929, *The last home of mysteries: adventures in Nepal together with accounts of Ceylon, British India, the Native States, the Persian Gulf, the Overland Desert Mail and the Baghdad Railway*. New York, The Century Co (4th reprint).
Preckel, Claudia, 2000, *The Begums of Bhopal*. New Delhi, Roli Books.
——, 2004, "Interpretations of Widow Remarriage and Divorce: Shah Jahan Begum's *Tahdhib an-Niswan* and the *Ahl-e hadith* Movement in 19th century Bhopal". *Pakistan Journal of Women's Studies: Alam-e Niswan*, 11, 1, pp. 41–51.
——, 2007, "Ahl-i ḥadīth", *Encyclopaedia of Islam*, Third Edition, 2007–3, Leiden, E. J. Brill pp. 92–97.
——, 2008, *Islamische Bildungsnetzwerke und Gelehrtenkultur im Indien des 19. Jahrhundert: Muḥammad Ṣiddīq Ḥasan Ḫān und die Entstehung der* Ahl-e ḥadīṯ-*Bewegung in Bhopal*. PhD Dissertation, Ruhr-University Bochum, 2005. (http://www-brs.ub.ruhr-uni bochum .de/netahtml/HSS/Diss/PreckelClaudia/diss.pdf)

Quaiser, Neshat, 2004, "Politics, Culture and Colonialism: Unani Debate with Doctory", in: B. Pati—M. Harrison, eds., *Health, Medicine and Empire: Perspectives on Colonial India.* New Delhi, Orient Longman, pp. 317–355.

Qureshi, M. Naem, 1999, *Pan-Islam in British-Indian Politics: a Study of the Khilafat Movement, 1918–1924*. Leiden, E. J. Brill.

"Registration of Midwives in Bhopal", 1920, *British Journal of Midwifery*, Supplement, July 24, p. 56.

*Report on the Political Administration of the Territories within the Central India Agency (1881–82).* Calcutta, Government Printing, 1883.

*Report on the Political Administration of the Territories within the Central India Agency (1883–84).* Calcutta, Government Printing, 1885.

Roberts, J. R., 1904, *Report on the Dispensaries, Jail Hospitals, on Vaccination, and on the Registration of Vital Statistics on the Central Indian Agency for 1903.* Calcutta, Government Printing.

——, 1910, *Report on the Dispensaries, Jail Hospitals, on Vaccination, and on the Registration of Vital Statistics on the Central Indian Agency for 1909*, Calcutta, Government Printing.

——, 1912, *Report on the Dispensaries, Jail Hospitals, on Vaccination, and on the Registration of Vital Statistics on the Central Indian Agency for 1911.* Calcutta, Government Printing.

Rubins, Adeline, 1926, "Labour complicated by a utero-vesical fistula". *British Medical Journal*, 1, 3394, January 16, p. 96.

Šāh Jahān Begum, 1876, *Tāj al-iqbāl*, English translation: *The Táj-ul Ikbál Tárikh Bhopal; or, the History of Bhopal*, H. C. Barstow, ed., Calcutta, Thacker & Spink.

——, 1970, *Tahḏīb al-niswān wa tarbiyat al-insān.* Lahore, Nuʿmānī Kutubḫāna.

*Selections from the Records of the Government of India, Foreign Department*, 1886. Calcutta, Government Press.

*Selections from the Records of the Government of India, Foreign Department*, 1912, Calcutta, Government Press.

Siddiqi, Tazimuddin 1980, "Nāẓim-i Jehān Ḥakīm Muḥammad Aʿẓam Khān". *Studies in History of Medicine*, IV, 4, pp. 229–279.

Speziale, Fabrizio, 2009a, "India xxxiii. Indo-Muslim Physicians". *Encyclopaedia Iranica* (on line version: www.iranica.com).

——, 2009b, "Ḥakīm Ajmal Khān". *Encyclopaedia of Islam*, Third Edition, 2009–1, Leiden, E. J. Brill, p. 56.

——, 2010, *Soufisme, religion et médecine en Islam indien*. Paris, Karthala.

Sulṭān Jahān Begum, 1328/ 1910, *Tuzuk-i Sulṭānī.* Bhopal, Maṭbaʿ-i Sulṭānī.

——, 1912, *Jawhar al-iqbāl*, English translation: *An Account of My Life I (Gohur-i-Ikbal)*, C. H. Payne, ed., London, John Murray.

——, 1913, *Baččūn kī parwariš.* N.p.

——, 1916, *Ḫānadārī kā dūsrā ḥiṣṣa.* Bhopal, Maṭbaʿ-i Sulṭānī.

——, 1918, *Ḥayāt-i Qudsī*, English translation: *Hayat-i Qudsi: life of the Nawab Gauhar Begum alias the Nawab Begum Qudsia of Bhopal.* London.

——, 1926, *Ḥayāt-i Šāh Jahānī*, English translation: *Hayat-i Shahjehani: life of Her Highness the late Nawab Shahjahan Begum of Bhopal*, B. Ghosal, ed., Bombay.

——, 1927, *Aḫtar al-iqbāl*, English translation: *An Account of My Life III (Akhtar Iqbal)*, C. H. Payne, ed., Bombay, The Times Press.

Tebb, William, 1893, *The Recrudescence of Leprosy and its Causation: A Popular Treatise.* London, Swan Sonnenschein.

The Society of Friends, 1897, *Report of the Proceedings of the Conference at Darlington on Foreign Missions, 1896.* London, West, Newman and Co.

Van Hollen, Cecilia Coale, 2003, *Birth on the Threshold: Childbirth and Modernity in South India.* Berkeley, University of California Press.

Zubairī, Muḥammad Amīn, 1918, *Begamāt-i Bhōpāl.* Bhopal, Maṭbaʿ-i Sulṭānī.

# HAMDARD, HOW TO SHARE PAIN IN A MUSLIM WAY

Anna Vanzan

## Introduction

When the Arabs came to the subcontinent they brought their medical school, which was the result of a combination of Greek, Persian, Indian and Syriac medicine put in the frame of Muslim ethics and philosophy, and which later became known as *yūnānī ṭibb*, "Greek medicine"[1]. This Greek-Arabic medicine thrived and often rivaled with the indigenous Ayurvedic medicine, but it can be said that mostly the two methods lived in a parallel way and that they were chosen according to the patients' cultural-religious background, i.e., *yūnānī* was preferred by Muslims while Ayurvedic was more popular with Hindus.

Both medical traditions received a blow from the rampant European (i.e., mainly British) conquest of the subcontinent: the newcomers were persuaded of their cultural superiority in every field including medicine, and looked down upon local medicine, though it was based on the same (Galenic) principles on which European medicine was practiced and in spite of the fact that Avicenna's treatises had remained in many European medical colleges syllabus as late as the 17th century. In addition, the fact that some European physicians (François Bernier, Nicolò Manucci, and John Fryer to name the most famous ones) had been summoned at the Mughal court in order to treat sultans and begums and therefore enjoyed a high rank, had increased the reputation of Western medicine at the expense of local ones.

In the 19th century *yūnānī* medicine was still popular with the Muslim community, because of its inexpensiveness and availability in comparison with the Western one, but it also enjoyed a privileged status among Muslim intellectuals and the leaders of the community, including the *nawāb* of places such as Lucknow, Rampur, Bhopal and other Muslim enclaves. *Yūnānī* medicine had been kept alive by influential families of physicians who had become the representatives of the Muslim community's

[1] On the *yūnānī* denomination see Speziale 2005.

social and cultural pride, and who were often aware of the stagnation in which *yūnānī* medicine had fallen; thus, they promoted its revival, mainly through the opening of formally organized schools where medicine could be learned and practiced. The first medical school of Delhi was opened in the late 1880s by Ḥakīm ʿAbd al-Majīd (d. 1901), a component of one of the most renowned families of physicians in the capital, the Šarīfī. At the turn of the century, the school could boast more than sixty graduates; and in 1906 another member of the family, Ḥakīm Ajmal Ḫān (1864–1927), managed to organize a Ṭibbī Conference in order to bring together the practitioners of the local medical traditions and to alert them on the need to reform both *yūnānī* and Ayurvedic medicine.

In those years, another innovative project in the field of *yūnānī* was rapidly maturing, i.e., Hamdard, which had to revolutionize the concept of the hospital itself. This paper aims to describe the role that Hamdard played within the history of *yūnānī* hospitals, not so much by illustrating the technical descriptions of the hospital structure *per se*, but rather by focusing on Hamdard's new perspective of the hospital. In Hamdard's view, in fact, the clinic was not only the heart of medical assistance, but also the center of multipurpose activities, from pharmacological research and production to the implementation of Islamic studies. Hamdard's new and peculiar vision puts the hospital at the core of a multidirectional effort that seeks to combine medical assistance and schooling with a more general and deep process of education which follows the tenets of Islam while keeping pace with the evolving world. Though the primary goal of any Hamdard hospital is the patients' recovery, its activities are harmonically entangled with a broader and wider project directed to maintain human wellbeing.

## The Beginning of Hamdard. The Role of the Hospital and Its Pharmacy in the Strategy of Medical Revival

1906 was an eventful year, as another famous practitioner of *yūnānī*, namely Ḥakīm Ḥāfiz ʿAbd al-Majīd (1883–1922), decided to open a *yūnānī* clinic in Delhi with the aim of revitalizing and improving the old tradition. ʿAbd al-Majīd's ancestors had migrated from Kashgar (nowadays in China) to Peshawar in the 17th century and then moved to Multan before establishing themselves in Delhi in the 19th century. Before setting up his own clinic Ḥakīm ʿAbd al-Majīd had worked in the Hindustānī dawāḫāna, the renowned *yūnānī* pharmacy established in early 20th century in Delhi by Ajmal Ḫān in order to develop the large-scale production of *yūnānī* drugs.

In the Muslim world, hospitals had been established since the Caliphs' time and became a typical feature of Muslim cities and of Muslim scientific civilization. India followed this tradition, and since the Tuġluq's era Delhi had become renowned for its hospital institutions. However, the general decline of the indigenous systems of medicine and the rise of Western hospitals introduced by the British had consequently caused the virtual disappearance of Muslim hospitals. Though *yūnānī* could continue to be practiced both at the physician's and at the patient's house, the establishment of a regular hospital side by side to the ones erected by the British had a double effect: to offer an extremely useful social service to the community and to affirm the validity of the indigenous treatment in spite of the rampant foreign one.

The first Hamdard hospital (*šifā-ḫāna*) was located in Asaf Ali Road, near the Turkman Gate in Old Delhi, and consisted of a few rooms located on one side of a courtyard in a building erected in perfect Mughal style, with cusped arches and a sparkling fountain, as a further affirmation of the Muslim character of this initiative and in contrast to the style the British has assumed for their medical buildings and displayed in the Medical College they had established in Calcutta in 1835. But though ʿAbd al-Majīd's place was small, it was meant to become a vehicle to find the grandeur of the past, when the hospital was just the core of a wide range of activities, from the *madrasa* to the Turkish bath, from the mosque to the guest house: in ʿAbd al-Majīd's mind, this hospital had to become the core of *yūnānī* renaissance, in which the educational institution had to play the most important role. Avicenna (980–1037) and Razes (850–925) had been great physicians, but, above all, they had been great teachers and scholars of medicine, therefore to revive their authority it was mandatory to re-establish their medical school. The new hospital had to become a center of both medical care and medical teaching, both undermined by the long period in which medicine had been exclusively taught at home: students had finally the proper setting to practice clinical observation, a reliable institution under quality control in order to isolate quacks and charlatans who had given *yūnānī* a bad name. In his hospital ʿAbd al-Majīd meant to promote *yūnānī* medicine as a science, while offering at the same time a better service to the Muslim community. ʿAbd al-Majīd's spirit and intent were very clear also through the name chosen for his newly born enterprise: Hamdard, i.e., "to share the pain", as if the *ḥakīm* was telling his patients "your pain is my pain".

The small Hamdard hospital had to develop very quickly; the patients had to be treated according to the main specialized branches of *yūnānī*, but the structure was apt to restore also the surgical tradition lost since colonial supremacy. The general misunderstanding that surgery was not part of *yūnānī* medicine had favored the total decline of *ḥakīms*' (*yūnānī* physicians) surgical skills, but Hamdard had to prove the it was possible and necessary to revive al-Zahrāwī's art (d. 1013),[2] and even to practice dissection of the human body. The hospital and the clinical experience were mandatory to this project and in a short time the Hamdard hospital began to integrate modern surgery with *yūnānī*; soon it would host anatomical rooms in order to promote the modernization of anatomical and physiological knowledge.

However, the new institution needed financial support: Ḥakīm 'Abd al-Majīd, following Ajmal Ḫān's example, believed that the large-scale manufacture of drugs would become the key in order to have a larger number of patients to benefit from the efficacy of *yūnānī* medicines. Therefore, a *dawā-ḫāna* (pharmacy) was opened and soon it gained a good reputation because of the quality and relative inexpensiveness of the drugs manufactured there. Once more, the pharmacy was not a separated corpus from the hospital, but an integrated part of Hamdard's concept, the obvious place in which to prepare medicines for the treated patients, both the hospitalized ones and those who would seek a medical opinion in the doctors' office and whose needs directed the research and production of the *dawā-ḫāna*. Hamdard reestablished the connection between clinic and pharmacy, a connection lost during the years of *ṭibb*'s decadence. While Hamdard was filling the lack of scientific pharmaceutical research, dealing a blow to charlatans and bazaar herbs sellers, it was simultaneously affirming that *yūnānī* doctrine could not substitute for clinical confirmation. Soon the new pharmaceutical enterprise proved to be a major success, so much so that its income turned out to be the main source not only for founding the hospital and its functioning, but also to subsidize a variety of projects connected with the hospital.

One of the first realizations of the new pharmacy, bound to become an overall and lasting success, was a *šarbat* (drink) called *rūḥ afzā*, "the one which enhances the soul". The way in which this product came into light and its name are indicative of the spirit with which 'Abd al-Majīd had

---

[2] Al- Zahrāwī, better known in Europe as Abulcasis, was the most famous Muslim surgeon.

embarked upon his venture. *Šarbat* is a drink made of sweetened fruit juice and water popular in North Africa, the Middle East and Central Asia, and it can be almost identified as the drink of the Muslim *umma* (community) to whom alcohol is prohibited. Its use in the subcontinent was encouraged by the Mughals who would send their emissaries as far as the Himalaya in order to get the ice to prepare the *šarbat*. Between 1907 and 1908 Ḥakīm ʿAbd al-Majīd introduced *rūḥ afzā* in the first list of drugs of Hamdard, as a drink whose qualities were mainly medicinal. Ḥakīm Ustād Ḥasan Ḫān, the first processor of *rūḥ afzā*, was a resident of Saharanpur in the state of Uttar Pradesh, a major center of Muslim cultural and political history especially after 1857, when the district became a center of activity of the Deoband School. Deoband represented opposition to British, supported reformist ideas and was responsible for Muslims' social and political awakening. The ulama of Deoband and of the connected Maẓāhir al-ʿUlūm school opened in Saharanpur were deeply involved in the process of reevaluation of *yūnānī* as they considered medicine a way of increasing their ties with their followers. So much so that at the end of the 19th century medicine became part of the curriculum at the Deoband academy.[3]

At Hamdard, Ḥakīm Ustād Ḥasan Ḫān and his collaborators came to the formula of the *rūḥ afzā* by integrating several drugs into the recipe of the *šarbat*. Among the drugs they included were *ḫurfa* seeds (*Portulacea oleracea*), *kāsnī* (Cichorium intybus), *munaqqā* (*Vitis vinifera*), *nilufar* (*Nymphae lotus*), *gāʾu-zabān* (*Borage officinalis*), *harā dhaniyā* (*Coriandrum sativum*) etc., which possessed wholly medicinal properties;[4] from among the fruits they chose orange, pineapple, carrot and watermelon, which contained higher medicinal qualities. Then they introduced a novelty by including in this formula some vegetables such as *pālak* (*Spinacia oleracea*), *pudina* (*Mentha arvensis*) and *harā ghiyā* (*Luffa cylindrica*). Besides those, they added rose and *keoṛā* (Garcinia Cambogia), the traditional flowers of the time, in addition to the use of flowers of juicy fruits like lemon and orange, roots with subtle aroma (like *ḫas, Andropogon muricatum*), and sweet-smelling woods like sandal. The result was an innovative product which had to become the drink *par excellence* of Muslims living in the subcontinent, not only for its therapeutic properties,

---

3 See Metcalf, 1983, p. 103 and Vanzan 2000, pp. 61–62.

4 On the medical properties of these and other plants see Nadkarni 1992 and Dastur 1988.

but also for its refreshing qualities, a crucial factor in the subcontinent climate. The red color of the *šarbat* and its evocative name, suggesting themes dear to Indian Muslims, increased its popularity. The name *rūḥ afzā*, in fact, came from books of ancient myths and legends, such as the *Maṯnawī gulzār-i nasīm*, first published in the 1830s: in this book, there is a character named Rūḥ Afzā, a daughter of Muẓaffar Šāh, the King of Firdaws (Heaven). Besides, Rūḥ Afzā was also the name of an Urdu weekly published in Jawnpur in the late 19th century. Thus *rūḥ afzā* imposed itself with a combination of inherent medical properties and the reminiscent power that its name and history awoke in Indian Muslims' collective consciousness.

## Difficult Times

While Hamdard was establishing itself, the Rāj was fighting against the indigenous medicines by passing a series of Medical Acts which aimed to preclude *ḥakīm*s and *vaidya*s (practitioners of Ayurvedic medicine) from the main stream of medical treatment in India. The 1912 and 1917 Medical Acts, in fact, debarred *ḥakīm*s and *vaidya*s from being registered in the newly instituted Provincial Medical Councils, to which only the practitioners of Western medicine could apply. The blow meant to weaken the prestige of local medicines and of their practitioners before their own people and to attract young Indians interested in studying medical sciences to Western medicine as the only option in order to find an employment. By the same token, to study English—the language in which Western medicine expressed itself (as did many other subjects)—was more preferable than to study Arabic or Persian, i.e., the main linguistic vehicles of *yūnānī* medicine.[5] In other words, the overall scheme was that of detaching the young Indian generations from the traditional subject matters, in order to address them towards the requirements of the British government.

However, many Indians resisted this plan: the common people continued to turn to *yūnānī* physicians, for a variety of reasons, including the inexpensiveness of its drugs, the availability of the physicians even in remote areas of the country, but also—and mainly—because *yūnānī* was an expression of Muslim culture and a symbol of resistance to the Westerners' (not only techno-scientific) supremacy. Also many *yūnānī*

---

[5] The same was true for Sanskrit, the language of Ayurvedic medicine.

physicians contributed to this struggle in order to assert the validity of the medical tradition they practiced, and also called to action Ayurvedic physicians with whom they strengthened an alliance, such as the All-India Ayurvedic and Ṭibbī Conference (1910). However, internal dissent was also a problem: many *yūnānī* practitioners resented the unwanted collaboration with the *vaidyas*; and many of them did not like some Conference leaders' insistence on the fact that *yūnānī* had to be open to some Western techniques, namely anatomy and surgery.[6] As we saw, Hamdard was in this vanguard, arguing that one of *yūnānī*'s pilasters, namely Galen, had outstandingly contributed to medical science by dissecting animal and human bodies.

The path towards an official recognition of *yūnānī* medicine was full of obstacles and *yūnānī* seemed to proceed one step forward and two back: when finally the Ayurvedic and Yūnānī Ṭibbiya College was opened in Delhi in 1921, Mahatma Gandhi, invited to the opening ceremony, explicitly criticized both *ḥakīms* and *vaidyas* for their lack of research spirit, the little investigation carried out and their "following formulas without question".[7]

In this quite controversial background Hamdard was building its reputation, when an unexpected event challenged its future: in 1922 Ḥakīm 'Abd al-Majīd died prematurely leaving two sons too young to administer the enterprise. The reins of Hamdard were taken into the hands of Ḥakīm 'Abd al-Majīd's wife, Mrs Rāb'ia, called Mādar-i Hamdard (Mother of Hamdard) who provided the first example of the capacities of the family's ladies in handling their business. Until her eldest son, Ḥakīm 'Abd al-Ḥamīd (1908–1999) came to the proper age and started to give Hamdard a new twist. In 1940 Ḥakīm Muḥammad Sa'īd (1920–1998), the younger brother, joined Hamdard and in the same year he graduated from the Ayurvedic and Yūnānī Ṭibbiya College. They were not destined to work together for a long time, because the Partition was on the way and ready to deeply affect everybody and everything in the subcontinent, including Hamdard.

---

6 See Metcalf, 1986, p. 302.

7 *Indian Medical Gazzette*, 1921, p. 189.

## Hamdard in India and in Pakistan

In August 1947 Pakistan was a reality. Ḥakīm Muḥammad Saʿīd left Delhi for Karachi, while the Hamdard institution in Delhi continued to be run by his elder brother. Here is his explanation of the reasons that drove him to such a choice:

> I was a sincere supporter of the Pakistan Movement. After the establishment of Pakistan, I felt my sympathies and loyalties should be directed toward Pakistan. Since Hamdard trust had been established in India, I thought it would not be correct, on principle, to transfer the Hamdard trust funds to Pakistan. My personal property was considerably larger than that of my elder brother, Hakim Abdul Hamid who had made self-denial and self-sacrifice his guiding principles. Now all this property was made over to him to enable him to devote his full time and energy to the building of great institutions such as the Indian Institute of Islamic Studies. I came over to Pakistan, almost devoid of funds. I stinted on meals and luxuries, and for seven months suffered deprivation and disappointment.[8]

Therefore Hamdard was split in two branches, and part of it remained in its original place, i.e., Delhi. The opportunity of such a choice was manifold: since the eve of independence, the indigenous medicines had gained considerable importance in India. Between 1946 and 1949 it was recognized that Indian traditional medicines had made significant contributions towards fulfilling Indian people's medical needs. In 1946 a national conference decided that adequate provision should be made for research in indigenous medical traditions. It was recommended to give impulse to educational and training institutions of these indigenous medicines, and to create post graduate courses in Indian traditional medicines for graduates in Western medicine. Besides, a number of committees were appointed by the Government of India with the task of drawing precise outlines for the development of local medicine. It was the signal that a new era had started, and that the Indian traditional medicines had been freed from the quarantine in which they had lingered. In this context, Hamdard had all the requirements in order to become a leading organization in the field. But there was also more than this: as a Muslim institution, Hamdard presence in the capital of an increasingly secular but at the same time mostly Hindu country was mandatory. Again, Hamdard was called on to hold the flag of Muslim culture. Hamdard was a medical/pharmaceutical institution,

---

[8] Extract of a speech given by Ḥakīm Muḥammad Saʿīd in 1953, *Hamdard Islamicus*, XXII, 4, 1999, p. 9.

but it was bound to become much more. Ḥakīm ʿAbd al-Ḥamīd gave impetus to Hamdard, by setting up new laboratories in which *yūnānī* drugs were to be tested according to modern, scientific criteria. Herbs and drugs which had been used for centuries were put under scrutiny in order to clinically establish their therapeutic efficacy: single and compound drugs of proven efficacy were standardized for the first time. As a further proof of Hamdard's humanitarian commitment, in 1953 it was converted from a commercial enterprise to a *waqf*, i.e., a pious endowment, and its scope and spheres of action additionally enlarged.

Both Hamdard in Delhi and its Pakistani sister in Karachi, while keeping the hospital at the core of their organizations, have been developing strategies in order to combine the development of *yūnānī* medicine and therapeutics with a broader concept of service and charity for the community. Thus, the two institutions have been doing their best in the ground of diversification and growth and have become two multi-dimensional organizations, and they have each founded a University system which comprises several faculties not only devoted to medicine and sciences, but also to Islamic Studies and Humanities; besides, they host libraries which offer bibliographical support to both Hamdard students and to foreign scholars. There are, though, some differences and peculiarities which differentiate the two institutions and which are dictated by local circumstances, by their respective trustees' different aims and by the historical and political issues of the two countries in which they are located, i.e., Pakistan and India.

For example, while Hamdard in Delhi was developing its hospitals and pharmaceutical laboratories in Old Delhi, it also established a variety of activities near the shrine of the Sufi saint Niẓām al-Dīn Awliyā (d. 1325), one of the Muslim hubs in the Indian capital which also hosts the mausoleum of the poet Amīr Ḫusraw (d. 1325): these enterprises included not only a medical office and a laboratory, but also a purely cultural center, namely, the Ġālib Academy. This cultural institution that primarily promotes literary activities, especially in Urdu (there are also classes in Urdu calligraphy), is entitled to a poet whose interest in *yūnānī* medicine was well known: not only had Ġālib (d. 1869) been trained in this medical tradition, as many of his verses prove, he was also very close to *yūnānī* practitioners who had distinguished themselves as the champions of Muslim culture in harsh the post-Mutiny days.[9]

---

[9] On Ġālib's relationship with influential *yūnānī* physicians see his letters edited by Rahbar, 1987; on his medical verses, see the article by Aʿẓmī, 2004, pp. 171–209. Hamdard's

It is noteworthy that Hamdard has been gradually developing a huge project in the Tughluqabad area (south Delhi), which comprises several educational institutions that prosper around what has been called Jāmiʿa Hamdard University and that comprises several faculties (including Science, Medicine, Pharmacy, Nursing). At the center of these activities there is the Majīdiya Hospital (so called in memory of the late Ḥakīm ʿAbd al-Majīd), now hosting about 150 beds, whose circular building is meant to facilitate the movement from one point to the other of doctors, nurses and patients alike. Among the other important institutions hosted in Tughluqabad, we also mention the Department of Islamic Studies whose researchers put particular emphasis on the problems faced by contemporary Muslim/Indian societies.

Likewise, Hamdard Pakistan has instituted the Madina al-Ḥikma—the City of Wisdom—in Karachi. Though the starting point was establishing a medical institution in which *yūnānī* could prosper, the Madina al-Ḥikma had been evolving as a comprehensive foundation which carried out various educational, religious, cultural, social, and academic activities. These range from the promotion and advancement of universal friendship (carried by its Bayt al-Amān branch), to the support of scholarly research in various fields (a task entrusted to the institution called Bayt al-ʿUlamā). Hamdard Pakistan puts particular emphasis on children and it has established two institutions for children, namely the Hamdard International Children's Club whose aim is that of promoting the general welfare of children of Pakistan, and the Nawnihāl Šahr (Children's city) for children's amusement, entertainment and education. Madina al-Ḥikma and its many branches is a realization of Hamdard Pakistan's founder, Ḥakīm Muḥammad Saʿīd, a figure whose multifaceted activities deserves to be focused on.

## Ḥakīm Muḥammad Saʿīd: Putting Knowledge into Practice

As seen above, as soon as the Partition created the new state of Pakistan, one of the heirs of Hamdard institution in Delhi, namely Ḥakīm Muḥammad Saʿīd, set out for Karachi where he founded a new Hamdard.

importance as a promoter of Muslims' education has been officially recognized, among others, by the late Rajiv Gandhi, who, by inaugurating Hamdard University, i.e., Jāmiʿa Hamdard (1989) declared that it was a major instrument to enable the Muslim minority to go forward.

The beginning was very tough: Pakistan was a poor country populated by people with no shelter, and Ḥakīm Muḥammad Saʿīd himself was without financial means and support. However, he had a great vision, that of building an institution with multiple aims: a) to revitalize *yūnānī* medicine and promote it not only amongst the people of Pakistan, but throughout the world; b) to treat the sick and the ailing by hospitalizing them in decent clinics; c) to promote scientific activities and encourage knowledge and education.

At first he received the help of some members of the Parsi community, who provided Ḥakīm Muḥammad Saʿīd with premises on Aram Bagh Road, where he established his first clinic and pharmacy: it was just one room, the used equipment was bought from Jodia Bazar and a bunch of beds were available, but the demand was such that Ḥakīm Muḥammad Saʿīd had to expand his facilities.

Pakistan Hamdard shared the same principles of its Indian sister, therefore no fees were charged to anyone for consultation, examination, tests or service. The clinics had to be financed by the drug laboratories that Ḥakīm Muḥammad Saʿīd had started with second hand copper equipment bought for a few hundred rupees. There was also a shortage of medicinal herbs, but in 1948 Hamdard Dawā-ḫāna was officially inaugurated, thus giving new strength to the hospital project.

In the meantime, the Hamdard hospital met such a great success that Ḥakīm Muḥammad Saʿīd had to expand it. More centers were required in Karachi, and soon he opened clinics in Firdaws Colony, Jahangir road, New Karachi, Landhi, as well as in other Pakistani towns, such as Peshawar, Lahore, Rawalpindi, Islamabad, Dacca, Faisalabad, Quetta, Multan and Sukkur. Hamdard activities required skilled physicians, therefore Ḥakīm Muḥammad Saʿīd summoned some *ḥakīms* from Delhi, such as Ṭabība Faḫr Jahān, who was a teacher at the Ayurvedic and Yūnānī Ṭibbiya College, founded in Delhi by the Šarīfī family, and who became the first lady physician of Pakistani Hamdard. There was a desperate need for female physicians,[10] as a Hamdard clinic was supposed to be run according to the following scheme: a male Assistant physician, a female Assistan physician, a Pathological Laboratory and a Radiological Unit. For patients who lived in far-flung areas, Hamdard provided mobile dispensaries, and a *ḥakīm* or *ḥakīma* (female physician) would reach their patients virtually everywhere. As time passed, even Pakistani migrants in the UK required a *yūnānī*

---

[10] Pakistan still faces the problem of a shortage of female physicians.

clinic, so a Hamdard unit was started in London: Ḥakīm Muḥammad Saʿīd used to go every fourth months to the UK to treat patients and supervise the management.

Concurrently, Hamdard was developing its pharmaceutical industry, creating conspicuous income to be channeled both into its clinics and in its philanthropic activities: the business volume was such that in 1953 Ḥakīm Muḥammad Saʿīd decided to convert the enterprise into a *waqf*. Moreover, he strove in order to establish a college of medicine in Karachi to be run on the same basis as its twin institution in Delhi. In 1958, the Hamdard College of Eastern Medicine was inaugurated in Karachi by Fāṭima Jinnāḥ (d. 1967), the Pakistan founder's sister, who shared Ḥakīm Muḥammad Saʿīd's concern for a qualified institutions of traditional medicine.

However, Ḥakīm Muḥammad Saʿīd aimed at a higher, broader recognition of the *yūnānī* medicine, therefore he began a policy of promotion of *ṭibb* at an international level, challenging the World Health Organization (WHO) by arguing that it had to recognize traditional medicines that are practiced by about half of the population of the globe. As he writes:

> I have been in constant touch with the World Health Organization from the time when Traditional Medicine was not included within the range and purview of WHO which harbored contradictory feelings about it. But I persevered in my insistence that a world body for health could hardly become universal in outlook with the absence of Eastern Medicine (that is, Arab Medicine, Chinese Medicine, Indian or Ayurvedic Medicine, and African Medicine). At long last my efforts did prevail in the face of utter indifference on the part of the so-called medical experts. It followed a gift of ten thousand US dollars, in token money, by the Hamdard Foundation Pakistan (of which I am President) for the establishment of a Division for Traditional Medicine which was eventually set up at the WHO headquarters in Geneva with my continued interest in it, participating in my capacity of adviser in meetings in several countries on behalf of WHO.[11]

In 1958 Ḥakīm Muḥammad Saʿīd founded the Society for the Promotion of Eastern Medicine whose members had the task to promote *yūnānī* internationally.[12] Hamdard tried especially to wake up those Muslim countries that, in spite of being the cradle of *yūnānī* medicine, had totally switched to Western medicine; such was the case of Kuwait, where, after a series

---

[11] Personal letter by Ḥakīm Muḥammad Saʿīd addressed to me on 10th January 1995.

[12] Among the activities undertaken by the Society for the Promotion of Eastern Medicine was a one month visit Ḥakīm Muḥammad Saʿīd made in 1963 in China to meet with the physicians of traditional Chinese medicine, on which see Saʿīd 1965; Alter 2008.

of Ḥakīm Muḥammad Saʿīd's visits, an Islamic Medical Center was established and studies of *ṭibb* enhanced.[13]

Among the many activities carried out by Hamdard, we cannot neglect its editorial activities. Perhaps because its promoter, Ḥakīm Muḥammad Saʿīd, was an extremely prolific writer,[14] Hamdard has engaged itself in a number of medical, religious, historical, literary publications. While journals, such as *Hamdard Medicus* (in English), spread knowledge and information about *yūnānī* medicine, *Hamdard Islamicus* (also in English) treats more general topics related to Muslim civilization. In conformity to its broad range of interests, Hamdard also edits some publications expressly dedicated to children, as well as the *Quarterly Journal of the Pakistan Historical Society*, whose articles explore the history of Muslims in South Asia.

Ḥakīm Muḥammad Saʿīd was not a politician and it was chiefly for his cultural and philanthropic merits that in 1993 he was appointed Governor of Sind, a charge that he held only until the following year. In spite of the positive impact that Ḥakīm Muḥammad Saʿīd had not only on the destiny of *yūnānī* medicine, but also on Pakistan cultural scene, quite inevitably his activities attracted enmity and dissent, to such an extent that he was assassinated, while walking into his clinic at Aram Bagh, in Karachi, at 6 a.m., on October 17th 1998. At his death the direction of the Hamdard remained in the hands of his family and it was taken by Muḥammad Saʿīd's daughter, Saʿdiya Rašīd.

## Conclusions

In an era in which indigenous Indian medicines were jeopardized by the colonial threat, Hamdard overcame the possible conflict with the Western system and integrated it in its hospitals which combined the more technical Western approach with the theoretical attitude of *yūnānī* medicine. Hamdard (re)proposed the old scheme of the *dār al-šifā* (hospital, lit. "house of healing") in which clinic went hand in hand with other scientific and humanistic branches of Muslim knowledge, thus constituting an

---

13 The Center suffered from the 1st Gulf war that took place in the early 1990s and was closed down, but it later merged into the Islamic Organization for Medical Sciences.

14 Ḥakīm Muḥammad Saʿīd wrote and edited quite a number of scientific publications on *ṭibb*, not only on its scientific-pharmacological aspects, but also on its history, ethics and sociology.

integrated system in which the hospital is the core of an articulated range of activities, a complex of educational institutions which develop different strategies for curing disease. Thus, since its very beginning, Hamdard affirmed the strategic, central importance of the hospital as the privileged place to practice medicine, as the engine of the approach in which clinical and therapeutic experiences combine in order to provide human well-being.

Hamdard actuated a true modernization in the field of medicine, by re-organizing existing institutions and adapting and justifying new ideas by drawing on tradition. The Hospital was modernized by invoking traditional values and thus promoting the social and political reinforcement of traditional forces, while accomplishing a radical integration of modern sciences. The implementation of hospitalization was Hamdard's underpinning process that illustrates how modern sciences were seen not only as an antagonist, but also as an impulse to reform traditional know-how.[15]

## Bibliography

Alter, Joseph S., 2008, "Rethinking the History of Medicine in Asia: Hakim Mohammed Said and the Society for the Promotion of Eastern Medicine". *Journal of Asian Studies*, 67, 4, pp. 1165–1186.

A'ẓmī, Alṭāf Aḥmad, 2004, *Dabistān-i Dillī ke tīn nām-war ṭabīb šā'ir*, in: A'ẓmī, Alṭāf Aḥmad, ed., *Ṭibb-i yūnānī awr urdū zabān wa adab*. Delhi, Centre for History of Medicine and Sciences, Jāmi'a Hamdard, pp. 171–209.

Dastur, J. F., 1988, *Medicinal Plants of India & Pakistan*. Bombay, D. B. Taraporevala sons & Co. (reprint of the 2nd edition).

*Deed of Declaration*, 1995. Karachi, Madinat al-Hikmah Trust.

Gupta, Narayan, 1981, *Delhi Between two Empires, 1803–1931. Society, Government and Urban Growth*. Delhi, Oxford University Press.

Heir, Patrick, 1923, *The Medical Profession in India*. London, Oxford Medical Publishing.

*Indian Medical Gazzette*, vol. 56, February 1921.

Metcalf, Barbara D., 1982, *Islamic Revival in British India: Deoband, 1860–1900*. Princeton, Princeton University Press.

——, 1986, "Hakim Ajmal Khan, *Rais* of Delhi and Muslim 'Leader' ", in: R. E. Frykenberg, ed., *Delhi through the Ages. Essays in Indian History, Culture and Society*. Delhi, Oxford University Press, pp, 299–315.

Nadkarni, K. M., 1992, *Indian Materia Medica*, 2 vols. Bombay, Popular Prakashan (5th reprint of the 3rd edition).

Qureishi, Ishtiaq Hussein, 1972, *Ulema in Politics*. Karachi, Ma'aref.

Rahbar, Daud, 1987, *Urdu Letters of Mirza Asadullah Khan Ghalib*, translated and annotated by D. Rahbar. New York, SUNY Press.

[15] The author acknowledges the hospitality and kindness that Hamdard institutions both in Delhi and in Karachi have showed her during her research.

Ranjha Shahid, Maqsood—Anusheh, Hussein, n. d., "Sexual Health Services for Adolescents at Sex Clinics in Rawalpindi, Pakistan". Islamabad, Sahil Organization.
Saʿīd, Ḥakīm Muḥammad, 1965, *Medicine in China*. Karachi, Hamdard Academy.
—— ed., 1969, *Hamdard Pharmacopoeia of Eastern Medicine*. Karachi, Hamdard Academy.
——, ed., 1973, *Al-Bīrūnī's book on pharmacy and Materia medica*, 2 vols., Karachi, Hamdard Academy.
——, 1975, *Traditional Greco-Arabic and Modern Western Medicine: Conflict or Symbiosis?* Karachi, Hamdard Academy.
——, 1982, *Diseases of the Liver: Greco-Arab Concepts*. Karachi, Hamdard Foundation Press.
——, 1983, *Greco-Arab Concepts on Cardiovascular Diseases*. Karachi, Hamdard Foundation Press.
——, 1983, *Avicenna's Tract on Cardial Drugs and Essays on Arab Cardiotherapy*. Karachi, Hamdard Foundation Press.
——, 1997, *Ethics for Medics*. Karachi, Hamdard Foundation Press.
Speziale, Fabrizio, 2005, "Linguistic strategies of de-Islamisation and Colonial science: Indo-Muslim physicians and the yūnānī denomination". *International Institute for Asian Studies Newsletter*, 37, p. 18. (available at http://www.iias.nl/nl/37/IIAS_NL37_18.pdf).
Vanzan, Anna, 1995, "Physicians and 'Ulama. Unani Medicine and Islamic Revival in British India". *Hamdard Medicus*, XXXVIII, July–September, n. 3, pp. 5–14.
——, 2000, "Medical Ethics of Muslim Women in Turn-of-the Century India. The 9th chapter of the *Bihistī Zewar*". *Journal of the Pakistan Historical Society*, XLVIII, January–March, n. 1, pp. 3–8.

## Websites

www.hamdard.com
www.jamiahamdard.edu
http://hakim-said.com.pk/Old/main.html

# GLOSSARY

*Afsar al-aṭibbā*: chief physician.
*Aṭibbā*: pl. of *ṭabīb* (q.v.).
*ʿAṭṭār-ḫāna*: lit. "house of the druggist", dispensary.
*Awqāf*: pl. of *vaqf* (q.v.).
*Bīmāristān*: lit. "place of the sick", hospital.
*Dāʾī*: traditional midwife.
*Dār al-majānīn*: lit. "house of the insane", mental hospital.
*Dār al-tašrīḥ*: anatomic room.
*Dār al-šifā*: lit. "house of healing", hospital.
*Dargāh*: Sufi shrine.
*Darmān*: medicine, remedy.
*Darmān-ḫāna*: lit. "house of the remedy", dispensary.
*Dāroġa*: head of a hospital, in Mughal India.
*Dārū*: drug, remedy.
*Dārū-ḫāna*: lit. "house of the remedy", pharmacy, dispensary.
*Davā, dawā*: medicine, remedy.
*Davā-ḫāna, dawā-ḫāna*: lit. "house of the remedy", dispensary, pharmacy.
*Farmān*: decree.
*Ḥakīm*: traditional physician.
*Jāgīr*: revenues of lands and villages.
*Madrasa-yi ṭibbiyya*: school of traditional medicine.
*Marīż-ḫāna*: lit. "house of the sick", hospital.
*Māristān*: a contraction of *Bīmāristān* (q.v.).
*Mutavallī, mutawallī*: administrator, of a *vaqf* (q.v.) or of an hospital.
*Nawāb*: viceroy, prince.
*Parhīzāna*: food given to the sick, dispensary.
*Pinjrāpol*: hospital for animals.
*Qanāt*: underground irrigation canal.
*Raʾīs al-aṭṭibā*: chief physician.
*Sanad*: certificate, diploma.
*Šarbat*: medicinal drink.
*Šarbat-ḫāna*: dispensary.
*Šifā-ḫāna*: lit. "house of healing", dispensary, hospital.
*Ṣiḥḥat-ḫāna*: dispensary.
*Ṭabīb*: physician.
*Ṭibb*: medicine.
*Tīmārčī-bāšī*: chief of a hospital, in Safavid Iran.
*Unani*: see *Yūnānī ṭibb*.
*Vaidya*: Ayurvedic physician.
*Vaqf, waqf*: pious endowment.
*Vaqf-nāma, waqf-nāma*: act of donation in *vaqf* (q.v.).
*Vāqif, wāqif*: donor of a *vaqf* (q.v.).
*Waqf*: see *vaqf*.
*Waqf-nāma*: see *vaqf-nāma*.
*Yūnānī ṭibb*: lit. "Greek medicine", traditional Avicennian medicine.
*Zanāna*: women apartments.

# LIST OF ABSTRACTS

## Avicennian Hospitals and Physicians in Safavid Iran (Hôpitaux et médecins avicenniens en Iran à l'époque safavide)

*Hasan Tadjbakhsh, University of Tehran, Tehran*

This chapter looks at the hospitals (*dār al-šifā*) established in Iran during the Safavid period (1501–1722). In Safavid Iran there were hospitals in the main Iranian cities and some of these establishments were part of bigger complexes including other buildings such as a mosque, a mausoleum or a caravanserai. Some eminent physicians and authors of medical books worked in these hospitals, and in particular ʿImād al-Dīn Maḥmūd Šīrāzī (16th century), who practiced at the hospital attached to the shrine of the Imam ʿAlī al-Riżā in Mashhad, and ʿAlī Afżal Qāṭiʿ (17th century), who worked in the *dār al-šifā* of Qazvin and mentioned in his books his medical practice at this hospital. It is especially during the period from the reign of Šāh Ṭahmāsp (r. 1524–1576) to the reign of Šāh ʿAbbās Ier (r. 1588–1629) that we find, practicing in these hospitals, some physicians who were also attached to the Safavid court, such as Mīrzā Muḥammad Šīrāzī, Ḥakīm Sayf al-Dīn Muẓaffar Kāšānī and Ḥakīm Šamsā Muḥammadā. There are no mentions of new hospitals established after the epoch of Šāh ʿAbbās Irst. However, we can presume that most of the existing hospitals remained opened during the late Safavid period, as it is also testified by the descriptions given by European travellers. The Europeans who visited Iran since the 30's of the 17th century give very negative descriptions of the conditions of Iranian hospitals, indicating that the state of these institutions had been deeply affected by the decline of the Safavid rule.

## Hospitals in Safavid and Qajar Iran: An Enquiry into Their Number, Growth and Importance

*Willem Floor, Independent Research Scholar, Bethesda*

The common wisdom is that the continuation of the institution of the Sasanian hospitals "was one of the most remarkable achievements in the Islamic East."[1] However remarkable the potential of the *dār al-šifā* was they did not deliver on their promise. For seen within the context of the size of the problem, neither the traditional *dār al-šifā* nor the nineteenth century modern European hospitals constituted an adequate response to the public health problem in Iran in view of their limited impact. To obtain a better understanding of the relative importance of hospitals I discuss their occurrence and activities in Iran. Given the scope of this publication, I have limited my remarks to the Safavid (1501–1722) and Qajar periods (1794–1925), but these remarks also apply to earlier periods. First, I raise

[1] Sajjādī 1990, pp. 257–259.

the question as to the significance of hospitals given their number in relation to the size of the population. Second, I discuss the introduction and development of European hospitals and dispensaries and what conclusions one may draw from that experience.

## Individuals Serving the People. The Role of *Vaqf* in the Establishment of Hospitals in Iran at the Beginning of the 20th Century

## (Des particuliers au service du peuple. Le rôle des *vaqf* dans la fondation d'hôpitaux en Iran au début du XX^e^ siècle)

*Omid Rezai, Institute for Humanities and Cultural Studies, Tehran*

This article explores the role of *vaqfs* (pious endowments) made by private individuals for the establishment of hospitals in Iran during the last part of the Qajar period. The cases presented here examine a period of about twenty years, starting from the beginning of the 20th century. This activity was not limited to the capital. Besides Tehran, *vaqfī* hospitals were established in Shiraz, Qazvin, Sari, Isfahan, Kerman and the village of Ḥiṣār. These *vaqfs* were made by local dignitaries and landlords with the religious milieu playing an important role. Among the factors that encouraged the deeds of these local dignitaries were the exhortations of the Iranian ulama to oppose the role of Western missionaries in the creation of health services in Iran. In these institutions founded through private *vaqfs* Western modern medicine was employed but from the point of view of the cultural dynamics of the epoch such activities of the Iranian dignitaries should not be interpreted just as the outcome of a modernising agenda. Some of these hospitals in particular were not the result of a cultural movement aiming to increase the influence of Western science in Iran, but a means to oppose the medical activities of the missionaries. The hospital of Kerman was established by a member of the *šayḫī* theological-mystical school and among the cases discussed here was the only one which had also a medical school attached to it. The texts of the *vaqf-nāma* (acts of donation in *vaqf*) concerning some of these hospitals are also presented.

## Together and Apart: Catholic Hospitals in Plural Goa

*Cristiana Bastos, Universidade de Lisboa, Lisbon*

In this paper we will examine the different depictions of the Royal Hospital of Goa, India, as either a wonder of the world, a place of decadence and mischief, the locus of creative encounters between different medical traditions, and the site of social segregation. The analysis will show that The Royal Hospital had different functions in different times, from an early moment of providing prime accommodation to European military men of the old Christian stock, to a later attempt to accommodate the needs of soldiers of different religious backgrounds. In parallel, a few other hospitals and institutions treated, hosted and converted other groups in Goa—civilians, women, the poor, the lower castes—in a process that involved merging and re-fashioning of goals through the centuries. The dynamics of healing, treating, and accommodating patients, as well as that of merging, renaming and moving the headquarters of the hospitals indicate that the healing institutions mirror a colonial order where the relationship between the European administration and the local agents and populations is far from being a simple opposition, and, rather, a complex intertwining of interests that at moments converge and often co-exist in tension.

## Tradition and Reform of the *dār al-šifā* in the Deccan (Tradition et réforme du *dār al-šifā* au Deccan)

*Fabrizio Speziale, Université Sorbonne Nouvelle—CNRS, Paris*

This chapter looks into the establishment of two hospitals of *yūnānī* medicine—as is called the Avicennian medical tradition in India—in Hyderabad. It analyses the evolution of this institution in the Deccan during the transition from the early-modern period to the colonial epoch. The first hospital (*dār al-šifā*) was built at the end of the 16th century by the sultan Muḥammad Qulī (r. 1580–1612), the founder of Hyderabad, the second was established by Mīr ʿUṯmān ʿAlī Ḫān (r. 1911–1948), the last ruler of the Niẓām dynasty. The first embodied the traditional Muslim model of the *dār al-šifā*, the hospital was part of a complex including other Muslim institutions: a mosque, a madrasa, a caravanserai and a *ḥammām*. Some scholars of Iranian origins are associated with the activities of this hospital. The adaptation to the scientific setting of Colonial India redefined the features of this institution. The new *yūnānī* hospital of Hyderabad, the Niẓāmiya ṣadr šifā-ḫāna, was part of a State plan of reforms aiming to regulate and modernize *yūnānī* institutions and practice. The Niẓāmiya ṣadr šifā-ḫāna was not based on the old model of the *dār al-šifā*, but presented new features reflecting the reformist trends of the colonial period which aimed to the renewal of the *yūnānī* tradition by incorporating elements of colonial medical institutions.

## Healing the People and the Princes: Hospitals, Ḥakīms and Doctors in Bhopal

*Claudia Preckel, Ruhr-Universität Bochum, Bochum*

The author analyses the development of hospitals in the princely state of Bhopal. During the 19th and early 20th centuries, Bhopal was ruled by four female rulers, the Begums, who enacted several reforms in the fields of administration, education and public health. These reforms were backed either by Islamic scholars at the court or by the British authorities, who supported the rule of the Begums. The Begums promoted the opening of modern medical institutions in Bhopal and at the same time they continued to offer patronage to Muslim traditional physicians who practiced *yūnānī ṭibb*. The Begums of Bhopal—such as the Niẓāms of Hyderabad—gave a considerable support towards the reform of *yūnānī* institutions and the creation of State run *yūnānī* dispensaries. However, all the hospitals founded in Bhopal during the Begums' rule were allopathic institutions. The main developments concerning hospital services were undertaken under the rule of Šāh Jahān (r. 1868–1901) and of her daughter Sulṭān Jahān (r. 1901–1926). Both were also active in the field of promoting women's education and women's healthcare and as a result a *zanāna* hospital was opened in the 1880s and a *yūnānī dawāḫāna* (dispensary) for the treatment of women was established in the beginning of the 20th century. While the Begums encouraged their subjects to be treated at hospitals, they and members of the ruling family abstained from being examined in hospitals, but were treated at home either by *ḥakīm*s or Western doctors.

## Hamdard, How to Share Pain in a Muslim Way

*Anna Vanzan, Università Statale di Milano, Milan*

In 1906 Ḥakīm Ḥāfiz ʿAbd al-Majīd (m. 1922), a famous *ḥakīm* (*yūnānī* physician) in Delhi, decided to open a small clinic of *yūnānī* medicine in the city. He named his enterprise Hamdard, i.e., "to share the pain". As time passed by, Hamdard was turned into a *waqf* and became a multi-dimensional organization that includes drug factories, hospitals, clinics and colleges. With its many branches both in India and in Pakistan, Hamdard foundation has become a leading institution of *yūnānī* medicine. While exploring the story of Hamdard, this paper looks at the figure of the founder of its Pakistani branch, i.e., Ḥakīm Muḥammad Saʿīd (1920–1998). Hamdard actuated a true modernization in the field of medicine, by reorganizing existing institutions and justifying new ideas and institutions by referring to tradition. The Hospital was modernized by invoking traditional values and thus promoting the reinforcement of traditional forces, while accomplishing a radical integration of modern medicine.

# INDEX

www.ingramcontent.com/pod-product-compliance
Lightning Source LLC
LaVergne TN
LVHW020652300926
849161LV00004B/912
*9789004228290*